# Workbook for Textbook of Diagnostic Sonography

*Eighth Edition*

**Sandra L. Hagen-Ansert, MS, RDMS, RDCS, FASE, FSDMS**
Cardiology Department
Manager, Echo Labs
Scripps Clinics and Scripps La Jolla Memorial Hospital
Torrey Pines, California

ELSEVIER

# ELSEVIER

3251 Riverport Lane
St. Louis, Missouri 63043

WORKBOOK FOR TEXTBOOK OF DIAGNOSTIC
SONOGRAPHY, EIGHTH EDITION

ISBN: 978-0-323-44183-4

---

**Notices**

Knowledge and best practice in this field are constantly changing. As new research and experience broaden our understanding, changes in research methods, professional practices, or medical treatment may become necessary.

Practitioners and researchers must always rely on their own experience and knowledge in evaluating and using any information, methods, compounds, or experiments described herein. In using such information or methods they should be mindful of their own safety and the safety of others, including parties for whom they have a professional responsibility.

With respect to any drug or pharmaceutical products identified, readers are advised to check the most current information provided (i) on procedures featured or (ii) by the manufacturer of each product to be administered, to verify the recommended dose or formula, the method and duration of administration, and contraindications. It is the responsibility of practitioners, relying on their own experience and knowledge of their patients, to make diagnoses, to determine dosages and the best treatment for each individual patient, and to take all appropriate safety precautions.

To the fullest extent of the law, neither the Publisher nor the authors, contributors, or editors, assume any liability for any injury and/or damage to persons or property as a matter of products liability, negligence or otherwise, or from any use or operation of any methods, products, instructions, or ideas contained in the material herein.

---

ISBN: 978-0-323-44183-4

*Content Strategist:* Sonya Seigafuse
*Content Development Manager:* Lisa Newton
*Content Development Specialist:* Betsy McCormac
*Publishing Services Manager:* Deepthi Unni
*Project Manager:* Maria Luisa Ordonio
*Design Direction:* Amy Buxton

Printed in the United States

Last digit is the print number: 9 8 7 6 5 4 3 2 1

# Preface

This workbook has been prepared to accompany Elsevier's *Textbook of Diagnostic Sonography*, Eighth Edition. The workbook chapters correlate with those in the primary textbook, and *Workbook for Textbook of Diagnostic Sonography* has been completely updated and expanded to keep pace with the eighth edition of the textbook.

The material serves both as a useful review of the textbook chapters and as a preparation tool for the national board examinations in diagnostic sonography. The workbook exercises provide the reader with a thorough review of terminology, anatomy, physiology, laboratory values, sonographic anatomy and technique, and pathology as it relates to diagnostic sonography. Each chapter begins with a review of the Key Terms that are bolded in the corresponding textbook chapter. A printable list of the key terms and their definitions may be found on the Evolve site. Each chapter also includes short answer questions, fill-in-the-blank exercises, and case reviews with images. Answers to all of the chapter exercises may be found at the back of the workbook.

**Four Reviews**—General Sonography, Pediatric, Cardiovascular Anatomy, and Obstetrics and Gynecology—are included at the end of the workbook. Students can test their knowledge here with the **hundreds of multiple choice questions**. In addition, a section of **Case Studies** with more than 30 new images from the textbook—and including all modalities—invites student sonographers to test their skills at identifying key anatomy and pathology and describing their sonographic findings. Answers to these additional reviews and case studies may also be found on the Evolve site.

**Sandra L. Hagen-Ansert, MS, RDMS, RDCS, FASE, FSDMS**

# Contents

1    Foundations of Clinical Sonography, 1

2    Essentials of Patient Care for the Sonographer, 7

3    Ergonomics and Musculoskeletal Issues in Sonography, 11

4    Anatomic and Physiologic Relationships within the Abdominopelvic Cavity, 15

5    Comparative Sectional Anatomy of the Abdominopelvic Cavity, 21

6    Basic Ultrasound Imaging: Techniques, Terminology & Tips, 31

7    Imaging and Doppler Artifacts, 35

8    Vascular System, 43

9    Liver, 53

10    Gallbladder and the Biliary System, 65

11    Spleen, 77

12    Pancreas, 85

13    Gastrointestinal Tract, 95

14    Peritoneal Cavity and Abdominal Wall, 107

15    Urinary System, 115

16    Retroperitoneum, 129

17    Abdominal Applications of Ultrasound Contrast Agents, 137

18    Ultrasound-Guided Interventional Techniques, 143

19    Emergent Ultrasound Procedures, 147

20    Sonographic Techniques in the Transplant Patient, 153

21    Breast, 163

22    Thyroid and Parathyroid Glands, 175

23    Scrotum, 181

24    Musculoskeletal System, 187

25    Neonatal and Pediatric Abdomen, 195

26    Neonatal and Pediatric Adrenal and Urinary System, 203

27    Neonatal and Infant Head, 211

28    Infant and Pediatric Hip, 223

29    Neonatal and Infant Spine, 231

30    Anatomic and Physiologic Relationships within the Thoracic Cavity, 239

31    Understanding Hemodynamics, 247

32    Introduction to Echocardiographic Techniques, Terminology and Tips, 251

33    Introduction to Clinical Echocardiography: Left-Sided Valvular Heart Disease, 259

34    Introduction to Clinical Echocardiography: Pericardial Disease, Cardiomyopathies, and Tumors, 267

35    Fetal Echocardiography: Beyond the Four Chambers, 275

**36** Fetal Echocardiography: Congenital Heart Disease, 283

**37** Extracranial Cerebrovascular Evaluation, 293

**38** Intracranial Cerebrovascular Evaluation, 299

**39** Peripheral Arterial Evaluation, 305

**40** Peripheral Venous Evaluation, 313

**41** Normal Anatomy and Physiology of the Female Pelvis, 323

**42** Sonographic and Doppler Evaluation of the Female Pelvis, 333

**43** Pathology of the Uterus, 339

**44** Pathology of the Ovaries, 345

**45** Pathology of the Adnexa, 353

**46** Role of Ultrasound in Evaluating Female Infertility, 357

**47** Role of Sonography in Obstetrics, 361

**48** Clinical Ethics for Obstetric Sonography, 367

**49** The Normal First Trimester, 369

**50** First-Trimester Complications, 377

**51** Sonography of the Second and Third Trimesters, 383

**52** Obstetric Measurements and Gestational Age, 393

**53** Fetal Growth Assessment by Sonography, 399

**54** Sonography and High-Risk Pregnancy, 403

**55** Prenatal Diagnosis of Congenital Anomalies, 411

**56** Placenta, 417

**57** Umbilical Cord, 425

**58** Amniotic Fluid and Fetal Membranes, 431

**59** Fetal Face and Neck, 437

**60** Fetal Neural Axis, 447

**61** Fetal Thorax, 453

**62** Fetal Anterior Abdominal Wall, 459

**63** Fetal Abdomen, 463

**64** Fetal Urogenital System, 469

**65** Fetal Skeleton, 479

**Cardiovascular Anatomy Review**, 487

**General Sonography Review**, 493

**Obstetrics and Gynecology Review**, 519

**Pediatric Review**, 543

**Case Studies**, 551

# 1 Foundations of Clinical Sonography

## KEY TERMS

### Exercise 1

*Match the following basic sonography terms with their definitions.*

_____ 1. acoustic impedance

_____ 2. angle of incidence

_____ 3. attenuation

_____ 4. axial resolution

_____ 5. compression

_____ 6. crystal

_____ 7. decibel (dB)

_____ 8. focal zone

_____ 9. frequency

_____ 10. intensity

_____ 11. interface

_____ 12. megahertz (MHz)

_____ 13. piezoelectric effect

_____ 14. power

_____ 15. refraction

_____ 16. resolution

_____ 17. transducer

_____ 18. wave

_____ 19. wavelength

_____ 20. resistance

A. Change in the direction of propagation of a sound wave transmitted across an interface where the speed of sound varies

B. Angle at which a sound beam strikes the interface between two types of tissue

C. Power per unit area

D. Special material in the transducer that has the ability to convert electric impulses into sound waves

E. Propagation of energy that moves back and forth or vibrates at a steady rate

F. Any device that converts energy from one form to another

G. Number of cycles per second that a periodic event or function undergoes

H. Measure of a material's resistance to the propagation of sound; expressed as the product of acoustic velocity of the medium and density of the medium

I. Generation of electric signals as the result of an incident sound beam on a material that has piezoelectric properties

J. Region over which the effective width of the sound beam is within some measure of its width at the focal distance

K. Reduction in amplitude and intensity of a sound wave as it propagates through a medium

L. Passive force in opposition to another, active force; occurs when tissue exerts pressure against the flow

M. Surface forming the boundary between media having different properties

N. Region of increased particle density

O. Distance over which a wave repeats itself during one period of oscillation

P. Refers to the minimum distance between two structures positioned along the axis of the beam where both structures can be visualized as separate objects

Q. Rate of energy flow over the entire beam of sound

R. Unit used to quantitatively express the ratio of two amplitudes or intensities

S. 1,000,000 Hz

T. Ability of the transducer to distinguish between two structures adjacent to one another

1

## Exercise 2

*Match the following sonography terms with their definitions.*

_____ 1. angle of reflection

_____ 2. velocity

_____ 3. cycle

_____ 4. Fraunhofer zone

_____ 5. hertz (Hz)

_____ 6. kilohertz (kHz)

_____ 7. lateral resolution

_____ 8. pulse duration

_____ 9. Fresnel zone

_____ 10. slice thickness

A. Time interval required for generating the transmitted pulse

B. Sequence of events occurring at regular intervals

C. Speed of the ultrasound wave; determined by tissue density

D. Minimum distance between two objects at which they still can be displayed as separate objects

E. Unit for frequency; equal to 1 cycle per second

F. Field closest to the transducer during formation of the sound beam

G. Angle of incidence at which the sound beam strikes the interface

H. 1000 Hz

I. Field farthest from the transducer during formation of the sound beam

J. Thickness of the section in a patient that contributes to echo signals on any one image

## Exercise 3

*Match the following instrumentation terms with their definitions.*

_____ 1. aliasing

_____ 2. amplitude

_____ 3. continuous wave (CW) Doppler

_____ 4. Doppler angle

_____ 5. Doppler shift

_____ 6. dynamic range

_____ 7. frame rate

_____ 8. gain

_____ 9. gray scale

_____ 10. laminar

_____ 11. Nyquist sampling limit

_____ 12. pulse repetition frequency (PRF)

_____ 13. pulsed wave (PW) Doppler

_____ 14. real time

_____ 15. spectral analysis

_____ 16. spectral broadening

_____ 17. temporal resolution

_____ 18. time gain compensation (TGC)

_____ 19. gate

_____ 20. frequency shift

A. Sound transmitted and received intermittently with one transducer

B. Ability to compensate for attenuation of the transmittal beam as the sound wave travels through tissue in the body

C. Change in frequency of a reflected wave; caused by motion between the reflector and the transducer's beam

D. One transducer continuously transmits sound, and one continuously receives sound; used in high-velocity flow patterns

E. Normal pattern of vessel flow; flow in the center of the vessel is faster than it is at the edges

F. Rate at which images are updated on the display; dependent on transducer frequency and depth selection

G. Analysis of the entire frequency spectrum

H. Technical artifact that occurs when the frequency change is so great that it exceeds the sampling view and pulse repetition frequency

I. In pulse-echo instruments, it is the number of pulses launched per second by the transducer

J. Ability of the system to accurately depict motion

K. Ratio of the largest to the smallest signals that an instrument or a component of an instrument can respond to without distortion

L. In pulsed Doppler, the Doppler signal must be sampled at least twice for each cycle in the wave if Doppler frequencies are to be detected accurately

M. Strength of the ultrasound wave measured in decibels

N. Measure of strength of the ultrasound signal

O. Echo fill-in of the spectral window that is proportional to the severity of stenosis

P. Ultrasound instrumentation that allows the image to be displayed many times per second to achieve a "real-time" image of anatomic structures and their motion patterns

Q. B-mode scanning technique that permits the brightness of the B-mode dots to be displayed in various shades of gray to represent different echo amplitudes

R. Amount of change in the returning frequency compared with the transmitting frequency when the sound wave hits a moving target such as blood in an artery

S. Sample site from which the signal is obtained with pulsed Doppler

T. Angle that the reflector path makes with the ultrasound beam; the most accurate velocity is recorded when the beam is parallel to flow

## HISTORY OF ACOUSTICS AND MEDICAL ULTRASOUND

**Exercise 4**

*Fill in the blank(s) with the word(s) that best completes the statements, or provide a short answer about the history of acoustics and medical use of ultrasound.*

1. Acoustics is the study of _____, _____, and _____ sound waves.

2. Ultrasound is defined as sound frequencies beyond the upper limits of human hearing, that is, greater than

    _____.

3. The terms _____ and _____ have been used to describe an imaging technique by which soft tissue structures of the body are visualized by recording the returning reflection of ultrasonic waves directed into the body.

4. The term that applies to the ultrasound evaluation of cardiac structures is _____.

5. One who performs ultrasound studies and gathers diagnostic data under the direct or indirect supervision of a

    physician is a _____.

6. List the qualities of a good sonographer.

    _____

    _____

    _____

## INSTRUMENTATION

**Exercise 5**

*Fill in the blank(s) with the word(s) that best completes the statements, or provide a short answer about ultrasound instrumentation.*

1. As the ceramic element vibrates, it periodically presses against and pulls away from the adjacent medium with

    resultant particle _____ and _____ in the medium.

2. A transducer converts _____ energy into _____ energy.

3. A propagation of energy that moves back and forth or vibrates at a steady rate is a _____.

4. The time required to produce each cycle depends on the _____ of the transducer.

**3**

5. The distance between two peaks over a period of time is the _____.

6. Wavelength is inversely related to frequency, which means that the higher the frequency, the

   _____ the wavelength.

7. As frequencies become higher, the pulse duration _____, yielding a decrease in the depth of field.

8. The rate at which energy is transmitted is referred to as the _____.

9. Power per unit area is defined as _____.

10. If you double the power, the intensity _____.

11. The piezoelectric effect was first described by the _____ brothers in 1880.

12. Air-filled structures, such as lungs and stomach, or gas-filled structures, such as bowel, _____ sound transmission.

13. Bone conducts sound at a _____ speed than soft tissue.

14. Normal transmission of sound through soft tissue travels at _____ m/sec.

15. Acoustic impedance is the product of the velocity of _____ in a medium and the density of that medium.

16. The angle of reflection is equal to the angle of _____.

17. If specular reflectors are aligned _____ to the direction of the transmitted pulse, they reflect sound directly back to the active crystal elements in the transducer and produce a strong signal.

18. The sum of acoustic energy losses resulting from absorption, scattering, and reflection is called

   _____.

19. Minimum reflector separation along the sound path required to produce separate echoes is _____ resolution.

20. The _____ resolution is the ability to produce separate echoes perpendicular to the sound path; it is affected by transducer diameter and focusing.

21. Lateral resolution is determined by beam _____.

22. _____ resolution refers to the ability to resolve objects that are the same distance from the transducer but are located perpendicular to the plane of imaging.

23. The number of pulses launched per second is the pulse repetition _____.

24. If the gain is set too _____, artifactual echo noise will be displayed throughout the image.

25. The condition of assigning each level of amplitude a particular shade of gray is referred to as the

   _____ scale.

26. The _____ mode displays time along the horizontal axis and depth along the vertical axis to depict movement, especially in cardiac structures.

27. With pulsed Doppler, for accurate detection of Doppler frequencies, the Doppler signal must be sampled at least

_____ for each cycle in the wave.

28. When the Nyquist limit is exceeded, an artifact called _____ occurs.

# 2 Essentials of Patient Care for the Sonographer

## KEY TERMS

### Exercise 1

*Match the following basic patient care terms with their definitions.*

_____ 1. patient-focused care (PFC)

_____ 2. vital signs

_____ 3. pulse

_____ 4. nasal cannula

_____ 5. bradycardia

_____ 6. oximetry

_____ 7. respiration

_____ 8. dyspnea

_____ 9. apnea

_____ 10. ostomy

_____ 11. isolated systolic hypertension

_____ 12. pulse pressure

_____ 13. intravenous (IV) therapy

_____ 14. body mechanics
_____ 15. standard precautions
_____ 16. nosocomial infection

A. An easy and effective way to measure heart rate; recorded as beats per minute (bpm)
B. Noninvasive method of monitoring oxygen levels in the blood
C. Refers to observable and measurable signs of life
D. Hospital-acquired infection
E. Shortness of breath or the feeling of not getting enough air, which may leave a person gasping
F. Difference between systolic and diastolic blood pressures
G. Spontaneous breathing that stops for any reason; it may be temporary, starting and stopping at intervals, or prolonged
H. Exists when systolic pressure is above 140 mmHg, while diastolic pressure remains below 90 mmHg
I. Represents a national movement to recapture the respect and goodwill of the American public
J. Heart rate of less than 60 bpm arising from disease in the heart's electrical conduction system
K. Process of inhaling and exhaling air
L. Surgical procedure to create an opening to allow passage of contents of the urinary bladder or bowel through the abdominal wall
M. The practice of giving liquid substances directly into a vein
N. Basic infection control guidelines used to reduce the risks of infection spread through these transmission modes: airborne infection, droplet infection, and contact infection
O. Refers to using the correct muscles to complete a task safely, efficiently, and without undue strain on any joints or muscles
P. Device for delivering oxygen by way of two small tubes inserted into the nostrils

## BASIC PATIENT CARE

### Exercise 2

*Fill in the blank(s) with the word(s) that best completes the statements, or provide a short answer.*

1. What is the most important facet of being a sonographer?

_____

2. Despite your personal or philosophical concerns, you must be considerate of the patient's _____, _____, _____, and _____.

3. Examples of vital signs include _____, _____, _____, and _____.

4. Strenuous exercise, coronary artery disease, and electrolyte imbalances in the blood can cause _____.

**7**

5. When a pulse is taken, which artery is usually palpated? _____

6. A normal pulse oximetry reading for a person breathing room air is _____.

7. Normal respiration occurs at a rate of 15 to _____ breaths per minute.

8. As blood travels away from the heart, the pressure of the circulating blood _____, spreading through arteries and capillaries and back toward the heart through the veins.

9. The primary function of respiration is to obtain oxygen for use by the body's cells and to eliminate the cells'

   production of _____.

10. In measuring blood pressure, the higher number is the _____ pressure, which occurs when the

    ventricles contract to pump blood to the body; the lower number is the _____ pressure, which occurs near the end of the cardiac cycle when the ventricles are filling with blood.

11. Describe the findings when a patient has an infiltrated IV tubing.

    _____

    _____

12. What is the purpose of an NG tube?

    _____

    _____

13. When catheterized patients are transferred from wheelchairs or stretchers to the scanning table, in what position should the collecting bag be placed?

    _____

## PATIENT TRANSFER TECHNIQUES

### Exercise 3

*Fill in the blanks with the word(s) that best completes the statements, or provide a short answer.*

1. List the four basic principles of body mechanics.

   a. _____

   b. _____

   c. _____

   d. _____

2. Lifting should be done using the _____ muscles, by lifting straight upward in one smooth motion.

3. Describe the method used to transfer a patient from a wheelchair to the bed when working alone.

   _____

   _____

   _____

   _____

   _____

## INFECTION CONTROL

### Exercise 4

*Fill in the blanks with the word(s) that best completes the statements, or provide a short answer.*

1. The most important weapon against the spread of infection is proper _____.

2. You should wash your hands whenever you come in contact with these five substances:

    a. _____

    b. _____

    c. _____

    d. _____

    e. _____

3. Is it acceptable to not wash your hands if gloves were used? _____

4. When should a mask be worn?

    _____

    _____

    _____

5. What should be used to clean the transducer? _____

6. Name four airborne diseases.

    a. _____

    b. _____

    c. _____

    d. _____

7. Name the six droplet diseases.

    a. _____

    b. _____

    c. _____

    d. _____

    e. _____

    f. _____

8. Name one of the most serious of contact diseases. _____

9. Describe the factors necessary to prepare a sterile field.

    _____

    _____

    _____

**Exercise 5**

*Reply to each question based on what you have learned in the chapter.*

1. List three rights that patients have in the medical setting.

   a. _____

   b. _____

   c. _____

2. List three responsibilities that the patient has.

   a. _____

   b. _____

   c. _____

3. What is HIPAA?

   _____

   _____

4. What does HIPAA mean for sonographers?

   _____

   _____

   _____

   _____

   _____

# 3 Ergonomics and Musculoskeletal Issues in Sonography

## KEY TERMS

**Exercise 1**

*Match the following terms with their definitions.*

_____ 1. work-related musculoskeletal disorders (WRMSDs)

_____ 2. tendinitis and tenosynovitis

_____ 3. de Quervain's disease

_____ 4. ergonomics

_____ 5. carpal tunnel

_____ 6. cubital tunnel

_____ 7. epicondylitis (lateral and medial)

_____ 8. thoracic outlet syndrome

_____ 9. Occupational Safety and Health Act

_____ 10. trigger finger

_____ 11. bursitis (shoulder)

_____ 12. rotator cuff injury

_____ 13. spinal degeneration

_____ 14. rotator cuff injury

A. Entrapment of the median nerve as it runs through the carpal bones of the wrist; results from repeated flexion and extension of the wrist and from mechanical pressure against the wrist

B. Nerve entrapment can occur at different levels, resulting in a variety of symptoms

C. The science of designing a job to fit the individual worker

D. Intervertebral disk degeneration resulting from bending and twisting and improper seating

E. Inflammation of the tendon and the sheath around the tendon; often occurs together

F. Inflammation of the periosteum in the area of the insertion of the biceps tendon into the distal humerus; can result from repeated twisting of the forearm

G. Inflammation of the shoulder bursa from repeated motion

H. Specific type of tendinitis involving the thumb; can result from gripping the transducer

I. Entrapment of the ulnar nerve as it runs through the elbow; can result from repeated twisting of the forearm and from mechanical pressure against the elbow when it is rested on the examination table during scanning

J. Repeated motion resulting in fraying of the rotator cuff muscle tendons; this injury increases with age and is even more prevalent when work-related stresses are added

K. Repeated arm abduction contributes to this injury by restricting blood flow to the soft tissues of the shoulder

L. Term currently used to describe occupational injury

M. Inflammation and swelling of the tendon sheath in a finger, entrapping the tendon and restricting motion of the finger

N. Federal law that ensures that every working man and woman in the United States has safe and healthful working conditions

**Exercise 2**

*Provide a short answer for the following questions.*

1. List the risk factors that may lead to musculoskeletal injury for sonographers.

_____

_____

2. Explain how accumulated exposure to one or more risk factors interferes with the muscles and joints.

_____

_____

_____

**BEST PRACTICES**

**Exercise 3**

*Provide a short answer for the following questions.*

1. Does the photo below demonstrate good or bad ergonomics? Explain your answer.

_____

_____

_____

2. Does the photo below demonstrate good or bad ergonomics? Explain your answer.

_____

_____

_____

3. Does the photo below demonstrate good or bad ergonomics? Explain your answer.

_____

_____

_____

# 4 Anatomic and Physiologic Relationships within the Abdominopelvic Cavity

## KEY TERMS

### Exercise 1

*Match the following general terms and terms related to abdominal planes with their definitions.*

_____ 1. homeostasis

_____ 2. intertubercular plane

_____ 3. metabolism

_____ 4. subcostal plane

_____ 5. transpyloric plane

A. Physical and chemical changes that occur within the body
B. Maintenance of normal body physiology
C. Lowest horizontal imaginary line that joins the tubercles on the iliac crests
D. Horizontal plane that passes through the pylorus, the duodenal junction, the neck of the pancreas, and the hilum of the kidneys
E. Upper horizontal imaginary line that joins the lowest point of the costal margin on each side of the body

### Exercise 2

*Match the following terms related to body cavities and abdominal structures with their definitions.*

_____ 1. diaphragm

_____ 2. inguinal ligament

_____ 3. lateral arcuate ligament

_____ 4. left crus of the diaphragm

_____ 5. linea alba

_____ 6. linea semilunaris

_____ 7. medial arcuate ligament

_____ 8. pelvic cavity

_____ 9. rectouterine space

_____10. rectus abdominis muscle

_____11. right crus of the diaphragm

_____12. scrotal cavity

_____13. superficial inguinal ring

_____14. vesicouterine pouch

_____15. viscera

A. Arises from the sides of the bodies of the first two lumbar vertebrae
B. Thickened upper margin of the fascia covering the anterior surface of the psoas muscle
C. Slightly curved line on the ventral abdominal wall that marks the lateral border of the rectus abdominis
D. Ligament between the anterior superior iliac spine and the pubic tubercle
E. Area in the pelvic cavity between the rectum and the uterus where free fluid may accumulate
F. Arises from the sides of the bodies of the first three lumbar vertebrae
G. Fibrous band of tissue that stretches from the xiphoid to the symphysis pubis
H. Formed by the deflection of the peritoneum from the bladder to the uterus
I. Broad muscle that separates the thoracic and abdominopelvic cavities and forms the floor of the thoracic cavity
J. Thickened upper margin of the fascia covering the anterior surface of the quadratus lumborum muscle
K. In the male, a small outpocket of the pelvic cavity containing the testes
L. Triangular opening in the external oblique aponeurosis
M. Lower portion of the abdominopelvic cavity that contains part of the large intestine, the rectum, urinary bladder, and reproductive organs
N. The internal organs
O. Muscle of the anterior abdominal wall

## Exercise 3

*Match the following terms related to abdominal membranes and ligaments, potential spaces in the body, and the retroperitoneum with their definitions.*

_____ 1. anterior pararenal space

_____ 2. ascites

_____ 3. epiploic foramen

_____ 4. falciform ligament

_____ 5. gastrosplenic ligament

_____ 6. greater omentum

_____ 7. greater sac

_____ 8. lesser omentum

_____ 9. lesser sac

_____ 10. lienorenal ligament

_____ 11. ligamentum teres

_____ 12. mesothelium

_____ 13. Morison's pouch

_____ 14. parietal peritoneum

_____ 15. perirenal space

_____ 16. peritoneal cavity

_____ 17. peritoneal recess

_____ 18. posterior pararenal space

_____ 19. visceral peritoneum

A. Attaches the liver to the anterior abdominal wall and undersurface of the diaphragm
B. Located between the anterior surface of the renal fascia and the posterior area of the peritoneum
C. Single layer of cells that forms the peritoneum
D. Primary compartment of the peritoneal cavity; extends across the anterior abdomen from the diaphragm to the pelvis
E. Ligament between the stomach and the spleen; helps support the stomach and spleen
F. Located directly around the kidney; completely enclosed by renal fascia
G. Accumulation of serous fluid in the peritoneal cavity
H. Membranous extension of the peritoneum that suspends the stomach and duodenum from the liver; helps support the lesser curvature of the stomach
I. Layer of the peritoneum that lines the abdominal wall
J. Ligament between the spleen and kidney
K. Found between the posterior renal fascia and the muscles of the posterior abdominal wall
L. Opening to the lesser sac
M. Double fold of the peritoneum attached to the duodenum, stomach, and large intestine; helps support the greater curve of the stomach
N. Right posterior subhepatic space located anterior to the kidney and inferior to the liver where fluid may accumulate
O. Slitlike spaces near the liver; potential space for fluid to accumulate
P. Potential space between the parietal and visceral peritoneal layers
Q. Layer of peritoneum that covers the abdominal organs
R. Peritoneal pouch located behind the lesser omentum and stomach
S. Termination of the falciform ligament; seen in the left lobe of the liver

## ANATOMIC DIRECTIONS

### Exercise 4

*Fill in the blank(s) with the word(s) that best completes the statements about the anatomic directions.*

1. The front (belly) surface of the body is _____.

2. When a structure is closer to the body midline or point of attachment to the trunk, it is described as

   _____.

3. The top of the head is the most _____ point of the body.

4. Structures located toward the surface of the body are _____.

5. The back surface of the body is _____.

6. The sphincter of Oddi is _____ to the common bile duct.

7. The bottom of the feet is the most _____ point of the body.

8. Structures located farther inward (away from the body surface) are _____.

9. The hepatic artery is _____ to the common duct.

10. Toward the head is _____.

11. The structure is _____ if it is toward the far side of the body.

12. Toward the tail, or _____, is sometimes used instead of inferior.

## ANATOMY AND PHYSIOLOGY

### Exercise 5

*Match the following anatomy terms with their region.*

_____ 1. thoracic

_____ 2. popliteal

_____ 3. perineal

_____ 4. pelvic

_____ 5. mammary

_____ 6. lumbar

_____ 7. leg

_____ 8. groin or inguinal

_____ 9. femoral

_____ 10. costal

_____ 11. cervical

_____ 12. celiac

_____ 13. brachial

_____ 14. axillary

_____ 15. abdominal

A. Loin; the region of the lower back and side, between the lowest rib and the pelvis
B. Pelvis; the bony ring that girdles the lower portion of the trunk
C. Thigh; the part of the lower extremity between the hip and the knee
D. Area behind the knee
E. Abdomen
F. Depressed region between the abdomen and the thigh
G. Breasts
H. Neck region
I. Lower extremity, especially from the knee to the foot
J. Ribs
K. Area of armpit
L. Region between the anus and the pubic arch; includes the region of the external reproductive structures
M. Arm
N. Portion of trunk below the diaphragm
O. Chest; the part of the trunk below the neck and above the diaphragm

### Exercise 6

*Fill in the blank(s) with the word(s) that best completes the statements about the body cavity or anatomic structure.*

1. The two principal body cavities are the _____ and the _____.

2. The bony dorsal cavity may be subdivided into the _____, which holds the brain, and the vertebral or spinal canal, which contains the spinal cord.

3. The _____ is located near the anterior body surface and is subdivided into the _____ cavity and the _____ cavity.

4. The thoracic and abdominopelvic cavities are separated by a broad muscle, the _____, which forms the floor of the thoracic cavity.

5. The thoracic cavity is divided into two _____, each containing a lung, with the mediastinum between them.

6. The heart is surrounded by another cavity called the _____.

Chapter **4** **Anatomic and Physiologic Relationships within the Abdominopelvic Cavity**

**Exercise 7**

*Fill in the blank(s) with the word(s) that best completes the statements about the abdominal cavity.*

1. The abdominal cavity is bounded superiorly by the _____; anteriorly by the _____ muscles; posteriorly by the vertebral column, ribs, and iliac fossa; and inferiorly by the _____.

2. The liver lies posterior to the lower ribs with the majority of the right lobe in the right _____ and in the _____; the left lobe lies in the _____ and the left _____.

3. The right kidney lies slightly _____ relative to the left kidney.

4. The aorta lies _____ to the spine, slightly to the _____ of the midline in the abdomen.

5. The inferior vena cava lies to the _____ of the spine.

6. The dome-shaped muscle that separates the thorax from the abdominal cavity is the _____.

7. The _____ crus of the diaphragm arises from the sides of the bodies of the first three lumbar vertebrae.

8. The medial borders of the two crura as they cross anterior to the aorta are connected by the _____.

9. The fibrous band that stretches from the xiphoid to the symphysis pubis is the _____.

10. A sheath formed by the aponeuroses of the muscles of the lateral group is the _____ muscle.

11. Part of the abdominal cavity proper and lying between the iliac fossae, superior to the pelvic brim, is the

    _____.

12. The _____ contains the pelvic cavity and is found inferior to the brim of the pelvis.

13. List the four organs contained within the pelvic cavity.

14. The peritoneum passes from the bladder to the uterus to form the _____ pouch.

15. Between the uterus and the rectum the peritoneum forms the deep _____ pouch.

16. The _____ tubes extend laterally from the fundus of the uterus and are enveloped by a fold of peritoneum known as the broad ligament.

17. A muscular "sling" composed of the _____ and _____ muscles forms the inferior boundary of the true pelvis and separates it from the perineum.

18. The muscles that lie along the posterior and lateral margins of the pelvis major are the _____ and

    _____.

19. The _____ muscles form the posterior pelvic wall.

20. The _____ peritoneum is the portion that lines the abdominal wall but does not cover a viscus; the _____ peritoneum is the portion that covers an organ.

21. The _____ omentum is attached to the greater curvature of the stomach and hangs down like an apron in the space between the small intestine and anterior abdominal wall.

22. An extensive peritoneal pouch located behind the lesser omentum and stomach is the _____ sac.

23. The opening to the lesser sac in the abdomen is the _____.

24. The peritoneal ligaments are two-layered folds of _____ that attach the lesser mobile solid viscera to the abdominal walls.

25. The liver is attached by the ligament to the _____ anterior abdominal wall and to the undersurface of the diaphragm.

26. The _____ lies in the free borders of this ligament.

27. The visceral peritoneum covers the spleen and is reflected onto the greater curvature of the stomach as the anterior layer of the _____ ligament.

## Exercise 8

*Fill in the blank(s) with the word(s) that best completes the statements about the potential spaces in the body.*

1. The right and left anterior _____ spaces lie between the diaphragm and the liver, one on each side of the falciform ligament.

2. The right posterior subphrenic space that lies between the right lobe of the liver, the right kidney, and the right colic flexure is also called _____.

3. The omental bursa normally has some empty places known as _____.

4. The _____ lateral paracolic gutter communicates with the right posterior subphrenic space.

5. The protrusion of part of the abdominal contents beyond the normal confines of the abdominal wall is called a

_____.

## Exercise 9

*Fill in the blank(s) with the word(s) that best completes the statements, or provide a short answer about the retroperitoneum.*

1. Name the 12 anatomic structures that are found in the retroperitoneal cavity.

_____

_____

_____

2. The _____ is located between the anterior surface of the renal fascia (Gerota's fascia) and the posterior area of the peritoneum.

3. The _____ is found between the posterior renal fascia and the muscles of the posterior abdominal wall.

4. The _____ space is located directly around the kidney and is completely enclosed by renal fascia.

## Exercise 10

*Fill in the blank(s) with the word(s) that best completes the statements.*

1. There are many areas of anatomy and physiology: _____ studies the body by dissection of tissue; _____ studies parts of the tissue under the microscope; _____ studies the development before birth; and _____ is the study of disease processes.

2. Within the human body, the next most complex basic unit of structure and function is a microscopic part called a

_____.

3. Cells are organized into layers or masses that have common functions, known as a _____.

4. The four primary types of tissues in the body are _____, _____, _____, and _____ tissues.

**19**

5. Groups of different tissues combine to form _____, which are complex structures with specialized functions, such as the liver, pancreas, or uterus.

6. A coordinated group of organs is arranged into _____ _____.

7. All of the physical and chemical changes that occur within the body are referred to as _____.

8. Taking vital signs includes measuring _____ and _____ and observing rates and types of _____ and _____ movements.

# 5  Comparative Sectional Anatomy of the Abdominopelvic Cavity

## KEY TERMS

### Exercise 1

*Match the following general terms and terms related to abdominal planes with their definitions.*

_____ 1. Transverse

_____ 2. Sagittal

_____ 3. Longitudinal

_____ 4. Coronal

A. A lengthwise plane running from front to back. It divides the body or any of its parts into right and left sides, or two equal halves.

B. A lengthwise plane running from side to side, dividing the body into anterior and posterior portions.

C. A plane that is horizontal to the body

D. A plane that is parallel to the long axis of the body or part.

## ANATOMY AND PHYSIOLOGY

### Exercise 2

*Label the following illustrations.*

1. Cross section of the abdomen at the level of the tenth intervertebral disk.

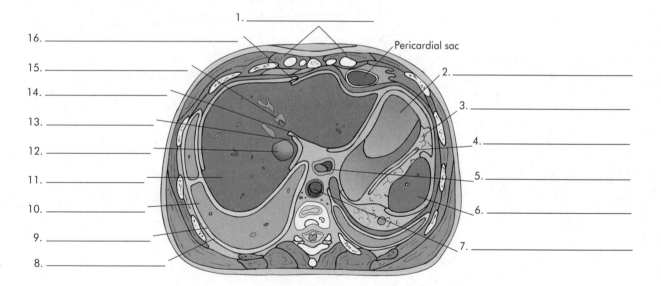

2. Cross section of the abdomen at the level of the eleventh thoracic disk.

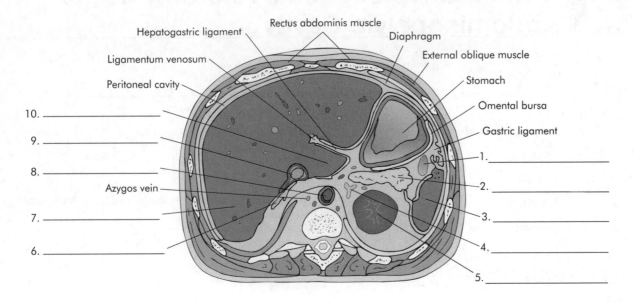

Hepatogastric ligament
Rectus abdominis muscle
Diaphragm
Ligamentum venosum
External oblique muscle
Peritoneal cavity
Stomach
Omental bursa
Gastric ligament

10. _____

9. _____

8. _____

Azygos vein

7. _____

6. _____

1. _____

2. _____

3. _____

4. _____

5. _____

3. Cross section of the abdomen at the level of the twelfth thoracic vertebra.

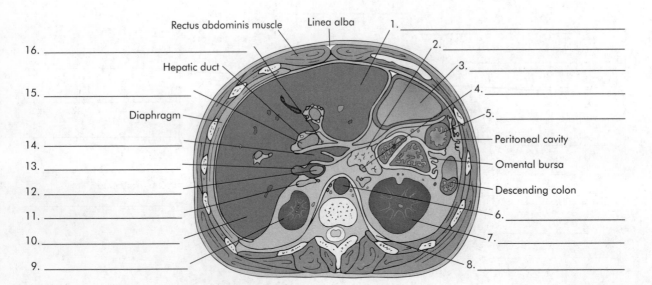

Rectus abdominis muscle
Linea alba

1. _____

16. _____

2. _____

Hepatic duct

3. _____

15. _____

4. _____

Diaphragm

5. _____

14. _____

Peritoneal cavity

13. _____

Omental bursa

12. _____

Descending colon

11. _____

6. _____

10. _____

7. _____

9. _____

8. _____

4. Cross section of the abdomen at the first lumbar vertebra.

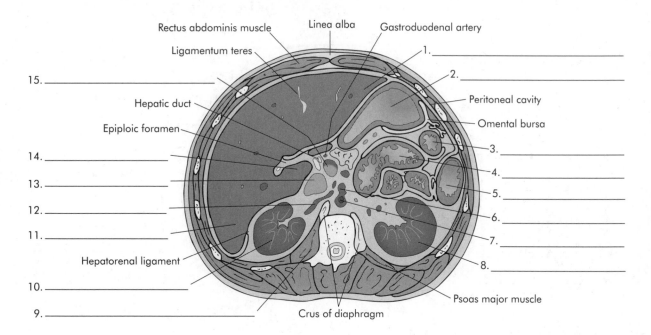

Rectus abdominis muscle    Linea alba    Gastroduodenal artery

Ligamentum teres

15. _____

Hepatic duct

Epiploic foramen

14. _____

13. _____

12. _____

11. _____

Hepatorenal ligament

10. _____

9. _____

1. _____

2. _____

Peritoneal cavity

Omental bursa

3. _____

4. _____

5. _____

6. _____

7. _____

8. _____

Psoas major muscle

Crus of diaphragm

5. Cross section of the abdomen at the level of the second lumbar vertebra.

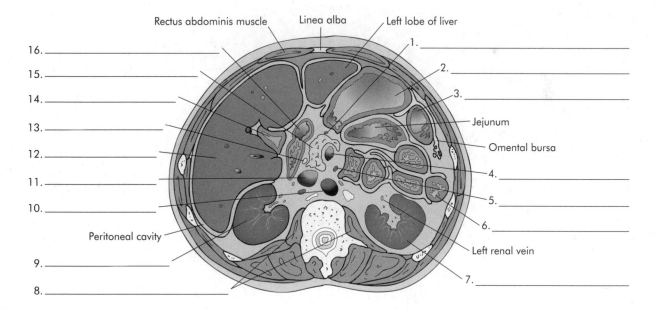

Rectus abdominis muscle    Linea alba    Left lobe of liver

16. _____

15. _____

14. _____

13. _____

12. _____

11. _____

10. _____

Peritoneal cavity

9. _____

8. _____

1. _____

2. _____

3. _____

Jejunum

Omental bursa

4. _____

5. _____

6. _____

Left renal vein

7. _____

Chapter 5  Comparative Sectional Anatomy of the Abdominopelvic Cavity

6. Cross section of the abdomen at the level of the third lumbar vertebra.

Rectus abdominis muscle    Linea alba    Rectus abdominis muscle
                                         Parietal peritoneum
Hepatocolic ligament                     1._____
12._____                   Transverse mesocolon
11._____                   Peritoneal cavity
10._____                   Jejunum
9._____                    Greater omentum
8._____                    2._____
7._____                    3._____
6._____                    4._____
                                         5._____

7. Cross section of the abdomen at the level of the third lumbar disk.

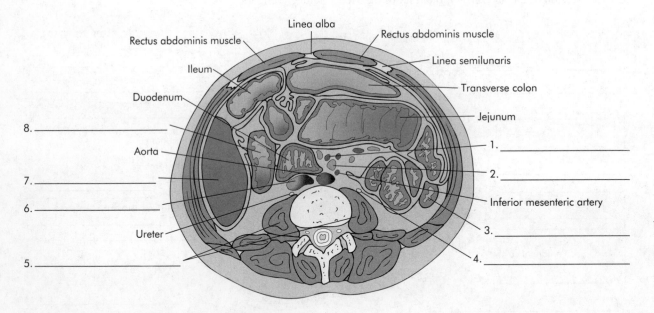

                          Linea alba
Rectus abdominis muscle              Rectus abdominis muscle
                                     Linea semilunaris
Ileum                                Transverse colon
Duodenum                             Jejunum
8._____                1._____
Aorta                                2._____
7._____                Inferior mesenteric artery
6._____                3._____
Ureter                               4._____
5._____

Chapter 5 **Comparative Sectional Anatomy of the Abdominopelvic Cavity**

8. Cross section of the pelvis taken at the lower margin of the fifth lumbar vertebra and disk.

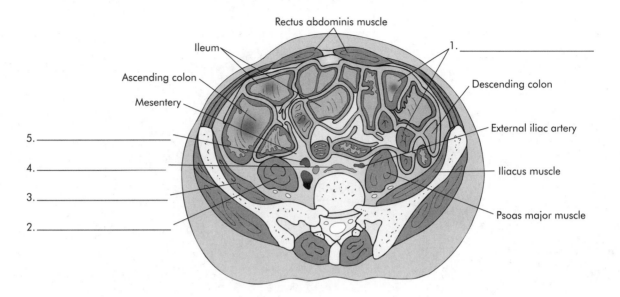

Rectus abdominis muscle

Ileum

Ascending colon

Mesentery

1. _____

Descending colon

External iliac artery

Iliacus muscle

Psoas major muscle

5. _____

4. _____

3. _____

2. _____

9. Cross section of the female pelvis just below the junction of the sacrum and coccyx.

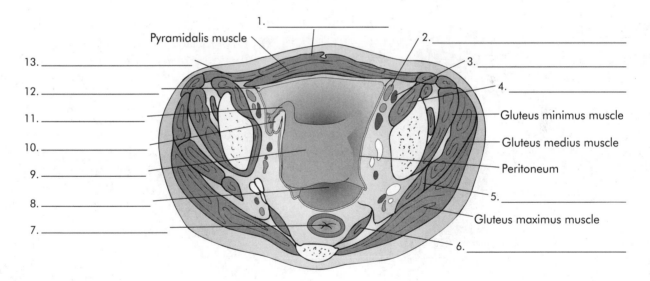

1. _____

Pyramidalis muscle

2. _____

3. _____

4. _____

13. _____

12. _____

11. _____

10. _____

9. _____

8. _____

7. _____

Gluteus minimus muscle

Gluteus medius muscle

Peritoneum

5. _____

Gluteus maximus muscle

6. _____

10. Cross section of the female pelvis taken through the lower part of the coccyx and the spine of the ischium.

Gluteus maximus muscle

Fascia of the pelvic diaphragm

Gluteus maximus muscle

11. Sagittal section of the abdomen taken along the right abdominal border.

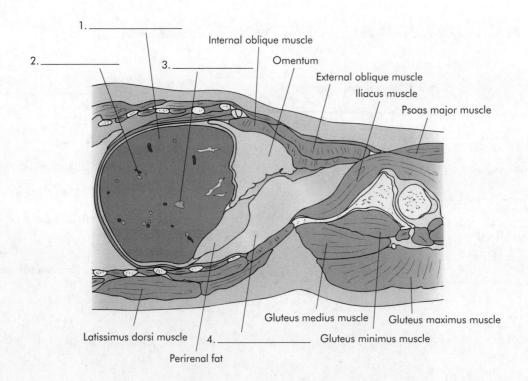

Internal oblique muscle

Omentum

External oblique muscle

Iliacus muscle

Psoas major muscle

Latissimus dorsi muscle

Perirenal fat

Gluteus medius muscle

Gluteus minimus muscle

Gluteus maximus muscle

12. Sagittal section of the abdomen 8 cm from the midline.

1. _____

6. _____

Hepatic flexure

5. _____

2. _____

3. _____

Cecum

Internal oblique muscle

Psoas major muscle

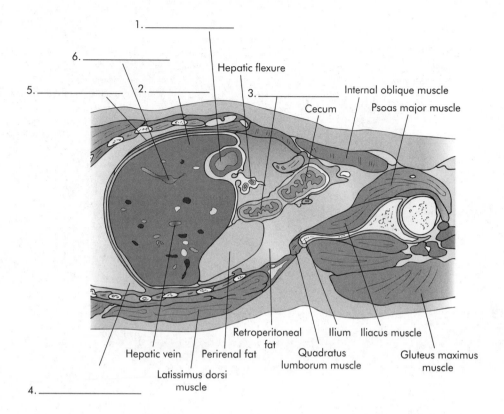

Retroperitoneal
fat

Ilium   Iliacus muscle

Hepatic vein    Perirenal fat

Quadratus
lumborum muscle

Gluteus maximus
muscle

Latissimus dorsi
muscle

4. _____

13. Sagittal section of the abdomen 7 cm from the midline.

2. _____

1. _____

5. _____

Transverse colon
Ascending colon

3. _____

4. _____

6. _____

Hepatic vein

Rectus sheath
Cecum

Small bowel
Mesentery

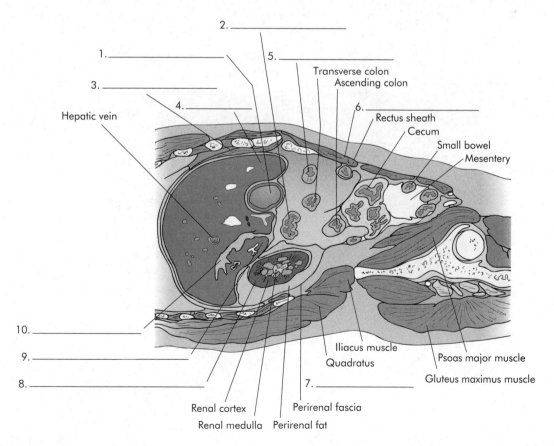

10. _____

9. _____

8. _____

Iliacus muscle
Quadratus

Psoas major muscle

Gluteus maximus muscle

7. _____

Renal cortex

Perirenal fascia

Renal medulla    Perirenal fat

14. Sagittal section of the abdomen 6 cm from the midline.

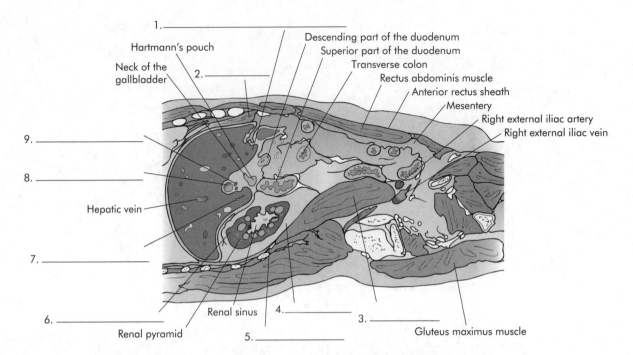

1. _____

Hartmann's pouch

Neck of the
gallbladder

2. _____

9. _____

8. _____

Hepatic vein

7. _____

6. _____

Renal pyramid

Renal sinus

4. _____

5. _____

3. _____

Descending part of the duodenum
Superior part of the duodenum
Transverse colon
Rectus abdominis muscle
Anterior rectus sheath
Mesentery
Right external iliac artery
Right external iliac vein

Gluteus maximus muscle

15. Sagittal section of the abdomen 3 cm from the midline.

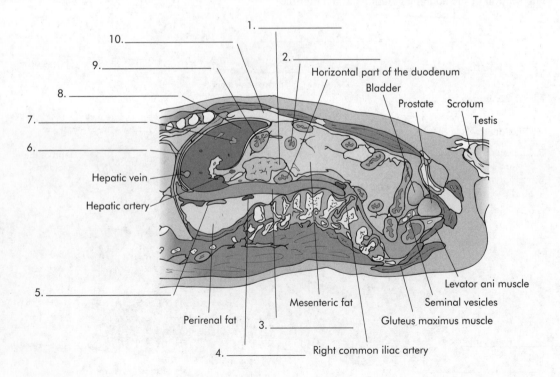

1. _____

10. _____

9. _____

8. _____

7. _____

6. _____

Hepatic vein

Hepatic artery

5. _____

Perirenal fat

Mesenteric fat

3. _____

4. _____

2. _____

Horizontal part of the duodenum
Bladder
Prostate    Scrotum
Testis

Levator ani muscle
Seminal vesicles
Gluteus maximus muscle

Right common iliac artery

16. Sagittal section of the abdomen 1 cm from the midline.

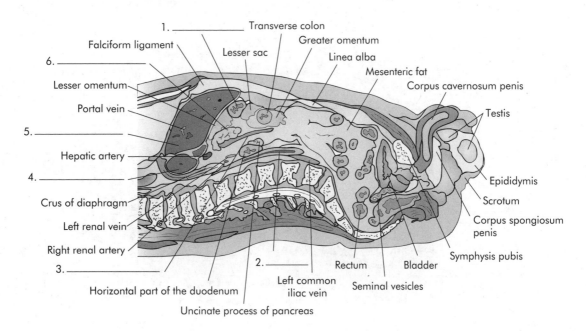

1. _____  Transverse colon
Falciform ligament  Greater omentum
6. _____  Lesser sac  Linea alba
Lesser omentum  Mesenteric fat
Portal vein  Corpus cavernosum penis
5. _____  Testis
Hepatic artery
4. _____  Epididymis
Crus of diaphragm  Scrotum
Left renal vein  Corpus spongiosum penis
Right renal artery  Symphysis pubis
3. _____  2. _____  Rectum  Bladder
Horizontal part of the duodenum  Left common iliac vein  Seminal vesicles
Uncinate process of pancreas

17. Midline sagittal section of the abdomen.

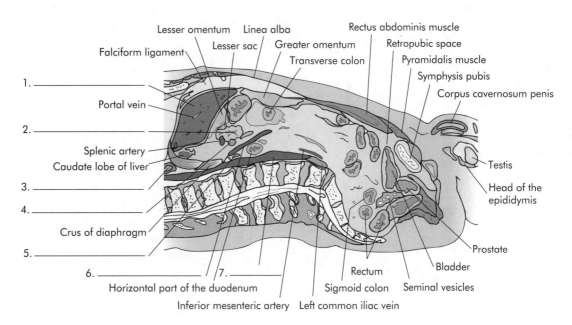

Lesser omentum  Linea alba  Rectus abdominis muscle
Falciform ligament  Lesser sac  Greater omentum  Retropubic space
Transverse colon  Pyramidalis muscle
Symphysis pubis
1. _____  Corpus cavernosum penis
Portal vein
2. _____
Splenic artery  Testis
Caudate lobe of liver  Head of the epididymis
3. _____
4. _____
Crus of diaphragm  Prostate
5. _____  Bladder
6. _____  7. _____  Rectum  Seminal vesicles
Horizontal part of the duodenum  Sigmoid colon
Inferior mesenteric artery  Left common iliac vein

18. Sagittal section of the abdomen along the left abdominal border.

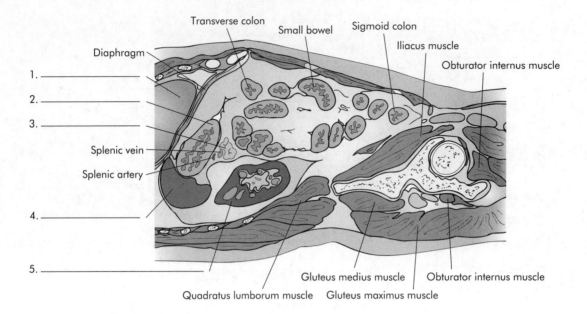

# 6 Basic Ultrasound Imaging: Techniques, Terminology & Tips

## Exercise 1

*Match the following arterial terms with their definitions.*

_____ 1. Curved array probe

_____ 2. Fan

_____ 3. Micro movement

_____ 4. Macro movement

_____ 5. Protocol

_____ 6. Rock

_____ 7. Rotate

_____ 8. Scan window

_____ 9. Sector array probe

_____10. Slide

_____11. Sweep

A. Standardization of specific anatomic structures that should be imaged in a complete or focused sonographic examination

B. Small-face transducer that allows adequate intercostal visualization, although the near field is reduced

C. This movement of the probe is used with the sweep and slight motion in which the probe is moved less than one centimeter.

D. This motion is used when the probe is physically moved along the area of interest.

E. Micro movement when the probe is minutely angled, pivoting on a point of interest

F. Motion used to navigate between the ribs or to change from transverse to longitudinal planes

G. The probe remains in one area while using a large wrist motion with the probe perpendicular to the skin surface to *sweep* through the area of interest.

H. This movement of the probe is used with the sweep and slight motion in which the probe is moved greater than one centimeter.

I. Large footprint that allows good near-field and far-field visualization with limited intercostal access

J. Probe is slowly angled back and forth in one place to image the area completely or to follow the anatomic structure.

K. Areas in the body that allow the sound beam to penetrate without obstruction

## SONOGRAPHIC EVALUATION

## Exercise 2

*Fill in the blank(s) with the word(s) that best completes the statements about abdominal scanning.*

1. All transverse supine scans are oriented with the liver on the _____ of the screen.

2. Longitudinal scans present the patient's head to the _____ and feet to the _____ of the screen and use the xiphoid, umbilicus, or symphysis to denote the midline of the scan plane.

3. The position of the patient should be described in relation to the _____.

4. Variations in the patient's respiration may also help eliminate _____ interference and improve image quality.

5. Patients should be instructed not to eat or drink anything for _____ hours before the abdominal ultrasound procedure.

6. Identify the structures that are included in a survey of the baseline upper abdominal ultrasound examination.

_____

_____

_____

7. In Doppler imaging, flow toward the transducer is positive, or _____, whereas flow away from the transducer is negative, or _____.

8. Arterial flow pulsates with the cardiac cycle and shows its maximal peak during the _____ part of the cycle.

9. A phasic pattern may be seen in the _____ (near the heart) that is associated with overload of the right ventricle.

10. Identify the following patient positions for ultrasound examinations.

1. _____

2. _____

3. _____

4. _____

## MEDICAL TERMS FOR THE SONOGRAPHER

### Exercise 3

*Match the following medical terms with their definitions.*

_____ 1. anechoic or sonolucent

_____ 2. echogenic or hyperechoic

_____ 3. enhancement, increased through transmission

_____ 4. fluid-fluid level

_____ 5. heterogeneous

_____ 6. homogeneous

_____ 7. hypoechoic

_____ 8. infiltrating

_____ 9. irregular borders

_____ 10. isoechoic

_____ 11. loculated mass

_____ 12. shadowing

A. Not uniform in texture or composition
B. Usually refers to a diffuse disease process or metastatic disease
C. Echo-producing structure; reflects sound with a brighter intensity
D. Interface between two fluids with different acoustic characteristics. This level will change with patient position.
E. Very close to the normal parenchymal echogenicity pattern
F. Sound that travels through an anechoic (fluid-filled) substance and is not attenuated. There is increased brightness directly beyond the posterior border of the anechoic structure as compared with the surrounding area.
G. Completely uniform in texture or composition
H. Borders are not well-defined, are ill-defined, or are not present.
I. Low-level echoes within a structure
J. Sound beam is attenuated by a solid or calcified object.
K. Well-defined borders with internal echoes; the septa may be thin (likely benign) or thick (likely malignant).
L. Without internal echoes; the structure is fluid filled and transmits sound easily.

**Exercise 4**

*Provide a short answer for each question about the criteria for identifying abnormalities.*

1. What three terms are used to describe various textures of the border of a structure?

   _____

2. What two terms may be used to identify the texture of a structure?

   _____

3. List the three terms that describe the transmission of sound.

   _____

4. List the five sonographic and medical terms that describe the characteristics of an organ or mass.

   _____

   _____

5. Describe the sonographic characteristics of a cystic mass.

   _____

   _____

6. Describe the sonographic characteristics of a solid mass.

   _____

   _____

7. Describe the sonographic characteristics of a complex mass.

   _____

   _____

# 7 Imaging and Doppler Artifacts

**Exercise 1**

*Match the following terms with their definitions.*

_____ 1. aliasing

_____ 2. anechoic

_____ 3. baseline shift

_____ 4. comet tail

_____ 5. cross talk

_____ 6. enhancement

_____ 7. hypoechoic

_____ 8. mirror image

_____ 9. multiple reflection

_____10. Nyquist limit

_____11. range ambiguity

_____12. resonance

_____13. reverberation

_____14. ring-down

_____15. section thickness

_____16. shadowing

_____17. speckle

_____18. speed error

A. Movement of the zero Doppler-shift frequency or zero flow speed line up or down on a spectral display

B. Increase in echo amplitude from reflectors that lie behind a weakly attenuating structure

C. Improper Doppler-shift information from a pulsed wave Doppler or color Doppler instrument when the true Doppler shift exceeds one half the pulse repetition frequency

D. Series of closely spaced reverberation echoes

E. Artifact produced when echoes are placed too close to the transducer because a second pulse was emitted before they were received

F. Echo-free

G. Leakage of strong signals in one direction channel of a Doppler receiver into the other channel; can produce the Doppler mirror-image artifact

H. Artifact resulting from a continuous stream of sound emanating from an anatomic site

I. Having relatively weak echoes

J. Condition where a driven mechanical vibration is of a frequency similar to a natural vibration frequency of the structure

K. Several reflections produced by a pulse encountering a pair of reflectors; reverberation

L. Artifactual gray-scale, color flow, or Doppler signal appearing on the opposite side (from the real structure or flow) of a strong reflector

M. Doppler-shift frequency above which aliasing occurs; one half the pulse repetition frequency

N. Multiple reflection

O. Granular appearance of images and spectral displays that is caused by the interference of echoes from the distribution of scatterers in tissue

P. Thickness of the scanned tissue volume perpendicular to the scan plane; also called slice thickness

Q. Propagation speed that is different from the assumed value (1.54 mm/ms)

R. Reduction in echo amplitude from reflectors that lie behind a strongly reflecting or attenuating structure

## Exercise 2

*Use each of the following terms once to describe the artifacts shown in the sonographic images.*

aliasing
banding
comet-tail
edge shadows
enhancement
grating lobe duplication
high gain produces a mirror image
interference

mirror image
range ambiguity
refraction
reverberation
ring-down
shadowing
slice thickness
speckle

1. _____

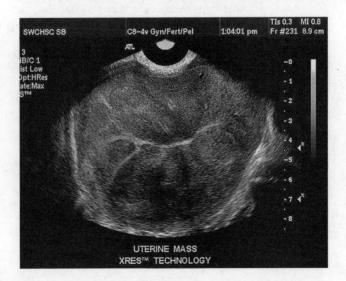

2. _____

Chapter **7**   **Imaging and Doppler Artifacts**

3. _____

4. _____

5. _____

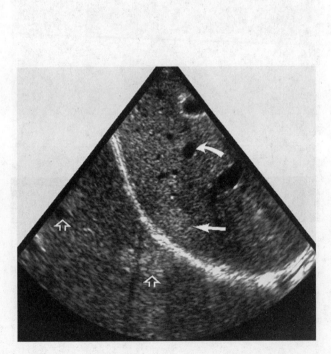

6. _____

Chapter **7** **Imaging and Doppler Artifacts**

7. _____

8. _____

9. _____

**39**

10. _____

11. _____

12. _____

13. _____

14. _____

15. _____

16. _____

# 8 Vascular System

## Exercise 1

*Match the following structural terms with their definitions.*

_____ 1. vasa vasorum

_____ 2. tunica media

_____ 3. tunica adventitia

_____ 4. tunica intima

_____ 5. anastomosis

_____ 6. capillaries

A. Tiny arteries and veins that supply the walls of blood vessels
B. Inner layer of the vascular system
C. Minute vessels that connect the arterial and venous systems
D. Communication between two blood vessels without any intervening capillary network
E. Outer layer of the vascular system, contains the vasa vasorum
F. Middle layer of the vascular system; veins have thinner tunica media than arteries

## Exercise 2

*Match the following arterial terms with their definitions.*

_____ 1. superior mesenteric artery

_____ 2. arteries

_____ 3. left hepatic artery

_____ 4. common iliac arteries

_____ 5. right renal artery

_____ 6. gastroduodenal artery

_____ 7. aorta

_____ 8. inferior mesenteric artery

_____ 9. left gastric artery

_____ 10. splenic artery

_____ 11. common hepatic artery

_____ 12. right hepatic artery

_____ 13. left renal artery

_____ 14. right gastric artery

A. Arises from the posterolateral wall of the aorta, travels posterior to the inferior vena cava to supply the kidney
B. Arises from the celiac axis to supply the stomach and lower third of the esophagus
C. Supplies the gallbladder via the cystic artery
D. Vascular structures that carry blood away from the heart
E. Arises from the celiac trunk to supply the liver
F. Supplies the stomach
G. Branch of the common hepatic artery that supplies the stomach and duodenum
H. Arises inferior to the celiac axis to supply the proximal half of the colon and the small intestine
I. The abdominal aorta bifurcates at the level of the umbilicus into these vessels, which supply blood to the lower extremities
J. Arises from the anterior aortic wall at the level of the third or fourth lumbar vertebra to supply the left transverse colon, descending colon, sigmoid colon, and rectum
K. Arises from the posterolateral wall of the aorta directly into the hilus of the kidney
L. Largest arterial structure in the body; arises from the left ventricle to supply blood to the head, upper and lower extremities, and abdominal-pelvic cavity and extremities
M. Small branch supplying the caudate and left lobes of the liver
N. Arises from the celiac axis to supply the spleen, pancreas, stomach, and greater omentum

**Exercise 3**

*Match the following venous terms with their definitions.*

_____1. splenic vein

_____2. hepatic veins

_____3. portal vein

_____4. right renal vein

_____5. veins

_____6. inferior mesenteric vein

_____7. left renal vein

_____8. superior mesenteric vein

_____9. inferior vena cava

A. Formed by the union of the superior mesenteric vein and splenic vein near the porta hepatis of the liver

B. Collapsible vascular structures that carry blood back to the heart

C. Drains the spleen; travels horizontally across abdomen (posterior to the pancreas) to join the superior mesenteric vein to form the portal vein

D. Drains the left third of the colon and upper colon and joins the splenic vein

E. Drains the proximal half of the colon and small intestine, travels vertically (anterior to the inferior vena cava) to join the splenic vein to form the portal veins

F. Three large veins that drain the liver and empty into the inferior vena cava at the level of the diaphragm

G. Leaves the renal hilum, travels anterior to the aorta and posterior to the superior mesenteric artery to enter the lateral wall of the inferior vena cava

H. Largest venous abdominal vessel that conveys blood from the body below the diaphragm to the right atrium of the heart

I. Leaves the renal hilum to enter the lateral wall of the inferior vena cava

**Exercise 4**

*Match the following pathology terms with their definitions.*

_____ 1. cystic medial necrosis

_____ 2. aneurysm

_____ 3. Budd-Chiari syndrome

_____ 4. arteriosclerosis

_____ 5. fusiform aneurysm

_____ 6. TIPS

_____ 7. saccular aneurysm

_____ 8. atherosclerosis

_____ 9. cavernous transformation of the portal vein

_____ 10. dissecting aneurysm

_____ 11. arteriovenous fistula

_____ 12. portal venous hypertension

_____ 13. pseudoaneurysm

_____ 14. Marfan syndrome

_____ 15. true aneurysm

A. Disease of the arterial vessels marked by thickening, hardening, and loss of elasticity in the arterial walls

B. Condition in which the aortic wall becomes irregular from plaque formation

C. Tear in the intima or media of the abdominal aorta

D. Permanent localized dilatation of an artery, with an increase of 1.5 times its normal diameter

E. Periportal collateral channels in patients with chronic portal vein obstruction

F. Circumferential enlargement of a vessel with tapering at both ends

G. Weakening of the arterial wall

H. Pulsatile hematoma that results from leakage of blood into soft tissue abutting the punctured artery with fibrous encapsulation and failure of the vessel wall to heal

I. Transjugular intrahepatic portosystemic shunt

J. Most commonly results from intrinsic liver disease; however, also results from obstruction of the portal vein, hepatic veins, inferior vena cava, or prolonged congestive heart failure; may cause flow reversal to the liver, thrombosis of the portal system, or cavernous transformation of the portal vein

K. Communication between an artery and a vein

L. Localized dilatation of the vessel

M. Permanent dilation of an artery that forms when tensile strength of the arterial wall decreases

N. Hereditary disorder of connective tissue, bones, muscles, ligaments, and skeletal structures

O. Thrombosis of the hepatic veins

## Exercise 5

*Match the following abdominal Doppler terms with their definitions.*

_____ 1. resistive

_____ 2. hepatopetal

_____ 3. nonresistive

_____ 4. resistive index

_____ 5. spectral broadening

_____ 6. hepatofugal

_____ 7. Doppler sample volume

A.  Vessels that have high diastolic component and supply organs that need constant perfusion (i.e., internal carotid artery, hepatic artery, and renal artery)
B.  Flow away from the liver
C.  Peak systole minus peak diastole divided by peak systole
D.  Flow toward the liver
E.  Vessels that have little or reversed flow in diastole and supply organs that do not need a constant blood supply (i.e., external carotid artery and brachial arteries)
F.  Increased turbulence is seen within the spectral tracing that indicates flow disturbance.
G.  Sonographer selects the exact site to record Doppler signals and sets the sample volume (gate) at this site.

## ANATOMY AND PHYSIOLOGY

### Exercise 6

*Label the following illustrations.*

1. The abdominal arterial vascular system and its tributaries.

1. _____

2. _____

3. _____

4. _____

5. _____

6. _____

7. _____

8. _____

9. _____

10. _____

11. _____

12. _____

13. _____

2. The celiac artery and its branches.

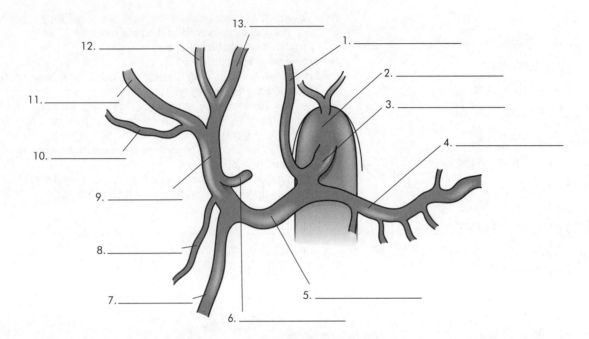

13. _____

12. _____

1. _____

2. _____

11. _____

3. _____

10. _____

4. _____

9. _____

8. _____

7. _____

5. _____

6. _____

3. The superior mesenteric artery.

17. _____

1. _____

16. _____

2. _____

15. _____

3. _____

14. _____

4. _____

13. _____

5. _____

12. _____

11. _____

6. _____

10. _____

7. _____

9. _____

8. _____

4. The abdominal venous system and its tributaries.

10. _____

1. _____

9. _____

2. _____

3. _____

8. _____

4. _____

7. _____

5. _____

6. _____

5. The portal vein.

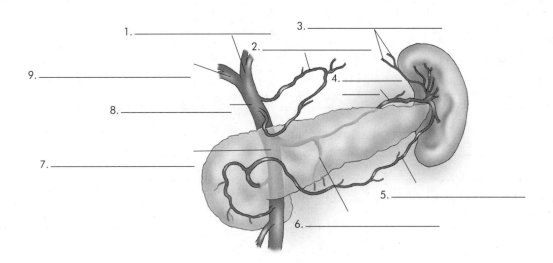

1. _____

3. _____

2. _____

9. _____

4. _____

8. _____

7. _____

5. _____

6. _____

**Exercise 7**

*Fill in the blank(s) with the word(s) that best completes the statements about the arterial and venous structures.*

1. The root of the aorta arises from the _____ outflow tract in the heart.

2. The _____ passes anterior to the third part of the duodenum and posterior to the neck of the pancreas, where it joins the splenic vein to form the main portal vein.

3. The _____ hepatic artery supplies the gallbladder via the cystic artery and the liver.

**47**

4. The aorta continues to flow in the _____ cavity anterior and slightly _____ of the vertebral column.

5. The _____ trunk is the first anterior branch of the aorta, arising 1 to 2 cm inferior to the diaphragm.

6. The _____ flows from the kidney posterior to the superior mesenteric artery and anterior to the aorta to enter the lateral wall of the inferior vena cava.

7. The diameter of the abdominal aorta measures approximately _____ cm, tapering to

   _____ cm after it proceeds inferiorly to the bifurcation into the iliac arteries.

8. The _____ is the second anterior branch, arising approximately 2 cm from the celiac trunk.

9. Portal veins become _____ as they progress into the liver from the porta hepatis.

10. The _____ renal artery courses from the aorta posterior to the inferior vena cava and anterior to the vertebral column in a posterior and slightly caudal direction to enter the hilum of the kidney.

11. The _____ artery courses along the upper border of the head of the pancreas, behind the posterior layer of the peritoneal bursa, to the upper margin of the superior part of the duodenum, which forms the lower boundary of the epiploic foramen.

12. Three arterial branches arise from the superior border of the aortic arch to supply the head, neck, and upper

    extremities: the _____, _____, and _____.

13. The _____ vein is formed posterior to the pancreas by the union of the superior mesenteric vein and splenic veins at the level of L2.

14. The _____ artery takes a somewhat tortuous course horizontally to the left as it forms the superior border of the pancreas.

15. The portion of the femoral artery posterior to the knee is the _____ artery.

16. The _____ veins originate in the liver and drain into the inferior vena cava at the level of the diaphragm.

## Exercise 8

*Provide a short answer for each anatomy and physiology question.*

1. List the five sections into which the aorta is divided.

   _____

   _____

   _____

   _____

2. Describe the specific differences between arteries and veins.

   _____

   _____

   _____

   _____

3. List the four branches of the aorta that supply other visceral organs and the mesentery.

   _____

   _____

   _____

   _____

Chapter **8** **Vascular System**

4. Describe the function of the circulatory system.

_____

_____

_____

_____

5. List the characteristics of a vein.

_____

_____

_____

_____

6. Describe how blood is transported from the artery and returned by the veins.

_____

_____

_____

_____

7. Define capillaries and describe their function.

_____

_____

_____

_____

## SONOGRAPHIC EVALUATION

### Exercise 9

*Fill in the blank(s) with the word(s) that best completes the statements, or provide a short answer about the vascular and abdominal sonographic evaluations.*

1. Describe how Doppler is used to distinguish the presence or absence of flow in a vessel from nonvascular structures.

_____

_____

_____

_____

2. A flow disturbance (increased velocity or obstruction of flow) may result from the formation of an atheroma, AV

fistula, _____, or aneurysmal dilation.

3. Describe the technique that should be used to image the inferior vena cava.

_____

_____

_____

_____

**49**

Chapter **8** **Vascular System**

4. Nonresistive vessels have a high _____ component and supply organs that need constant perfusion, such as the internal carotid artery, the hepatic artery, and the renal artery.

5. Resistive vessels have very little or even reversed flow in diastole and supply organs that do not need a constant blood supply, such as the _____ carotid and the iliac and brachial arteries.

6. Explain how to differentiate the inferior vena cava from the aorta.

_____

_____

_____

_____

7. _____ is a pattern of blood flow, typically seen in large arteries, in which most cells are moving at the same velocity across the entire diameter of the vessel. In other vessels the different velocities are the result of friction between the cells and arterial walls.

8. Doppler records accurate velocity patterns only when the beam is _____ to the flow.

9. The flow pattern of the proximal abdominal aorta above the renal arteries shows a high _____ peak and a relatively low _____ component.

10. The main renal artery has a(n) _____ impedance (nonresistive) pattern with significant diastolic flow—usually 303% to 50% of peak systole.

11. During rejection, the vascular impedance _____, resulting in a decrease or even reversal of the diastolic flow.

12. The portal vein shows a relatively _____ flow at low velocities, which may vary slightly with respirations.

13. Cavernous transformation of the portal vein demonstrates _____ collateral channels in patients with chronic portal vein obstruction.

14. With a recanalized _____ vein, the main portal vein and the left portal vein show normal flow, but the flow in the right portal vein is reversed.

## PATHOLOGY

### Exercise 10

*Fill in the blank(s) with the word(s) that best completes the statements, or provide a short answer about vascular pathology.*

1. The most common causes of aneurysms are _____ and _____.

2. The large aneurysm may rupture into the peritoneal cavity or retroperitoneum, causing _____ and a drop in _____.

3. The normal measurement for an adult abdominal aorta is less than 3 cm, measuring from _____ to _____ walls.

4. Thrombus usually occurs along the _____ or _____ wall.

5. A(n) _____ is a pulsatile hematoma that results from the leakage of blood into the soft tissue abutting the punctured artery, with subsequent fibrous encapsulation and failure of the vessel wall defect to heal.

6. What are the clinical findings in a patient with a dissecting aneurysm?

_____

_____

_____

_____

7. Describe the three locations where a dissection of the aorta may occur.

_____

_____

_____

_____

8. Describe other pseudopulsatile abdominal masses that may simulate an aortic aneurysm.

_____

_____

_____

_____

9. In patients with right ventricular failure, the inferior vena cava does not collapse with _____.

10. Describe the complications of inferior vena caval thrombosis.

_____

_____

_____

_____

11. The most common origin of pulmonary emboli is venous thrombosis from the _____ extremities.

**Exercise 11**

*Provide a short answer for each question after evaluating the images.*

1. A patient presents with a pulsatile abdominal mass. What does this longitudinal image of the abdomen demonstrate?

A                                    B

_____

_____

2. How can the sonographer determine that the inferior vena cava is dilated?

_____

_____

3. Which renal vessel is demonstrated in this image?

_____

_____

# 9 Liver

## KEY TERMS

### Exercise 1

*Match the following anatomy terms with their definitions.*

__C__ 1. bare area

__A__ 2. caudate lobe

__N__ 3. epigastrium

__G__ 4. falciform ligament

__M__ 5. left hypochondrium

__D__ 6. left lobe of the liver

__H__ 7. left portal vein

__I__ 8. ligamentum teres

__B__ 9. ligamentum venosum

__F__ 10. main lobar fissure

__J__ 11. main portal vein

__K__ 12. right hypochondrium

__E__ 13. right lobe of the liver

__L__ 14. right portal vein

A. Smallest lobe of the liver situated on the posterosuperior surface of the left lobe; the ligamentum venosum is the anterior border

B. Separates left lobe from caudate lobe; shown as echogenic line on the transverse and sagittal images

C. Area superior to the liver that is not covered by peritoneum so that inferior vena cava may enter the chest

D. Lies in the epigastrium and left hypochondrium

E. Largest lobe of the liver

F. Boundary between the right and left lobes of the liver; seen as hyperechoic line on the sagittal image extending from the portal vein to the neck of the gallbladder

G. Extends from the umbilicus to the diaphragm in a sagittal plane and contains the ligamentum teres

H. Supplies the left lobe of the liver

I. Appears as bright echogenic foci on transverse image; along with falciform ligament, it divides medial and lateral segments of left lobe of the liver

J. Enters the liver at the porta hepatis

K. Right upper quadrant of the abdomen that contains the liver and gallbladder

L. Supplies the right lobe of the liver; branches into anterior and posterior segments

M. Left upper quadrant of the abdomen that contains the left lobe of the liver, spleen, and stomach

N. Area between the right and left hypochondrium

### Exercise 2

*Match the following physiology and laboratory terms with their definitions.*

__H__ 1. alkaline phosphatase

__E__ 2. ALT

__D__ 3. AST

__A__ 4. bilirubin

__J__ 5. BUN

__I__ 6. hepatocellular disease

__F__ 7. hepatocyte

__C__ 8. liver function tests

__K__ 9. obstructive disease

__G__ 10. hyperglycemia

__B__ 11. hypoglycemia

A. Yellow pigment in bile formed by the breakdown of red blood cells; excreted by liver and stored in the gallbladder

B. Deficiency in blood glucose levels

C. Specific laboratory tests that look at liver function (aspartate or alanine aminotransferase, lactic acid dehydrogenase, alkaline phosphatase, and bilirubin)

D. Aspartate aminotransferase—enzyme of the liver

E. Alanine aminotransferase—enzyme of the liver

F. Parenchymal liver cell that performs all functions ascribed to the liver

G. Uncontrolled increase in blood glucose levels

H. Enzyme of the liver

I. Classification of liver disease where hepatocytes are the primary problem

J. Blood urea nitrogen; laboratory measurement of the amount of nitrogenous waste and creatinine in the blood

K. Classification of liver disease where the main problem is blocked bile excretion within the liver or biliary system

## Exercise 3

*Match the following pathology terms with their definitions.*

B  1. bull's-eye (target) lesion
H  2. collateral circulation
F  3. diffuse hepatocellular disease
A  4. extrahepatic
D  5. intrahepatic
E  6. metastatic disease
C  7. neoplasm
G  8. pyogenic abscess

A. Outside the liver
B. Hypoechoic mass with an echogenic central core (abscess, metastases)
C. Any new growth (benign or malignant)
D. Within the liver
E. Most common form of neoplasm of the liver; primary sites are colon, breast, and lung
F. Affects hepatocytes and interferes with liver function
G. Pus-forming collection of fluid
H. Develops when normal venous channels become obstructed

## ANATOMY AND PHYSIOLOGY

### Exercise 4

*Label the following illustrations.*

1. Anterior view of the liver.

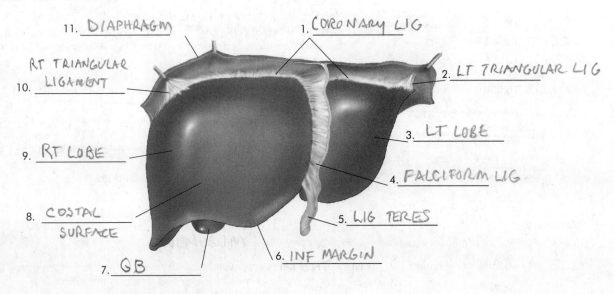

11. DIAPHRAGM
1. CORONARY LIG
10. RT TRIANGULAR LIGAMENT
2. LT TRIANGULAR LIG
9. RT LOBE
3. LT LOBE
8. COSTAL SURFACE
4. FALCIFORM LIG
7. GB
5. LIG TERES
6. INF MARGIN

2. Superior view of the liver.

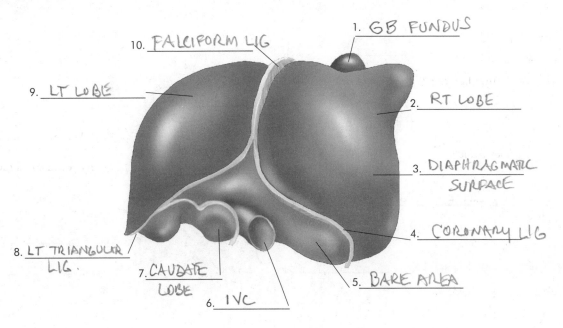

10. _FALCIFORM LIG_

1. _GB FUNDUS_

9. _LT LOBE_

2. _RT LOBE_

3. _DIAPHRAGMATIC SURFACE_

4. _CORONARY LIG_

8. _LT TRIANGULAR LIG._

7. _CAUDATE LOBE_

6. _IVC_

5. _BARE AREA_

3. Interior view of the visceral surface of the liver.

20. _GB_

19. _CYSTIC DUCT_

18. _COLIC IMPRESSION_

17. _DUODENAL IMPRESS._

16. _RENAL IMPRESSION_

15. _RT LOBE_

14. _RT TRIANGULAR LIG._

13. _BARE AREA_

12. _CORONARY LIG_

11. _IVC_

10. _CAUDATE LOBE_

1. _MEDIAL LT LOBE_

2. _PYLORIC AREA_

3. _LIG TERES_

4. _HEPATIC AA_

5. _LT LOBE_

6. _PORTAL VEIN_

7. _GASTRIC IMPRESSION_

8. _ESOPHAGEAL IMPRESSION_

9. _LIG VENOSUM_

**55**

4. Posterior view of the diaphragmatic surface of the liver.

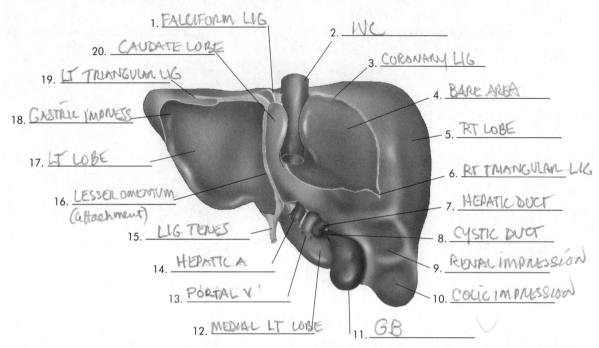

1. FALCIFORM LIG
20. CAUDATE LOBE
19. LT TRIANGULAR LIG
18. GASTRIC IMPRESS
17. LT LOBE
16. LESSER OMENTUM (attachment)
15. LIG TERES
14. HEPATIC A
13. PORTAL V
12. MEDIAL LT LOBE
11. GB
2. IVC
3. CORONARY LIG
4. BARE AREA
5. RT LOBE
6. RT TRIANGULAR LIG
7. HEPATIC DUCT
8. CYSTIC DUCT
9. RENAL IMPRESSION
10. COLIC IMPRESSION

**Exercise 5**

*Fill in the blank(s) with the word(s) that best completes the statements about the anatomy and physiology of the liver.*

1. A congenital variant, REIDEL'S lobe, can sometimes be seen as an anterior projection of the liver and may extend inferiorly as far as the iliac crest.

2. The liver is covered by a thin connective tissue layer called GLISGON'S capsule.

3. The MAIN LOBAR fissure is the boundary between the right and left lobes of the liver.

4. The FALCIFORM ligament extends from the umbilicus to the diaphragm in a parasagittal plane and contains the ligamentum teres.

5. The ligamentum TERES appears as a bright echogenic focus on the sonogram and is seen as the rounded termination of the falciform ligament.

6. The fissure for the ligamentum VENOSUM separates the left lobe from the caudate lobe.

7. The hepatic veins are divided into three components: RIGHT, MI, MIDDLE, and LEFT.

8. The liver is a major center of METABOLISM, which may be defined as the physical and chemical process whereby foodstuffs are synthesized into complex elements.

9. Through the process of DIGESTION, the liver expels these waste products from the body via its excretory product, bile, which also plays an important role in fat absorption.

10. A pigment released when the red blood cells are broken down is BILIRUBIN.

11. The liver is a(n) STORAGE site for several compounds used in a variety of physiologic activities throughout the body.

12. The liver is also a center for DETOXIFICATION of the waste products of metabolism accumulated from other sources in the body and foreign chemicals that enter the body.

13. Diseases affecting the liver may be classified as HEPATOCELLULAR when the liver cells or hepatocytes are the immediate problem, or as OBSTRUCTIVE when bile excretion is blocked.

**56**

14. Raw materials in the form of ___C HO___, ___FATS___, and ___AAs___ are absorbed from the intestine and transported to the liver via the circulatory system.

15. Sugars may be absorbed from the blood in several forms, but only ___GLUCOSE___ can be used by cells throughout the body as a source of energy.

16. Dietary fats are converted in the hepatocytes to ___LIPOPROTEINS___, in which form fats are transported throughout the body to sites where they are used by other organs or stored.

17. The accompanying loss of ohcotic pressure in the vascular system allows fluid to migrate into the interstitial space, resulting in ___EDEMA___ in dependent areas.

18. Because the liver is a major center of metabolism, large quantities of ___ENZYMES___ are present in hepatocytes, and these leak into the bloodstream when the liver cells are damaged or destroyed by disease.

19. In severe hepatocellular destruction, such as acute viral or toxic hepatitis, striking elevation of ___AST/SGOT___ and ___ALT/SGPT___ may be seen.

20. Marked elevation of ___ALK PHOS___ is typically associated with biliary obstruction or the presence of mass lesions in the liver.

21. Hemoglobin released from the red cells is converted to ___BILIRUBIN___ within the reticuloendothelial system and is then released into the bloodstream.

22. Elevation of serum bilirubin results in ___JAUNDICE___, which is a yellow coloration of the skin, sclerae, and body secretions.

**Exercise 6**

*Provide a short answer for each anatomy and physiology question.*

1. Name the landmarks of the liver.

_____

_____

_____

_____

2. Identify at least three characteristics of the right lobe of the liver.

_____

_____

_____

_____

3. Identify at least three characteristics of the left lobe of the liver.

_____

_____

_____

_____

4. Name the ligaments and fissures found within the hepatic parenchyma.

_____

_____

5. Explain how to distinguish hepatic veins from portal veins.

_____

_____

_____

_____

6. List the seven liver function tests established to analyze how the liver is performing under normal and diseased conditions.

_____

_____

_____

## SONOGRAPHIC EVALUATION

### Exercise 7

*Fill in the blank(s) with the word(s) that best completes the statements, or provide a short answer about the sonographic techniques used for liver examination.*

1. Explain why the evaluation of the hepatic structures is one of the most important procedures in sonography.

_____

_____

_____

_____

2. Within the homogeneous parenchyma lie the thin-walled _____ veins, the brightly reflective _____ veins, the _____ arteries, and the _____ duct.

3. The portal flow is shown to be _____ (toward the liver), whereas the hepatic venous flow is _____ (away from the liver).

4. Near the porta hepatis, the hepatic duct can be seen along the lateral _____ border of the portal vein, whereas the hepatic artery can be seen along the anterior _____ border.

5. How should time gain compensation be adjusted to balance the far-gain and the near-gain echo signals?

_____

_____

_____

_____

6. Generally a wider pie sector or curved linear array transducer is the most appropriate to optimally image the _____ of the abdomen.

7. To image the far field better, a(n) _____ array transducer with a longer focal zone is used.

**Exercise 8**

*Fill in the blank(s) with the word(s) that best completes the statements, or provide a short answer about the pathology of the liver.*

1. List the four criteria assessed when evaluating the liver parenchyma.
   SIZE - CONFIGURATION - HOMOGENEITY - CONTOUR

2. Hepatocellular disease affects the HEPATOCYTES and interferes with liver function enzymes.

3. The hepatic enzyme levels are elevated with CELL (hepatocyte) necrosis.

4. Fatty infiltration implies increased LIPID accumulation in the hepatocytes and results from significant injury to the liver or a systemic disorder leading to impaired or excessive metabolism of fat.

5. Describe the sonographic findings for fatty infiltration of the liver.
   INCREASED ECHOGENICITY (moderate to severe fatty infiltration)
   ENLARGEMENT OF AFFECTED LOBE(S)
   PORTAL VEINS HARD TO VISUALIZE (d/t increased attenuation of US)
   DECREASED PENETRATION OF SOUND BEAM / FOCAL SPARING

6. In focal sparing, the most common affected areas are anterior to the GALL BLADDER or the portal vein and the posterior portion of the CAUDATE LOBE of the liver. (LEFT LOBE)

7. On ultrasound examination, the liver parenchyma in chronic hepatitis is COARSE with DECREASED brightness of the portal triads, but the degree of attenuation is not as great as seen in fatty infiltration.

8. Cirrhosis is a chronic degeneration of the liver in which the lobes are covered with fibrous tissue, the parenchyma DEGENERATES, and the lobules are infiltrated with FAT.

9. Glycogen storage disease is associated with HEPATIC ADENOMAS, focal nodular HYPERPLASIA, and hepatomegaly.

10. List the criteria that the sonographer should use to determine whether the mass is extrahepatic or intrahepatic.
    INTRAHEPATIC: displacement of hepatic vascular radicles, external bulging of liver capsule; posterior shift of IVC
    EXTRAHEPATIC: internal invagination or discontinuity of liver capsule; formation of triangular fat wedge; anteromedial shift of IVC, ant. displaced right kidney

11. List the signs and symptoms of a patient who has inflammatory disease of the liver.
    FEVER, ↑ wbc's, RUQ PAIN

12. A(n) NEOPLASM is any new growth of new tissue, either benign or malignant.

13. A(n) HEMANGIOMA is a benign congenital tumor consisting of large, blood-filled cystic spaces.

14. The pathogenesis of hepatocellular carcinoma is related to CIRRHOSIS, chronic HEP B virus infection, and hepatocarcinogens in food.

15. Describe the pathologic patterns seen in carcinoma of the liver.
    SOLITARY MASSIVE TUMOR; MULTIPLE NODULES THROUGHOUT LIVER; n
    DIFFUSE INFILTRATIVE MASSES IN LIVER

**59**

16. The liver is the third most common organ injured in the abdomen after the __SPLEEN__ and the __KIDNEY__.

17. An increase in portal venous pressure or hepatic venous gradient is defined as __PORTAL HTN__.

18. Portal hypertension may also develop when hepatopetal flow is impeded by __THROMBUS__ or __TUMOR__ invasion. (OBSTRUCTION)

19. The umbilical vein may become __RECANALIZED__ secondary to portal hypertension.

20. The pulse repetition frequency allows one to record lower velocities as the PRF is __DECREASED__.

21. The Doppler sample volume should be __SMALLER__ than the diameter of the lumen.

22. Explain what color Doppler velocity is dependent on. __DIRECTION OF FLOW, VELOCITY; ANGLE TO FLOW__

23. Acute abdominal pain, massive ascites, and hepatomegaly secondary to thrombosis of the hepatic veins or inferior vena cava characterize __BUDD-CHIARI__ syndrome, which has a poor prognosis.

**Exercise 9**

*Provide a short answer for each question after evaluating the images.*

A  B

C

1. What liver disease is present in these images? __FATTY INFILTRATION__

2. Describe the abnormality in this image.

ACUTE HEPATITIS - PORTAL VEIN BORDERS SLIGHTLY MORE ECHOGENIC
THAN NORMAL
- "STARRY SKY" PATTERN

A

B

C

3. Multiple images over the right upper quadrant are shown. What liver abnormality is demonstrated? ~~Is this velocity flow pattern high resistance or low resistance?~~

POLYCYSTIC LIVER DISEASE (LIVER AND KIDNEY CYSTS)

4. Describe the lesion seen in the right upper quadrant, and list the most likely differentials in this asymptomatic patient.

CAVERNOUS HEMANGIOMA

DDx: METASTASIS, HEPATOMA (HCC), ADENOMA, FOCAL NODULAR
      HYPERPLASIA

A                                                    B

5. A patient with an incidental finding on ultrasound during the evaluation of the liver. What is your differential?

LARGE SOLID MASS IN RT LOBE, LIKELY HEPATOCELLULAR CARCINOMA
- note ascites, pleural effusion
DDx: metastatic disease

# 10 Gallbladder and the Biliary System

## KEY TERMS

### Exercise 1

*Match the following anatomy and physiology terms with their definitions.*

C 1. ampulla of Vater
L 2. bilirubin
M 3. cholecystectomy
A 4. common bile duct
F 5. common duct
O 6. common hepatic duct
G 7. cystic duct
B 8. gallbladder
I 9. Hartmann's pouch
E 10. Heister's valve
D 11. hydrops
J 12. pancreatic duct
N 13. phrygian cap
H 14. porta hepatis
K 15. sphincter of Oddi

A. Extends from the point where the common hepatic duct meets the cystic duct; drains into the duodenum after it joins with the main pancreatic duct
B. Storage pouch for bile
C. Small opening in the duodenum in which the pancreatic and common bile ducts enter to release secretions
D. Massive enlargement of the gallbladder
E. Tiny valves found within the cystic duct
F. Refers to common bile and hepatic ducts when cystic duct is not seen
G. Connects the gallbladder to the common hepatic duct
H. Central area of the liver where the portal vein, common duct, and hepatic artery enter
I. Small part of the gallbladder that lies near the cystic duct where stones may collect
J. Travels horizontally through the pancreas to join the common bile duct at the ampulla of Vater
K. Small muscle that guards the ampulla of Vater
L. Yellow pigment in bile formed by the breakdown of red blood cells
M. Removal of the gallbladder
N. Gallbladder variant in which part of the fundus is bent back on itself
O. Bile duct system that drains the liver into the common bile duct

### Exercise 2

*Match the following sonographic evaluation and pathology terms with their definitions.*

E 1. adenomyomatosis
C 2. cholangitis
K 3. cholecystitis
I 4. cholecystokinin
L 5. choledochal cyst
O 6. choledocholithiasis
A 7. cholelithiasis
J 8. cholesterolosis

A. Gallstones in the gallbladder
B. Calcification of the gallbladder wall
C. Inflammation of the bile duct
D. Excessive bilirubin accumulation causes yellow pigmentation of the skin; first seen in the whites of the eyes
E. Small polypoid projections from the gallbladder wall
F. Sonographic pattern found when the gallbladder is packed with stones
G. Cancer at the bifurcation of the hepatic ducts; may cause asymmetrical obstruction of the biliary tree
H. Low-level echoes found along the posterior margin of the gallbladder; move with change in position

<table>
<tr><td>D</td><td>9. jaundice</td></tr>
<tr><td>M</td><td>10. junctional fold</td></tr>
<tr><td>G</td><td>11. Klatskin's tumor</td></tr>
<tr><td>P</td><td>12. Murphy's sign</td></tr>
<tr><td>N</td><td>13. polyp</td></tr>
<tr><td>B</td><td>14. porcelain gallbladder</td></tr>
<tr><td>H</td><td>15. sludge</td></tr>
<tr><td>F</td><td>16. wall echo shadow (WES) sign</td></tr>
</table>

I. Hormone secreted into the blood by the mucosa of the upper small intestine; stimulates contraction of the gallbladder and pancreatic secretion of enzymes
J. Variant of adenomyomatosis; cholesterol polyps
K. Inflammation of the gallbladder; may be acute or chronic
L. Cystic growth on the common duct that may cause obstruction
M. Small septum within the gallbladder, usually arising from the posterior wall
N. Small, well-defined soft tissue projection from the gallbladder wall
O. Stones in the bile duct
P. Positive sign implies exquisite tenderness over the area of the gallbladder upon palpation

## ANATOMY AND PHYSIOLOGY

### Exercise 3

*Label the following illustrations.*

1. Gallbladder and biliary system.

12. VALVE OF HEISTER
11. NECK
10. HARTMANN'S POUCH
9. BODY
8. FUNDUS
7. AMPULLA of VATER

1. RT HEPATIC DUCT
2. LT HEPATIC DUCT
3. COMMON HEPATIC DUCT
4. CYSTIC DUCT
5. COMMON BILE DUCT
6. PANCREATIC DUCT

2. Relationships within the porta hepatis.

1. _RT + LT HEPATIC DUCTS_
2. _RT + LT HEPATIC ARTERIES_
3. _COMMON HEPATIC DUCT_
4. _PROPER HEPATIC A_
5. _RT GASTRIC A_
6. _PANCREAS_
7. _DUODENUM_
8. _COLON_
9. _GALLBLADDER_
10. _LIVER_
11. _CBD_
12. _CYSTIC DUCT_
13. _CYSTIC A_

## Exercise 4

*Fill in the blank(s) with the word(s) that best completes the statements, or provide a short answer about the anatomy and physiology of the gallbladder.*

1. The gallbladder serves as a reservoir for __BILE__ that is drained from the hepatic ducts in the liver.

2. The common hepatic duct is joined by the cystic duct to form the __COMMON BILE__ duct.

3. The main pancreatic duct joins the common bile duct, and together they open through a small ampulla (the ampulla of __VATER__) into the duodenal wall.

4. The end parts of the common bile duct and main pancreatic duct and the ampulla are surrounded by circular muscle fibers known as the sphincter of __ODDI__.

5. The arterial supply of the gallbladder is from the __CYSTIC__ artery, which is a branch of the right hepatic artery.

6. List the two primary functions of the extrahepatic biliary tract.
   __TRANSPORT BILE FROM LIVER TO INTESTINE ; REGULATION OF BILE FLOW__

## Exercise 5

*Fill in the blank(s) with the word(s) that best completes the statements, or provide a short answer about the anatomy and physiology of the gallbladder.*

1. Describe the normal function of the gallbladder during digestion.
   __CONCENTRATION OF BILE DURING FASTING__
   __FOOD (FATTY) IN DUODENUM → RELEASE OF CCK FROM MUCOSA OF UPPER SI INTO__
   __BLOODSTREAM → GB CONTRACTS → BILE INTO DUODENUM__

2. Bile is the principal medium for excretion of bilirubin, __CHOLESTEROL__.

3. The bile salts from the small intestine stimulate the liver to make more bile, which activates __INTESTINAL__ and __PANCREATIC__ enzymes.

4. The sign that indicates an extrahepatic mass compressing the common bile duct, which can produce an enlarged gallbladder, is called __COURVOISIER'S SIGN__.

5. Sonographically, the common duct lies _ANTERIOR_ and to the _RIGHT_ of the portal vein in the region of the porta hepatis and gastrohepatic ligament.

6. The hepatic artery lies _ANTERIOR_ and to the _LEFT_ of the portal vein.

## SONOGRAPHIC EVALUATION

### Exercise 6

*Fill in the blank(s) with the word(s) that best completes the statements about the sonographic evaluation of the biliary system.*

1. To ensure maximum dilation of the gallbladder, the patient should be given nothing to eat for at least _(6?) 8_ hours before the ultrasound examination.

2. The patient is initially examined with ultrasound in full _INSPIRATION_.

3. The patient should also be rolled into a steep _DECUBITUS (LLD)_ or upright position (to ensure there are no stones within the gallbladder) in an attempt to separate small stones from the gallbladder wall or cystic duct.

4. The gallbladder may be identified as a(n) _ANECHOIC_ oblong structure located anterior to the right kidney, lateral to the head of the pancreas and duodenum.

5. The gallbladder commonly resides in a(n) _FOSSA_ on the medial aspect of the liver.

6. Because of _FIBROUS/FAT_ tissue within the main lobar fissure of the liver (which lies between the gallbladder and the right portal vein), this bright linear reflector is a reliable indicator of the location of the gallbladder.

7. A small _JUNCTIONAL_ _ECHOGENIC?_ fold has been reported to occur along the posterior wall of the gallbladder at the junction of the body and infundibulum.

8. On a transverse scan, the common duct, hepatic artery, and portal vein have been referred to as the _MICKEY MOUSE_ sign.

9. To obtain a cross section of the portal triad, the transducer must be directed in a slightly _OBLIQUE_ path from the left shoulder to the right hip.

※ 10. On sagittal scans, the right branch of the hepatic artery usually passes _POSTERIOR_ to the common duct.

11. The common duct is seen just _ANTERIOR_ to the portal vein before it dips posteriorly to enter the head of the pancreas.

12. When the right subcostal approach is used, the common hepatic duct is seen as a tubular structure anterior to the portal vein. The right branch of the _HEPATIC_ artery can be seen between the duct and the portal vein as a small circular structure.

## PATHOLOGY

### Exercise 7

*Fill in the blank(s) with the word(s) that best completes the statements, or provide a short answer about the pathology of the gallbladder and biliary system.*

1. The most classic symptom of gallbladder disease is _RUQ_ pain, usually occurring after ingestion of greasy foods.

2. A gallbladder attack may cause pain in the _RIGHT_ shoulder.

3. The normal wall thickness of the gallbladder is less than _3_ mm.

4. List the six biliary causes of gallbladder wall thickening.
   _CHOLECYSTITIS_

5. Clinically the patient with acute cholecystitis presents with these symptoms:
   ACUTE RUQ PAIN ( ⊕ MURPHY'S SIGN) , FEVER , LEUKOCYTOSIS

6. The ___WES___ sign is described as a contracted bright gallbladder with posterior shadowing caused by a packed bag of stones.

7. A fairly rare complication of acute cholecystitis associated with the presence of gas-forming bacteria in the gallbladder wall and lumen with extension into the biliary ducts is called ___PYOGENIC___ cholecystitis.

8. Clinically the patient falls under the five "F"s:___FAT___, ___FORTYs___, ___FERTILE___, ___FAIR___, and ___FEMALE___. (FLATULENT)

9. Explain why the patient's position should be shifted during the ultrasound examination.

   _____

   _____

   _____

   _____

10. Describe the factors that produce a shadow in the gallbladder.

    _____

    _____

    _____

    _____

11. _____ cysts may be the result of pancreatic juices refluxing into the bile duct because of an anomalous junction of the pancreatic duct into the distal common bile duct, causing duct wall abnormality, weakness, and outpouching of the ductal walls.

12. A hyperplastic change in the gallbladder wall is _____.

13. The differential for a porcelain gallbladder would include a packed bag or _____ sign.

14. What is the most notable sonographic finding with carcinoma of the gallbladder?

    _____

15. The most common cause of biliary ductal system obstruction is the presence of a(n) _____ or _____ within the ductal system.

16. The job of the sonographer is to localize the level and cause of the obstruction. List the three primary areas where obstruction occurs.

    _____

    _____

17. An uncommon cause of extrahepatic biliary obstruction as a result of an impacted stone in the cystic duct creating extrinsic mechanical compression of the common hepatic duct is ___MIRIZZI___ syndrome.

18. _____ causes increasing pressure in the biliary tree with pus accumulation.

19. The majority of stones in the common bile duct have migrated from the gallbladder. Common duct stones are usually associated with _____ cholecystitis.

20. <u>AIR OR GAS</u> within the duodenum may also give rise to a dirty shadow in the right upper quadrant.

21. On ultrasound, multiple cystic structures that converge toward the porta hepatis are seen in _____ disease.

## Exercise 8

*Provide a short answer for each question after evaluating the images.*

A — 7-224 CHOLELITHIASIS / SLUDGE

B — 7-223 CHOLELITHIASIS / SLUDGE

C — 7-196 GALLBLADDER SLUDGEBALL

D — 7-174 GALLBLADDER SLUDGEBALL

E — 7-220 GALLBLADDER SLUDGE

F — 7-140

1. What maneuvers may be performed to be sure the sludge in the gallbladder is not a tumor?

<u>SLUDGE SHOULD MOVE WITH CHANGE OF POSITION; DUE TO HIGH VISCOSITY,</u>

<u>MAY BE SLOW</u>

2. Describe the clinical signs and sonographic findings of the patient with acute cholecystitis as shown on these images. What complications should the sonographer be aware of?

_____

_____

_____

3. What anechoic structure(s) surround the gallbladder that may lead to confusion during the examination?

_____

_____

_____

Chapter **10** **Gallbladder and the Biliary System**

4. This scan over the right upper quadrant was made in a patient with a history of chronic pain. These sonographic images are representative of what disease?

W·E·S WALL ECHO SHADOW SIGN ; GB PACKED WITH STONES

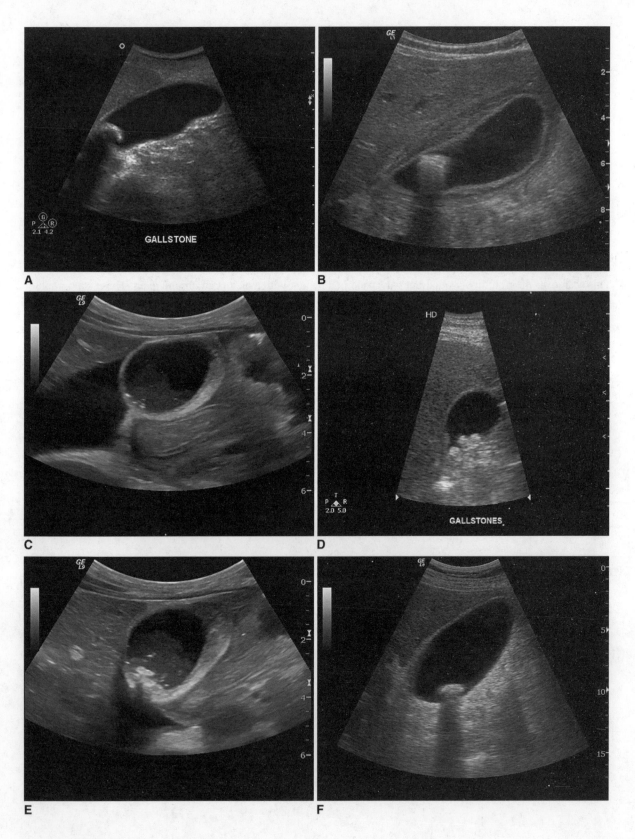

5. Describe the sonographic characteristics of these images.

_____

_____

6. Describe the sonographic findings in these images.

_____

_____

_____

A

B

C

7. A 60-year-old female presents with a history of cholecystectomy several years ago. The patient was known to have had previous hepatic calculi and now presents with right upper quadrant pain. What questions should the sonographer ask before starting the examination? Describe the sonographic findings and specify what additional organ(s) should be imaged.

_____

_____

_____

_____

# 11 Spleen

KEY TERMS

## Exercise 1

*Match the following anatomy terms with their definitions.*

_____ 1. accessory spleen

_____ 2. gastrosplenic ligament

_____ 3. intraperitoneal

_____ 4. left hypochondrium

_____ 5. lienorenal ligament

_____ 6. lymph

_____ 7. phrenocolic ligament

_____ 8. polysplenia

_____ 9. reticuloendothelial

_____10. splenic agenesis

_____11. splenic artery

_____12. splenic hilum

_____13. splenic vein

_____14. wandering spleen

A. Ligament between the spleen and the splenic flexure of the colon
B. Within the peritoneal cavity
C. Complete absence of the spleen
D. Condition where there is more than one spleen
E. Results from the failure of fusion of separate splenic masses forming on the dorsal mesogastrium; most commonly found in the splenic hilum or along the splenic vessels or associated ligaments
F. Leaves the splenic hilum, travels transversely through the upper abdomen to join with the superior mesenteric vein to form the main portal vein; serves as the posterior medial border of the pancreas
G. Located in the middle of the spleen; site where vessels and lymph nodes enter and exit the spleen
H. Spleen that has migrated from its normal location in the left upper quadrant
I. One of the ligaments between the stomach and spleen that helps to hold the spleen in place
J. Alkaline fluid found in the lymphatic vessels
K. Ligament between the spleen and kidney that helps support the greater curvature of the stomach
L. Certain phagocytic cells (found in the liver and spleen) make up the reticuloendothelial system (RES); plays a role in the synthesis of blood proteins and hematopoiesis
M. Left upper quadrant of the abdomen that contains the left lobe of the liver, spleen, and stomach
N. Branch of the celiac axis; tortuous course toward the spleen; serves as the superior border of the pancreas

## Exercise 2

*Match the following physiology terms with their definitions.*

_____ 1. culling

_____ 2. erythrocyte

_____ 3. hematopoiesis

_____ 4. hemoglobin

_____ 5. hemosiderin

_____ 6. leukopenia

_____ 7. malpighian corpuscles

_____ 8. phagocytosis

_____ 9. pitting

_____10. red pulp

_____11. splenic sinuses

_____12. white blood cells

_____13. white pulp

A. Follicles in the white pulp of the spleen, containing many lymphocytes
B. Pigment released from hemoglobin process
C. Blood cell production
D. Defend the body by destroying invading microorganisms and their toxins
E. Consists of reticular cells and fibers (cords of Billroth); surrounds the splenic sinuses
F. Red blood cell
G. Abnormal decrease of white blood corpuscles; may be drug induced
H. Consists of lymphatic tissue and lymphatic follicles
I. Process by which the spleen removes nuclei from blood cells without destroying the erythrocytes
J. Process by which the spleen removes abnormal red blood cells as they pass through
K. Oxygen-binding protein found in red blood cells
L. Long irregular channels lined by endothelial cells or flattened reticular cells
M. Process by which the red pulp destroys the degenerating red blood cells

## Exercise 3

*Match the following pathology terms with their definitions.*

_____ 1. amyloidosis

_____ 2. autoimmune hemolytic anemia

_____ 3. Gaucher's disease

_____ 4. hemolytic anemia

_____ 5. Hodgkin disease

_____ 6. infarction

_____ 7. mononucleosis

_____ 8. non-Hodgkin lymphoma

_____ 9. polycythemia

_____10. polycythemia vera

_____11. sickle cell anemia

_____12. sickle cell crisis

_____13. spherocytosis

_____14. splenomegaly

_____15. thalassemia

A. Interruption in the blood supply to an area that may lead to necrosis of the area

B. Chronic, life-shortening condition of unknown cause involving bone marrow elements; characterized by an increase in red blood cell mass and hemoglobin concentration

C. Acute infection caused by the Epstein-Barr virus that most commonly affects teenagers and young adults; symptoms include fever, sore throat, enlarged lymph nodes, abnormal lymphocysts, and hepatosplenomegaly

D. Malignant disease of lymphoid tissue seen in increased frequency in individuals more than 50 years of age

E. Group of hereditary anemias occurring in Asian and Mediterranean populations

F. Hereditary condition in which erythrocytes assume a spheroid shape

G. One of the storage diseases in which fat and proteins are deposited abnormally in the body

H. Excess of red blood cells

I. Malignant disease that involves lymphoid tissue

J. Condition in sickle cell anemia in which the sickled cells interfere with oxygen transport, obstruct capillary blood flow, and cause fever and severe pain in the joints and abdomen

K. Metabolic disorder marked by amyloid deposits in organs and tissue

L. Enlargement of the spleen

M. Inherited disorder transmitted as an autosomal recessive trait that causes an abnormality of the globin genes in hemoglobin

N. Anemia resulting from hemolysis of red blood cells

O. Anemia caused by antibodies produced by the patient's own immune system

## ANATOMY AND PHYSIOLOGY

### Exercise 4

*Label the following illustrations.*

1. Sagittal plane of the spleen and left kidney.

1. _____

11. _____

10. _____

9. _____

8. _____

7. _____

6. _____

5. _____

4. _____

3. _____

2. _____ Sigmoid colon

Iliacus muscle

Obturator internus muscle

Gluteus medius muscle

Gluteus maximus muscle

Obturator internus muscle

2. Anterior view of the spleen as it lies in the left hypochondrium.

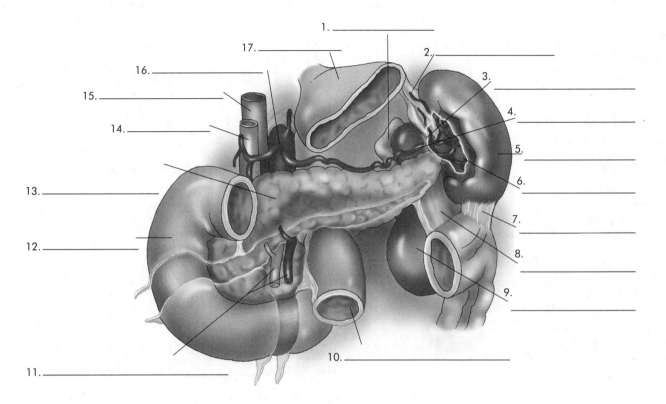

1. _____

17. _____

16. _____

15. _____

14. _____

13. _____

12. _____

11. _____

2. _____

3. _____

4. _____

5. _____

6. _____

7. _____

8. _____

9. _____

10. _____

3. The splenic vein leaves the hilum of the spleen.

1. _____

7. _____

6. _____

5. _____

3. _____

2. _____

4. _____

**Exercise 5**

*Fill in the blank(s) with the word(s) that best completes the statements about the anatomy and physiology of the spleen.*

1. The spleen is part of the reticuloendothelial system and is the largest single mass of _____ tissue in the body.

2. The spleen is a(n) _____ organ, covered with peritoneum over its entire extent except for a small area at its hilum, where the vascular structures and lymph nodes are located.

3. The spleen is normally measured with ultrasound on a longitudinal image from the _____ margin

   to the _____ margin at the long axis.

4. Splenic _____ may occur as part of asplenic or polysplenia syndromes in association with complex cardiac malformations, bronchopulmonary abnormalities, or visceral heterotaxis.

5. A(n) _____ spleen is usually found near the hilum or inferior border of the spleen but has been reported elsewhere in the abdominal cavity.

6. The _____ indicates the percentage of red blood cells per volume of blood.

7. The term _____ indicates bacteria in the bloodstream.

8. The increase in the number of white blood cells present in the blood that is a typical finding of infection

   is called _____.

## SONOGRAPHIC EVALUATION

**Exercise 6**

*Fill in the blank(s) with the word(s) that best completes the statements about the sonographic evaluation of the spleen.*

1. Sonographically the splenic parenchyma should have a fine homogeneous _____, as is seen within the liver parenchyma.

2. Systemic venous congestion is found in cardiac decompensation involving the _____ side of the heart.

3. In infants and children in crisis, in the earlier stage of _____ anemia, the spleen is enlarged with marked congestion of the red pulp.

4. Patients with hepatosplenic _____ may show irregular masses within the spleen, the "wheels-within-wheels" pattern, with the outer wheel representing the ring of fibrosis surrounding the inner echogenic wheel of inflammatory cells and a central hypoechoic area.

5. If the patient has severe left upper quadrant pain secondary to trauma, a splenic _____

   or a(n) _____ hematoma should be considered.

**Exercise 7**

*Provide a short answer for each question after evaluating the images.*

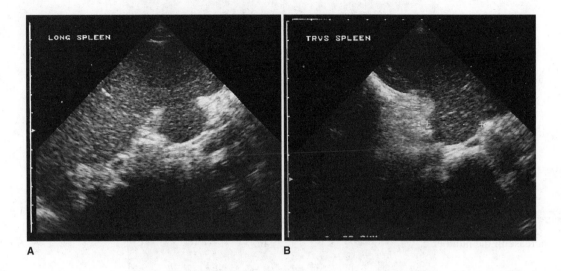

A      B

1. A young male presented with vague epigastric pain. Ultrasound revealed an anomaly. In the scan over the left upper quadrant, what is the sonographic finding?

---

2. This patient had left upper quadrant pain and fever for 1 week before ultrasound examination. What is the sonographic finding?

---

3. These images over the left upper quadrant demonstrate which feature?

_____

4. Describe the abnormality in the spleen in this patient with fever and chills for 3 weeks.

_____

5. A 20-year-old presents to the ER after a bicycle accident. Based on this image, what are your sonographic findings?

_____

6. Is this image taken of the liver or spleen? How would you know?

_____

# 12 Pancreas

## KEY TERMS

### Exercise 1

*Match the following anatomy terms with their definitions.*

E ___ 1. body of the pancreas
A ___ 2. caudal pancreatic artery
G ___ 3. C-loop of the duodenum
J ___ 4. common hepatic artery
O ___ 5. dorsal pancreatic artery
N ___ 6. duct of Santorini
K ___ 7. duct of Wirsung
L ___ 8. head of the pancreas
H ___ 9. neck of the pancreas
D ___ 10. pancreaticoduodenal arteries
C ___ 11. portal-splenic confluence
M ___ 12. superior mesenteric artery
I ___ 13. superior mesenteric vein
B ___ 14. tail of the pancreas
F ___ 15. uncinate process

A. Branch of splenic artery that supplies the tail of the pancreas
B. Tapered end of the pancreas that lies in the left hypochondrium near the hilus of the spleen and upper pole of the left kidney
C. Junction of the splenic and main portal veins; posterior border of the body of the pancreas
D. Helps supply blood to the pancreas along with the splenic artery
E. Lies in the midepigastrium anterior to the superior mesenteric artery and vein, aorta, and inferior vena cava
F. Small, curved tip of the pancreatic head that lies posterior to the superior mesenteric vein
G. Forms the lateral border of the head of the pancreas
H. Small area of the pancreas between the head and the body; anterior to the superior mesenteric vein
I. Lies posterior to the neck or body of the pancreas and anterior to the uncinate process of the gland
J. Forms the right superior border of the body and head of the pancreas and gives rise to the gastroduodenal artery
K. Largest duct of the pancreas that drains the tail, body, and head of the gland; it joins the common bile duct to enter the duodenum through the ampulla of Vater
L. Lies in the C-loop of the duodenum; the gastroduodenal artery is the anterolateral border, and the common bile duct is the posterolateral border
M. Serves as the posterior border to the body of the pancreas
N. Small accessory duct of the pancreas found in the head of the gland
O. Branch of the splenic artery that supplies the body of the pancreas

### Exercise 2

*Match the following physiology terms with their definitions.*

F ___ 1. acini cells
I ___ 2. amylase
A ___ 3. endocrine
D ___ 4. exocrine
C ___ 5. glucagons
G ___ 6. insulin
B ___ 7. islets of Langerhans
H ___ 8. lipase
E ___ 9. serum amylase

A. The kind of pancreatic function that involves the production of the hormone insulin
B. Portion of the pancreas that has an endocrine function and produces insulin, glucagon, and somatostatin
C. Stimulates the liver to convert the glycogen to glucose; produced by alpha cells
D. The kind of pancreatic function that involves the production and digestion of pancreatic juice
E. Pancreatic enzyme that is elevated during pancreatitis
F. Cells that perform exocrine function
G. Hormone that causes glycogen formation from glucose in the liver and that allows circulating glucose to enter tissue cells
H. Pancreatic enzyme that breaks down fats; enzyme is elevated in pancreatitis and remains increased longer than amylase
I. Enzyme secreted by the pancreas to aid in the digestion of carbohydrates

**Exercise 3**

*Match the following pathology terms with their definitions.*

___I___ 1. Courvoisier's gallbladder

___L___ 2. cystic fibrosis

___J___ 3. hypercalcemia

___A___ 4. hyperlipidemia

___D___ 5. ileus

___H___ 6. leukocytosis

___C___ 7. lymphoma

___B___ 8. obstructive jaundice

___K___ 9. pancreatic ascites

___G___ 10. pancreatic pseudocyst

___F___ 11. pancreatitis

___E___ 12. pseudocyst

A. Congenital condition in which elevated fat levels cause pancreatitis
B. Excessive bilirubin in the bloodstream caused by an obstruction of bile from the liver; characterized by a yellow discoloration of the sclera of the eye, skin, and mucous membranes
C. Malignant neoplasm that arises from the lymphoid tissues
D. Dilated loops of bowel without peristalsis; associated with various abdominal problems, including pancreatitis, sickle cell crisis, and bowel obstruction
E. Space or cavity that contains fluid but has no true endothelial lining membrane
F. Inflammation of the pancreas; may be acute or chronic
G. "Sterile abscess" collection of pancreatic enzymes that accumulate in the available space in the abdomen, usually in or near the pancreas
H. Abnormal increase in white blood cells caused by infections
I. Enlargement of the gallbladder caused by a slow, progressive obstruction of the distal common bile duct from an external mass, such as adenocarcinoma of the pancreatic head
J. Elevated levels of calcium in the blood
K. Fluid accumulation caused by a rupture of a pancreatic pseudocyst into the abdomen; free-floating pancreatic enzymes are very dangerous to surrounding structures
L. Hereditary disease that causes excessive production of thick mucus by the endocrine glands

## ANATOMY AND PHYSIOLOGY

**Exercise 4**

*Label the following illustrations.*

1. The aorta and inferior vena cava are the posterior landmarks of the pancreas.

2. Sagittal planes of the pancreas.

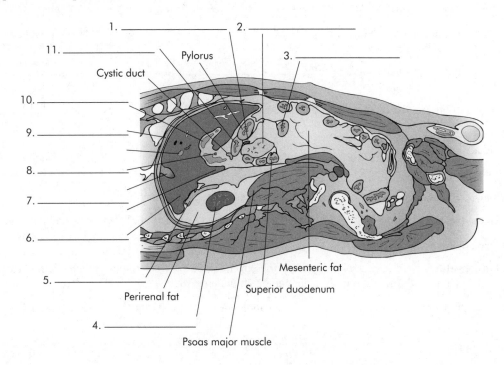

1. _____    2. _____

11. _____

Pylorus

3. _____

Cystic duct

10. _____

9. _____

8. _____

7. _____

6. _____

5. _____

Perirenal fat

4. _____

Psoas major muscle

Mesenteric fat

Superior duodenum

3. The portal venous system is the posterior border of the pancreas.

14. _____

13. _____

12. _____

11. _____

10. _____

9. _____

1. _____

2. _____

3. _____

4. _____

5. _____

6. _____

7. _____

8. _____

**Exercise 5**

*Fill in the blank(s) with the word(s) that best completes the statements about the anatomy of the pancreas.*

1. The pancreas is located in the ___RETROPERITONEAL___ cavity posterior to the stomach, duodenum, and proximal jejunum of the small bowel.

2. The pancreatic gland appears sonographically ___ISO-___ to slightly more ___HYPERECHOIC___ than the hepatic parenchyma.

3. The major posterior vascular landmarks of the pancreas are the ___AORTA___ and ___IVC___.

4. The head of the pancreas lies ___ANTERIOR___ to the inferior vena cava.

5. The ___SUPERIOR MES.___ vein crosses anterior to the uncinate process of the head of the gland and posterior to the neck and body.

6. The tortuous ___SPLENIC___ artery is the superior border of the pancreas.

7. The tail of the pancreas is more difficult to image because it lies anterior to the left kidney and posterior to the left ___SPLENIC/COLIC___ flexure and ___TRANSVERSE___ colon.

8. The duct of ___WIRSUNG___ receives tributaries from lobules at right angles and enters the medial second part of the duodenum with the common bile duct at the ampulla of Vater.

9. The blood supply for the pancreas is from the ___SPLENIC___ artery and the ___PANCREATICO DUODENAL___ arteries.

10. The ___GDA___ artery is seen along the anterolateral border of the pancreas as it travels a short distance along the anterior aspect of the pancreatic head.

11. The ___CBD___ duct crosses the anterior aspect of the portal vein to the right of the proper hepatic artery.

12. The portal vein is ___ANT___ to the inferior vena cava.

**Exercise 6**

*Fill in the blank(s) with the word(s) that best completes the statements about the physiology of the pancreas.*

1. The pancreas is both a digestive (___EXOCRINE___) and a hormonal (___ENDOCRINE___) gland.

2. Failure of the pancreas to furnish sufficient insulin leads to _____.

3. Exocrine function is performed by _____ of the pancreas.

4. The _____ is a muscle surrounding the ampulla of Vater that relaxes to allow pancreatic juice and bile to empty into the duodenum.

5. The endocrine function is located in the islets of _____ in the pancreas.

6. The beta cells are most prevalent and produce _____, a hormone that causes glycogen formation from glucose in the liver.

7. Alpha cells produce _____, a hormone that causes the cells to release glucose to meet the energy needs of the body.

8. Delta cells are the smallest composition of endocrine tissue and produce _____.

9. There are specific enzymes of the pancreas that may become altered in pancreatic disease, namely _____ and _____.

10. Both amylase and lipase rise at the same rate, but the elevation in _____ concentration persists for a longer period in pancreatitis.

11. _____ controls the blood sugar level in the body.

### Exercise 7

*Provide a short answer that best completes the statements about the sonographic evaluation of the pancreas.*

1. Explain how fat influences the echogenicity of the pancreas on ultrasound.

   _____

   _____

   _____

   _____

2. Name the structures that should be identified as landmarks to locate the pancreas.

   _____

   _____

   _____

   _____

3. Describe the water technique used to image the pancreas with ultrasound.

   _____

   _____

   _____

   _____

4. When the pancreas is enlarged, the anterior border of the _____IVC_____ may depict a slight indentation.

## PATHOLOGY

### Exercise 8

*Fill in the blank(s) with the word(s) that best completes the statements, or provide a short answer about the pathology of the pancreas.*

1. When the pancreas becomes damaged and malfunctions as a result of increased secretion and blockage of ducts,

   _____ occurs.

2. An acute attack of pancreatitis is commonly related to _____ and _____ disease.

3. The patient with pancreatitis typically presents with moderate to severe tenderness in the _____

   radiating to the _____.

4. When swelling does occur, the gland is hypoechoic to anechoic and is less echogenic than the liver because of the

   increased prominence of _____ and congested _____.

5. The pancreatic duct may be obstructed in acute pancreatitis as a result of _____,

   _____, _____, _____, and _____.

6. Fluid collections around the pancreatic _____, along the _____ spaces, within

   the _____ pouch, and around the _____ may be present in a patient with acute pancreatitis.

7. Patients with acute pancreatitis may develop complications, such as _____, _____,

   _____, _____, and _____ obstruction.

8. Necrosis of the blood vessels results in the development of hemorrhagic areas referred to as

_____ sign.

9. An inflammatory process that spreads along fascial pathways, causing localized areas of diffuse inflammatory edema of soft tissue, is known as _____.

10. The _____ ducts become obstructed with a buildup of protein plugs with resultant calcifications along the duct in _____ pancreatitis.

11. Describe how a pseudocyst develops.

_____

_____

_____

_____

12. The most common location of a pseudocyst is in the _____, anterior to the pancreas and posterior to the stomach.

13. A pseudocyst develops when pancreatic _____ escape from the gland and break down tissue to form a sterile abscess somewhere in the abdomen.

14. The most common primary neoplasm of the pancreas is _____.

15. List the clinical findings in a patient with carcinoma of the pancreas.

_____

16. The most frequent parapancreatic neoplasm is _____.

**Exercise 9**

*Provide a short answer for each question.*

1. To which vascular structure are the arrows pointing in this image?

_____

2. Identify whether this image is transverse or longitudinal and what the arrows are pointing to.

_____

3. Identify the anatomic structure that the arrows are pointing to in this image.

_____

4. What is the signal arrow pointing to?

_____

5. What is the arrowhead pointing to?

_____

6. A 45-year-old male presents with midepigastric pain, elevated amylase and lipase levels, and tenderness. Identify the sonographic findings.

_____

_____

**A**

**B**

**C**

7. A patient with known acute pancreatitis presents with continued pain. Describe the sonographic findings.

_____

_____

8. A 56-year-old male with a 1-week history of jaundice and pain has reported a 3-month history of nausea, vomiting, weight loss, and diarrhea. Given this information, what are the sonographic findings?

_____

_____

# 13 Gastrointestinal Tract

## KEY TERMS

### Exercise 1

*Match the following anatomy terms with their definitions.*

_____ 1. alimentary canal

_____ 2. cardiac orifice

_____ 3. duodenal bulb

_____ 4. gastrohepatic ligament

_____ 5. gastrophrenic, gastrosplenic, and lienorenal ligaments

_____ 6. greater omentum

_____ 7. haustra

_____ 8. hepatic flexure

_____ 9. lesser omentum

_____ 10. mesentery

_____ 11. mesothelium

_____ 12. mucosa

_____ 13. muscularis

_____ 14. pyloric canal

_____ 15. rugae

_____ 16. serosa

_____ 17. splenic flexure

_____ 18. submucosa

_____ 19. valvulae conniventes

_____ 20. villi

A. Ascending colon arises from the right lower quadrant to bend at this point to form the transverse colon
B. First part of the duodenum
C. Double fold of the peritoneum attached to the duodenum, stomach, and large intestine; helps support the greater curvature of the stomach; known as the "fatty apron"
D. Help support the greater curvature of the stomach
E. Fold from the parietal peritoneum that attaches to the small intestine, anchoring it to the posterior abdominal wall
F. Also known as the digestive tract; includes the mouth, pharynx, esophagus, stomach, duodenum, and small and large intestine
G. Inner folds of the small intestine
H. Entrance of the esophagus into the stomach
I. First layer of bowel
J. Helps support the lesser curvature of the stomach
K. The transverse colon travels horizontally across the abdomen and bends at this point to form the descending colon
L. One of the layers of the bowel, under the mucosal layer; contains blood vessels and lymph channels
M. Normal segmentation of the wall of the colon
N. Suspends the stomach and duodenum from the liver; helps to support the lesser curvature of the stomach
O. Muscle that connects the stomach to the proximal duodenum
P. Fourth layer of bowel; thin, loose layer of connective tissue, surrounded by mesothelium covering the intraperitoneal bowel loops
Q. Third layer of bowel
R. Normal segmentation of the small bowel
S. Inner folds of the stomach wall
T. Fifth layer of bowel

## Exercise 2

*Match the following physiology and sonographic evaluation terms with their definitions.*

_____1. abscess

_____2. absorption

_____3. cholecystokinin

_____4. gastrin

_____5. McBurney's point

_____6. peristalsis

_____7. secretin

A. Hormone secreted into the blood by the mucosa of the upper small intestine; stimulates contraction of the gallbladder and pancreatic secretion of enzymes

B. Rhythmic dilation and contraction of the gastrointestinal tract as food is propelled through it

C. Located by drawing a line from the right anterosuperior iliac spine to the umbilicus; at approximately the midpoint of this line lies the root of the appendix

D. Process of nutrient molecules passing through the wall of the intestine into the blood or lymph system

E. Endocrine hormone released from the stomach; stimulates secretion of gastric acid

F. Localized collection of pus surrounded by inflamed tissue

G. Released from small bowel as antacid; stimulates secretion of bicarbonate

## Exercise 3

*Match the following pathology terms with their definitions.*

_____ 1. appendicolith

_____ 2. ascites

_____ 3. Crohn's disease

_____ 4. diverticulum

_____ 5. fecalith

_____ 6. hemorrhage

_____ 7. lymphoma

_____ 8. McBurney's sign

_____ 9. Meckel's diverticulum

_____10. paralytic ileus

_____11. polyp

_____12. target sign

A. Calcified deposit within the appendix; appendicitis can develop when the appendix becomes blocked by hard fecal matter

B. Pouchlike herniation through the muscular wall of a tubular organ that occurs in the stomach, the small intestine, or, most commonly, the colon

C. Malignancy of the lymph nodes, spleen, or liver

D. Dilated fluid-filled bowel loops without peristalsis

E. Characteristic of gastrointestinal wall thickening consisting of an echogenic center and a hypoechoic rim

F. Collection of blood

G. Site of maximal tenderness in the right lower quadrant; usually with appendicitis

H. Accumulation of serous fluid in the abdomen

I. Congenital sac or blind pouch found in the lower portion of the ileum

J. Fecalith or calcification located in the appendix

K. Small tumorlike growth that projects from a mucous membrane surface

L. Inflammation of the bowel, accompanied by abscess and bowel wall thickening

**Exercise 4**

*Label the following illustrations.*

1. The digestive system.

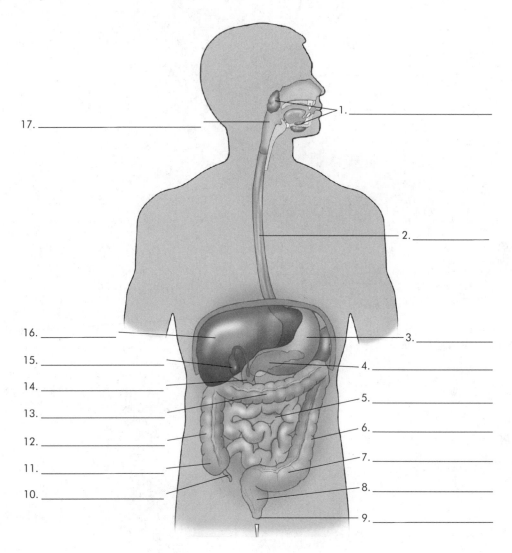

17. _____

1. _____

2. _____

16. _____

15. _____

14. _____

13. _____

12. _____

11. _____

10. _____

3. _____

4. _____

5. _____

6. _____

7. _____

8. _____

9. _____

2. The stomach.

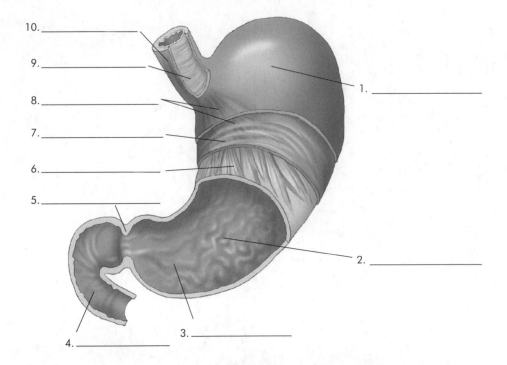

10. _____

9. _____

8. _____

7. _____

6. _____

5. _____

4. _____

3. _____

1. _____

2. _____

3. Vascular supply to the stomach.

15. _____

14. _____

13. _____

12. _____

11. _____

10. _____

9. _____

8. _____

7. _____

1. _____

2. _____

3. _____

4. _____

5. _____

6. _____

4. The superior mesenteric artery.

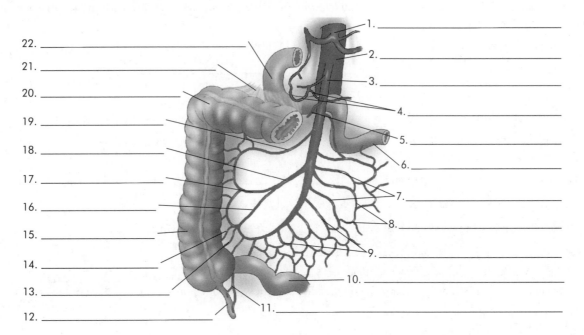

22. _____
21. _____
20. _____
19. _____
18. _____
17. _____
16. _____
15. _____
14. _____
13. _____
12. _____
11. _____

1. _____
2. _____
3. _____
4. _____
5. _____
6. _____
7. _____
8. _____
9. _____
10. _____

5. The inferior mesenteric artery.

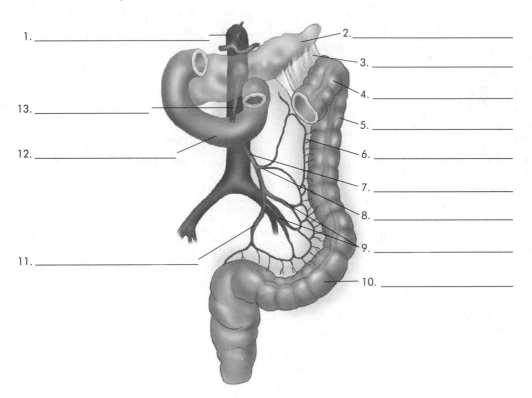

1. _____
13. _____
12. _____
11. _____

2. _____
3. _____
4. _____
5. _____
6. _____
7. _____
8. _____
9. _____
10. _____

**Exercise 5**

*Fill in the blank(s) with the word(s) that best completes the statements or provide a short answer about the anatomy and physiology of the gastrointestinal tract.*

1. List the sequential parts of the digestive system.

   _____

   _____

2. The lower end of the esophagus is a circular muscle that acts as a sphincter, constricting the tube so that the

   entrance to the stomach, at the _____, is generally closed. This helps to prevent gastric acid from moving up into the esophagus.

3. The pylorus is further subdivided into the _____, the _____ canal, and the

   _____ sphincter.

4. The duodenum is subdivided into four segments: (1) _____, (2) _____,

   (3) _____, and (4) _____.

5. The duodenal bulb is peritoneal, supported by the hepatoduodenal ligament, and passes _____ to the common bile duct, gastroduodenal artery, common hepatic artery, hepatic portal vein, and head of the pancreas.

6. The common bile duct joins the pancreatic duct to enter the _____.

7. The arteries that supply the esophagus include the inferior _____ branch of the

   _____ artery that supplies the upper esophagus; the descending _____ aorta

   that supplies the midesophagus; and the _____ branch of the celiac axis and the left inferior

   _____ artery of the abdominal aorta that supplies the lower end of the esophagus.

8. The _____ outlines the small intestine and contains the superior mesenteric vessels, nerves, lymphatic glands, and fat between its two layers.

9. The nutrients are transported to the liver after they are absorbed by the _____; the liver processes and stores the nutrients.

10. The three layers of smooth muscle in the wall enable the stomach to mash and churn food and move it along with

    _____.

11. Gastric glands secrete gastric juice containing _____ acid and _____.

12. The hormone _____, which is released by the stomach mucosa, stimulates gastric acid secretion.

13. Gastrointestinal hormones include _____ and _____.

14. _____ within the large intestine devour the chyme and in turn produce vitamins that can be absorbed and used by the body.

15. The most common laboratory data the sonographer may come across in a patient with gastrointestinal disease

    relate to the presence of _____ in the stool.

16. As a result of chronic blood loss, _____ may be present.

## SONOGRAPHIC EVALUATION

### Exercise 6

*Fill in the blank(s) with the word(s) that best completes the statements, or provide a short answer about the sonographic evaluation of the gastrointestinal tract.*

1. Describe the technique sonographers use to observe the upper gastrointestinal tract.

   _____

   _____

   _____

2. The _____ junction is seen on the sagittal scan to the left of the midline as a bull's-eye or target-shaped structure anterior to the aorta, posterior to the left lobe of the liver, and inferior to the hemidiaphragm.

3. The gastric _____ can be seen as a target shape in the midline.

4. Describe the measures that should be taken if a patient presents with a "cystic" mass in the left upper quadrant.

   _____

   _____

   _____

5. The sonographer usually cannot see the small bowel with ultrasound; the valvulae conniventes may be seen as

   linear echo densities spaced 3 to 5 mm apart. This is called the "_____" sign and can be seen in the duodenum and jejunum.

6. The appendix is located on the abdominal wall under _____ point.

## PATHOLOGY

### Exercise 7

*Fill in the blank(s) with the word(s) that best completes the statements about pathology of the gastrointestinal tract.*

1. Movable intraluminal masses of congealed ingested materials that are seen on upper gastrointestinal radiographs

   are known as gastric _____.

2. A gastric _____ is an outgrowth of tissue from the wall.

3. The most common tumor of the stomach is the _____.

4. Acute _____ is the result of luminal obstruction and inflammation, leading to ischemia of the vermiform appendix.

5. The normal appendix can occasionally be visualized with gradual _____ on sonography.

6. The ultrasound pattern of acute appendicitis is characterized by a(n) _____ appearance of the appendix in transverse view.

7. A(n) _____ designates gross enlargement of the appendix from accumulation of mucoid substance within the lumen.

8. _____ disease is regional enteritis, a recurrent granulomatous inflammatory disease that affects the terminal ileum, colon, or both at any level.

## Exercise 8

*Provide a short answer for each question after evaluating the images.*

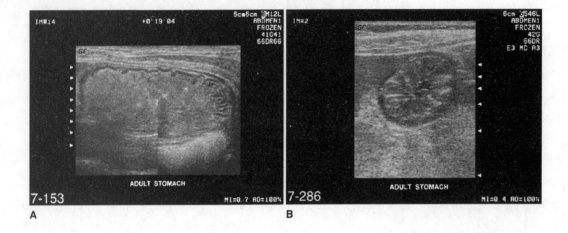

1. Identify the internal structures that are demonstrated in these images of the stomach.

_____

2. This image represents what structure?

_____

3. Identify the anatomic structure signified by the arrows.

_____

4. Identify the anatomy that is demonstrated in these images of the small bowel.

_____

A

B

BOWEL

C

D

BOWEL AND INFLAMMATORY REACTION

5. Identify the structure demonstrated in the images recorded over the right lower quadrant.

_____

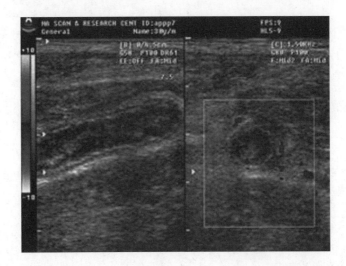

6. Young patient presents with exquisite tenderness over the right lower quadrant. What are the sonographic findings?

_____

# 14 Peritoneal Cavity and Abdominal Wall

## Exercise 1

*Match the following anatomy terms with their definitions.*

_____1. mesentery

_____2. Morison's pouch

_____3. omentum

_____4. subhepatic

_____5. subphrenic

A. Loops of the digestive tract are anchored to the posterior wall of the abdominal cavity by this large double fold of peritoneal tissue
B. Inferior to the liver
C. Pouchlike extension of the visceral peritoneum from the lower edge of the stomach, part of the duodenum, and the transverse colon
D. Below the diaphragm
E. Space anterior to the right kidney and posterior to the inferior border of the liver where ascites or fluid may accumulate or an abscess may develop

## Exercise 2

*Match the following pathology terms with their definitions.*

_____ 1. abscess

_____ 2. ascites

_____ 3. gutters

_____ 4. hemorrhage

_____ 5. leukocytosis

_____ 6. peritonitis

_____ 7. pyogenic

_____ 8. sandwich sign

_____ 9. sepsis

_____10. septicemia

_____11. urinoma

A. Sonographic sign that you see when a vessel or organ is surrounded by a tumor on either side
B. Most dependent areas in the flanks of the abdomen and pelvis where fluid collections may accumulate
C. Inflammation of the peritoneum
D. Accumulation of serous fluid in the peritoneal cavity
E. Infection in the blood
F. Increase in the number of leukocytes (white blood cells)
G. Spread of an infection from its initial site to the bloodstream
H. Localized collection of pus
I. Pus producing
J. Cyst containing urine
K. Collection of blood

**Exercise 3**

*Label the following illustrations.*

1. Transverse view of the subphrenic spaces.

8. _____    1. _____

7. _____    2. _____

6. _____    3. _____

5. _____    4. _____

2. Transverse view of the retroperitoneal space.

10. _____    1. _____

9. _____     2. _____

8. _____     3. _____

7. _____     4. _____

6. _____     5. _____

3. Transverse view of the subhepatic spaces and Morison's pouch.

10. _____    1. _____

9. _____     2. _____

8. _____     3. _____

7. _____     4. _____

6. _____     5. _____

4. Sagittal view of the abdomen delineating the peritoneal cavity.

1. _____
22. _____
21. _____
20. _____
19. _____
18. _____
17. _____
16. _____
15. _____
14. _____
13. _____
12. _____
11. _____

2. _____
3. _____
4. _____
5. _____
6. _____
7. _____
8. _____
9. _____
10. _____

5. The muscles of the anterior and lateral abdominal walls.

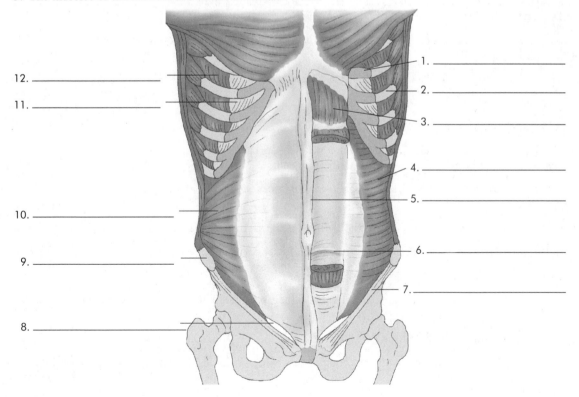

12. _____
11. _____
10. _____
9. _____
8. _____

1. _____
2. _____
3. _____
4. _____
5. _____
6. _____
7. _____

**Exercise 4**

*Fill in the blank(s) with the word(s) that best completes the statements about the determination of intraperitoneal location.*

1. Because of the _____ ligament attachments, collections in the right posterior subphrenic space cannot extend between the bare area of the liver and the diaphragm.

2. The pleural fluid tends to distribute _____ in the chest.

3. Subcapsular liver and splenic collections are seen when they are _____ to the diaphragm unilaterally and conform to the shape of an organ capsule.

4. A mass is confirmed to be within the retroperitoneal cavity when anterior renal displacement or anterior displacement of the dilated _____ can be documented.

5. The mass interposed _____ or superiorly to kidneys can be located either intraperitoneally or retroperitoneally.

6. Fatty and collagenous connective tissues in the perirenal or anterior pararenal space produce echoes that are best demonstrated on _____ scans.

7. Retroperitoneal lesions displace echoes _____ and cranially.

8. Hepatic and subhepatic lesions produce _____ and posterior displacement.

9. A large right-sided retroperitoneal mass rotates the intrahepatic portal veins to the _____.

**Exercise 5**

*Fill in the blank(s) with the word(s) that best completes the statements about the anatomy and sonographic evaluation of the peritoneal cavity and abdominal wall.*

1. The peritoneal cavity is made up of multiple peritoneal ligaments and folds that connect the _____ to each other and to the abdominal-pelvic _____.

2. Within the cavity are found the lesser and greater _____, the _____, and multiple fluid spaces (lesser sac, perihepatic and subphrenic spaces).

3. The _____ is a smooth membrane that lines the entire abdominal cavity and is reflected over the contained organs.

4. The part that lines the walls of the cavity is the _____ peritoneum, whereas the part covering the abdominal organs to a greater or lesser extent is the _____ peritoneum.

5. The general peritoneal cavity is known as the _____ sac of the peritoneum.

6. With the development of the stomach and the spleen, a smaller sac, called the _____ sac (omental bursa), is the peritoneal recess posterior to the stomach.

7. This sac communicates with the greater sac through a small vertical opening known as the _____ foramen.

8. When the patient is lying supine, the lowest part of the body is the _____.

9. A double layer of peritoneum extending from the liver to the lesser curvature of the stomach is known as the _____ omentum.

10. The _____ omentum is an apronlike fold of peritoneum that hangs from the greater curvature of the stomach.

11. Ligaments on the right side of the liver form the _____ and _____ spaces.

12. The subphrenic space is divided into right and left components by the _____ ligaments.

13. The _____ teres ascends from the umbilicus to the umbilical notch of the liver within the free margin of the falciform ligament before coursing within the liver.

14. The paired _____ abdominis muscles are delineated medially in the midline of the body by the linea alba.

## PATHOLOGY

### Exercise 6

*Fill in the blank(s) with the word(s) that best completes the statements, or provide a short answer about the pathology of the peritoneal cavity.*

1. The amount of intraperitoneal fluid depends on the _____, _____, and patient

   _____.

2. The ascitic fluid first fills the pouch of _____, then the lateral paravesical recesses before it ascends to both paracolic gutters.

3. The small bowel loops _____ or _____ in the surrounding ascitic fluid, depending on relative gas content and amount of fat in the mesentery.

4. Inflammatory or malignant ascites appears with _____ echoes; loculation; unusual distribution, matting, or clumping of bowel loops; and thickening of interfaces between the fluid and neighboring structures.

5. A cavity formed by necrosis within a solid tissue or a circumscribed collection of purulent material is a(n)

   _____.

6. Name the five major pathways through which bacteria can enter the liver and cause abscess formation.

   _____

   _____

   _____

7. Extrahepatic loculated collections of bile that may develop because of iatrogenic, traumatic, or spontaneous rupture

   of the biliary tree are _____.

8. An abscess that forms within the renal parenchyma is a(n) renal _____. Clinical symptoms vary from none to fever, leukocytosis, and flank pain.

9. The most common abdominal pathologic process is _____ that requires immediate surgery.

### Exercise 7

*Fill in the blank(s) with the word(s) that best completes the statements, or provide a short answer about the pathology of the mesentery, omentum, and peritoneum.*

1. A mass or lesion within the mesentery and omentum may have solid or cystic characteristics, whereas a mass

   within the peritoneum may show a(n) _____ pattern.

2. Mesenteric and omental cysts may be uniloculated or _____ with smooth walls and thin internal septations.

3. An incomplete regression of the urachus during development is a(n) _____ cyst.

4. An encapsulated collection of urine, or _____, may result from a closed renal injury or from surgical intervention, or it may arise spontaneously secondary to an obstructing lesion.

5. The most common primary sites of peritoneal metastases are the _____, _____,

   and _____.

6. The _____ sign of lymphoma represents a mass infiltrating the mesenteric leaves and encasing the superior mesenteric artery.

**111**

7. A key factor in determining whether an abdominal wall mass is present is the _____ of the rectus sheath muscles.

8. A collection of fluid that occurs after surgery in the pelvis, retroperitoneum, or recess cavities is known as a(n)

_____.

9. Extraperitoneal rectus sheath _____ are acute or chronic collections of blood lying either within the rectus muscle or between the muscle and its sheath.

10. An abdominal _____ is the protrusion of a peritoneal-lined sac through a defect in the weakened abdominal wall.

11. A variant of the ventral hernia that is found more laterally in the abdominal wall is a(n) _____ hernia.

12. List the four sonographic criteria for a hernia.

_____

_____

_____

## Exercise 8

*Provide a short answer for each question after evaluating the images.*

A

B

C

D

1. Describe the fluid collection.

_____

2. Which abnormality does this longitudinal image demonstrate in this patient with trauma from a football injury?

_____

3. A patient 2 days after surgery for a kidney transplant was imaged post op. Describe what this image shows.

_____

_____

_____

4. This mass was noted between the umbilicus and the bladder and most likely represents a

   _____.

# 15 Urinary System

---

**KEY TERMS**

---

**Exercise 1**

*Match the following anatomy terms with their definitions.*

_____ 1. afferent arteriole

_____ 2. Bowman's capsule

_____ 3. cortex

_____ 4. Gerota's fascia

_____ 5. hilus

_____ 6. major calyces

_____ 7. minor calyces

_____ 8. nephron

_____ 9. renal corpuscle

_____ 10. renal pelvis

_____ 11. retroperitoneum

_____ 12. urethra

A.  Area of kidney where vessels, ureter, and lymphatics enter and exit
B.  Another term for the renal fascia; the kidney is covered by the renal capsule, perirenal fat, Gerota's fascia, and pararenal fat
C.  Functional unit of the kidney; includes a renal corpuscle and a renal tubule
D.  Carries blood into the glomerulus of the nephron
E.  Receive urine from the renal pyramids; form the border of the renal sinus
F.  Part of the nephron that consists of Bowman's capsule and the glomerulus
G.  Area in the midportion of the kidney that collects urine before entering the ureter
H.  Site of filtration in the kidney; contains water, salts, glucose, urea, and amino acids
I.  Receives urine from the minor calyces to convey to the renal pelvis
J.  Outer parenchyma of the kidney that contains the renal corpuscle and proximal and distal convoluted tubules of the nephron
K.  Small, membranous canal that excretes urine from the urinary bladder
L.  Space behind the peritoneal lining of the abdominal cavity

---

**Exercise 2**

*Match the following anatomy and physiology terms with their definitions.*

_____ 1. arcuate arteries

_____ 2. blood urea nitrogen (BUN)

_____ 3. calyx

_____ 4. creatinine

_____ 5. efferent arteriole

_____ 6. glomerulus

_____ 7. homeostasis

_____ 8. loop of Henle

_____ 9. medulla

_____ 10. Morison's pouch

_____ 11. renal pyramid

_____ 12. renal hilum

_____ 13. renal sinus

A.  Portion of a renal tubule lying between the proximal and distal convoluted portions; reabsorption of fluid, sodium, and chloride occurs here and in the proximal convoluted tubule
B.  One of several conical masses of tissue that form the kidney medulla; each consists of the loops of Henle and the collecting tubules of the nephrons
C.  Retroperitoneal structures that exit the kidney to carry urine to the urinary bladder
D.  Inner portion of the renal parenchyma that contains the loop of Henle
E.  Small vessels found at the base of the renal pyramids; appear as echogenic structures
F.  Muscular retroperitoneal organ that serves as a reservoir for urine
G.  Part of the collecting system adjacent to the pyramid that collects urine and is connected to the major calyx
H.  Network of capillaries that are part of the filtration process in the kidney
I.  Central area of the kidney that includes the calyces, renal pelvis, renal vessels, fat, nerves, and lymphatics
J.  Right posterior subhepatic space located anterior to the kidney and inferior to the liver where fluid may accumulate
K.  Small vessel that carries blood from the glomerulus of the nephron and conducts blood to the peritubular capillaries that surround the renal tubule

_____14. specific gravity

_____15. ureters

_____16. urinary bladder

L.  Area in the midportion of the kidney where the renal vessels and ureter enter and exit
M.  Laboratory measurement of the amount of nitrogenous waste and creatinine in the blood
N.  A product of metabolism; laboratory test that measures the ability of the kidney to get rid of waste
O.  Maintenance of normal body physiology
P.  Laboratory tests that measure how much dissolved material is present in the urine

## Exercise 3

_Match the following terms related to pathology and sonographic evaluation with their definitions._

_____1. columns of Bertin

_____2. dromedary hump

_____3. ectopic kidney

_____4. horseshoe kidney

_____5. hydronephrosis

_____6. renal agenesis

_____7. renal capsule

_____8. urolithiasis

A.  Normal variant that occurs on the left kidney as a bulge on the lateral border
B.  Located outside of the normal position, most often in the pelvic cavity
C.  Stone within the urinary system
D.  First layer adjacent to the kidney that forms a tough, fibrous covering
E.  Bands of cortical tissue that separate the renal pyramids; may mimic a renal mass on ultrasound
F.  Dilation of the renal collecting system
G.  Congenital malformation in which both kidneys are joined together by an isthmus, most commonly at the lower poles
H.  Interruption in the normal development of the kidney resulting in absence of the kidney; may be unilateral or bilateral

## ANATOMY AND PHYSIOLOGY

## Exercise 4

_Label the following illustrations._

1. The kidney cut longitudinally.

1. _____
2. _____
3. _____
4. _____
5. _____
6. _____
7. _____
8. _____
9. _____
10. _____
11. _____
12. _____
13. _____
14. _____
15. _____
16. _____
17. _____
18. _____

2. Anatomic structures related to the anterior surfaces of the kidneys.

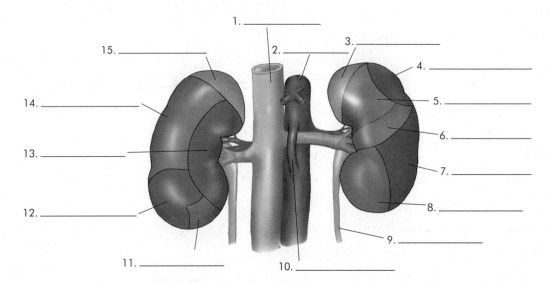

3. Vascular relationship of the great vessels and their tributaries to the kidneys.

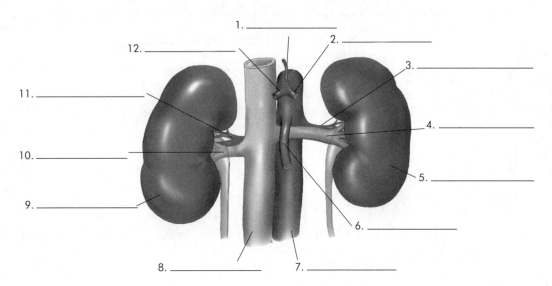

**Exercise 5**

*Fill in the blank(s) with the word(s) that best completes the statements, or provide a short answer about the anatomy of the kidney.*

1. The urinary system has two principal functions: excreting _____ and regulating the composition

   of _____.

2. The right kidney lies slightly _____ than the left kidney because the large right lobe of the

   _____ pushes it _____.

3. The kidneys move with respiration; on deep inspiration, both kidneys move _____ approximately
   1 inch.

4. Within the hilus of the kidney are other _____ structures, a ureter, and the _____.

5. A fibrous capsule called the _____ surrounds the kidney.

6. Outside of this fibrous capsule is a covering of _____.

7. The _____ fascia surrounds the perinephric fat and encloses the kidneys and adrenal glands.

8. The renal fascia, known as _____ fascia, surrounds the true capsule and perinephric fat.

9. The medullary substance consists of a series of striated conical masses, called the renal _____.

10. A nephron consists of two main structures, a renal _____ and a renal _____.

11. Nephrons _____ the blood and produce _____.

12. The renal corpuscle consists of a network of capillaries, called the _____, which is surrounded by a cuplike structure known as _____.

13. Blood flows into the glomerulus through a small _____ arteriole and leaves the glomerulus through a(n) _____ arteriole.

14. There are three constrictions along the ureter's course: (1) _____, (2) _____, and (3) _____.

15. The main renal artery is a lateral branch of the aorta and arises just inferior to the _____ artery.

16. The renal vein drains into the _____ of the inferior vena cava.

## Exercise 6

*Fill in the blank(s) with the word(s) that best completes the statements, or provide a short answer about the physiology of the kidney.*

1. The urinary system is located posterior to the peritoneum lining the abdominal cavity in an area called the

   _____.

2. The kidneys adjust the amounts of _____ and _____ leaving the body so that these equal the amounts of substances entering the body.

3. The principal metabolic waste products are _____, _____, and nitrogenous wastes.

4. Both urea and uric acid are carried away from the liver into the kidneys by the _____ system.

5. The presence of an acute infection causes _____, which is _____ in the urine; pyuria means there is _____ in the urine.

6. The pH refers to the strength of the urine as a partly _____ or _____ solution.

7. The _____ is the measurement of the kidney's ability to concentrate urine.

8. The specific gravity is especially _____ in cases of renal failure, glomerular nephritis, and pyelonephritis.

9. A decreased _____ occurs with acute hemorrhagic processes secondary to disease or blunt trauma.

10. Impairment of renal function and increased protein catabolism result in BUN _____ that is relative to the degree of renal impairment and rate of urea nitrogen excreted by the kidneys.

### Exercise 7

*Fill in the blank(s) with the word(s) that best completes the statements, or provide a short answer about the sonographic evaluation of the kidney.*

1. The renal parenchyma surrounds the fatty central renal sinus, which contains these five structures:

   _____

   _____

2. Dilation of the collecting system has also been noted in _____ patients, especially the right kidney.

3. The _____ is the area from the renal sinus to the outer renal surface.

4. The _____ and _____ arteries are best demonstrated as intense specular echoes in cross section or oblique section at the corticomedullary junction.

5. The _____ generally is echo producing, whereas the medullary pyramids are _____.

6. The cortex and medullary pyramids are separated from each other by bands of cortical tissue, called

   _____, that extend inward to the renal sinus.

7. The _____ lie posterior to the renal arteries and should be identified by their lack of pulsations and absence of Doppler flow.

8. The _____ of the pyramid points toward the sinus, and the _____ lies adjacent to the renal cortex.

9. The _____ is a cortical bulge that occurs on the lateral border of the kidney, typically more on the left side.

10. A(n) _____ is a triangular, echogenic area in the upper pole of the renal parenchyma that can be seen during normal scanning.

11. In a patient with a(n) _____, there is fusion of the kidneys during fetal development that almost

    invariably involves the _____ poles.

12. A cystic mass presents sonographically with several characteristic features:

    _____

    _____

13. A cystlike enlargement of the lower end of the ureter is called a(n) _____.

## PATHOLOGY

### Exercise 8

*Fill in the blank(s) with the word(s) that best completes the statements, or provide a short answer about the pathology of the kidney.*

1. Sonographically, it is difficult to differentiate between a(n) _____ cyst and a small adjacent cortical cyst.

2. The parapelvic cyst is found in the _____ but does not communicate with the renal collecting system.

3. Name the four forms of autosomal recessive polycystic kidney disease.

   _____

**119**

4. Discuss the characteristics of autosomal dominant polycystic kidney disease.

_____

_____

_____

_____

5. Usually a(n) _____ renal contour is the first finding that a mass may be present and require further investigation.

6. Define the characteristics of renal cell carcinoma.

_____

_____

_____

_____

7. One of the most common benign renal tumors is called _____.

8. An uncommon benign renal tumor composed mainly of fat cells and commonly found in the renal cortex is

_____.

9. A(n) _____ appears as a well-defined echogenic mass, found more often in females.

10. Sonographic findings include one or more fluid spaces at the _____ junction that corresponds to the distribution of the renal pyramids.

11. Although the kidneys appear enlarged with a highly echogenic renal sinus, the intrarenal anatomy is preserved with

uniform loss of renal tissue in patients with _____.

12. The most common medical renal disease that produces acute renal failure is _____.

13. Chronic renal disease is loss of renal _____ as a result of disease, most commonly parenchymal disease.

14. There are three primary types of chronic renal failure: _____, _____, and

_____.

15. _____ is when the dilated pyelocalyceal system appears as separation of the renal sinus echoes by fluid-filled areas that conform anatomically to the infundibula, calyces, and renal pelvis.

16. A localized hydronephrosis occurs as a result of _____, calculi, _____, or the

_____.

17. Hydronephrosis with a dilated ureter and bladder indicates obstruction of the _____ junction or

of the _____.

18. If hydronephrosis is suspected, the sonographer should evaluate the _____.

19. Name two conditions that might mimic hydronephrosis.

_____

20. Describe the sonographic findings in acute obstruction.

_____

_____

_____

21. Ureteral jets are best visualized by _____ imaging.

22. When pus is found within the obstructed renal system, the condition is called _____.

23. _____ is characterized by diffuse foci of calcium deposits that are usually located in the medulla but infrequently can be seen also in the renal cortex.

24. A renal _____ occurs when part of the tissue undergoes necrosis after the cessation of the blood supply, usually as a result of artery occlusion.

## Exercise 9

*Fill in the blank(s) with the word(s) that best completes the statements, or provide a short answer about renal transplantation.*

1. The major problem encountered with renal transplantation is _____.

2. Early after surgery, a baseline sonographic examination is performed to determine _____, _____, and _____.

3. Perirenal fluid collections such as _____, _____, _____, or _____ can be diagnosed reliably and differentiated from acute rejection.

4. _____ rejection occurs within hours of transplantation and is caused by vasculitis leading to thrombosis and usually the loss of the graft.

5. _____ rejection occurs within days to months after transplant.

6. _____ rejection causes include preformed antibodies, immune complexes, and cell-mediated responses.

7. _____ rejection can occur months after transplantation with gradual onset.

8. When using ultrasound to help diagnose rejection, care must be taken to visualize these five things:

   _____

   _____

   _____

9. The incidence of acute tubular necrosis is usually higher in _____ transplants than in _____ transplants.

10. Early signs of obstruction are _____ or severe _____ in a patient with satisfactory renal volumes.

11. Renal artery stenosis exhibits a(n) _____ jet with distal turbulence.

12. _____ Doppler is not angle dependent and has a greater sensitivity to detect blood flow.

## Exercise 10

*Fill in the blank(s) with the word(s) that best completes the statements, or provide a short answer about urolithiasis and bladder pathology.*

1. The initial clinical sign of a kidney stone is extreme _____, typically followed by cramping on the side where the stone is located; nausea and vomiting may also occur.

2. Renal stones have very _____ foci with posterior acoustic shadowing.

3. If the stone causes obstruction, there will be _____ and, depending on the location of the stone, the ureter may be dilated _____ to the level of obstruction.

4. _____ entails herniation of all layers of the bladder wall and is located in the posterior angle of the trigone.

5. _____ diverticula are herniations of only the two inner layers through the muscle layer.

6. _____ is usually secondary to another condition that causes stasis of urine in the bladder.

7. The majority of bladder tumors in adults are _____ carcinoma.

**Exercise 11**

*Provide a short answer for each question after evaluating the images.*

1. List the anatomic structures shown to arise from the inferior vena cava in this coronal image.

_____

2. What anatomic structure do the arrows point to?

_____

3. What anatomic variation of the kidney are the arrows pointing to?

_____

4. Identify the anatomic variant demonstrated in this image.

_____

5. Name the structure that the arrow is pointing to along the anterior wall of the kidney.

_____

Chapter **15** **Urinary System**

A    B

6. Describe the sonographic finding in this transverse and longitudinal image of the kidney.

_____

CLA/3.5MI/40
-8 dB
160 mm
60  dg    17 fps
S CURVE
          FF TP 46%

SAGITTAL
RIGHT

+D 55.7 mm
xD 24.6 mm

A    B

RIGHT TRANS            8fps    12cm

7. What pathology is demonstrated on these longitudinal scans of both kidneys of a young adult male?

_____

_____

A    B

8. A 66-year-old male presents with an incidental finding on his abdominal ultrasound. What pathology do the images demonstrate?

_____

A

B

C

D

9. A 14-month-old child presents with a palpable right-sided mass, decreased appetite, and lethargy. What is the sonographic finding?

_____

10. A 6-year-old male presents with chronic urinary tract infections. What is the ultrasound finding?

_____

11. Does this patient have hydronephrosis? Explain why or why not.

_____

_____

A        B

12. A young adult male presents with flank pain after renal transplant surgery. What are the sonographic findings?

_____

# 16 Retroperitoneum

## KEY TERMS

### Exercise 1

*Match the following anatomy and physiology terms with their definitions.*

___D___ 1. adrenocorticotropic hormone (ACTH)

___A___ 2. cortex

___B___ 3. false pelvis

___E___ 4. hyperplasia

___C___ 5. medulla

A. Outer parenchyma of the adrenal gland that secretes steroid hormones commonly called corticoids
B. Portion of the pelvic cavity that is above the pelvic brim, bounded posteriorly by the lumbar vertebrae, laterally by the iliac fossae and iliacus muscles, and anteriorly by the lower anterior abdominal wall
C. Central tissue of the adrenal gland that secretes epinephrine and norepinephrine
D. Hormone secreted by the pituitary gland
E. An increase in the number of cells of a body part that results from an increased rate of cellular division

### Exercise 2

*Match the following pathology terms to their definitions.*

___D___ 1. adenoma

___A___ 2. Addison's disease

___F___ 3. Cushing's syndrome

___E___ 4. lymphoma

___C___ 5. neuroectodermal tissue

___B___ 6. neuroblastoma

___H___ 7. pheochromocytoma

___G___ 8. lymphadenopathy

A. Condition caused by hyposecretion of hormones from the adrenal cortex
B. Malignant adrenal mass that is seen in pediatric patients
C. Early embryonic tissue that will eventually develop into the brain and spinal cord
D. Smooth, round, homogeneous benign tumor of the adrenal cortex associated with Cushing's syndrome
E. Malignancy that primarily affects the lymph nodes, spleen, or liver
F. Condition caused by hypersecretion of hormones from the adrenal cortex
G. Any disorder characterized by enlargement of the lymph nodes or lymph vessels
H. Benign adrenal tumor that secretes hormones that produce hypertension

## Exercise 3

*Label the following illustrations.*

1. The psoas muscle extends from the mediastinum to the thigh.

13. IVC
12. RT CRUS
11. RT PHRENIC N
10. MEDIAN ARUATE LIG
9. Medial ARCUATE LIG
8. LAT ARCUATE LIG

1. CENTRAL TENDON
2. LT PHRENIC N
3. LT CRUS
4. ESOPHAGUS
5. AORTA
6. PSOAS M
7. QL

2. The quadratus lumborum muscle originates from the iliolumbar ligament.

7. CENTRAL TENDON
6. DIAPHRAGM

1. IVC
2. ESOPHAGUS
3. AORTA
4. QL M.
5. ILIOPSOAS M.

Chapter **16** **Retroperitoneum**

3. Identify the structures on this diagram.

10. TRANSVERSALIS FASCIA
9. PERITONEUM
8. DUODENUM
7. ANT RENAL FASCIA
6. ASC COLON
5. POST RENAL FASCIA

1. SKIN
2. PANCREAS
3. _____
4. DESC COLON

4. The right crus of the diaphragm passes posterior to the inferior vena cava.

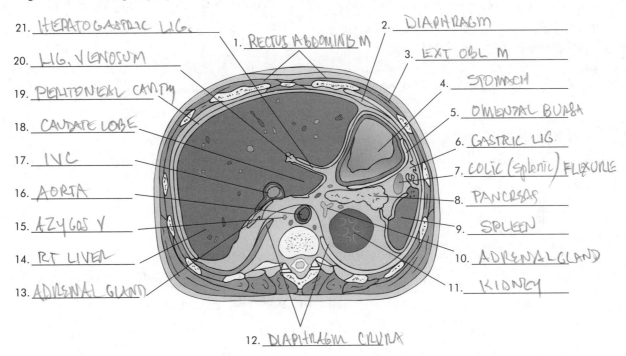

21. HEPATOGASTRIC LIG.
20. LIG. VENOSUM
19. PERITONEAL CAVITY
18. CAUDATE LOBE
17. IVC
16. AORTA
15. AZYGOS V
14. RT LIVER
13. ADRENAL GLAND

1. RECTUS ABDOMINIS M

2. DIAPHRAGM
3. EXT OBL M
4. STOMACH
5. OMENTAL BURSA
6. GASTRIC LIG.
7. COLIC (splenic) FLEXURE
8. PANCREAS
9. SPLEEN
10. ADRENAL GLAND
11. KIDNEY

12. DIAPHRAGM CRURA

RT

**Exercise 4**

*Fill in the blank(s) with the word(s) that best completes the statements, or provide a short answer about the anatomy of the retroperitoneum.*

1. The retroperitoneal space is the area between the posterior portion of the ___PARIETAL PERIT.___ and the ___POSTERIOR___ abdominal wall muscles.

2. The retroperitoneal space is subdivided into three spaces: the anterior ___PARARENAL___ space, the ___PERIRENAL___ space, and the posterior ___PARARENAL___ space.

3. The ___PERIRENAL___ space surrounds the kidney, adrenal, and perirenal fat.

4. The anterior ___PARARENAL___ space includes the duodenum, pancreas, and ascending and transverse colon.

5. The posterior ___PARARENAL___ space includes the iliopsoas muscle, ureter, and branches of the inferior vena cava and their lymphatics.

6. The right adrenal is more ___SUPERIOR___ to the kidney, whereas the left adrenal is more ___MEDIAL___ to the kidney.

7. The right renal artery crosses ___ANTERIOR___ to the crus and ___POSTERIOR___ to the inferior vena cava at the level of the right kidney.

8. The ___PSOAS___ muscle, the fascia of which merges with the posterior transversalis fascia, makes up the medial border of this posterior space.

**Exercise 5**

*Fill in the blank(s) with the word(s) that best completes the statements about the physiology of the retroperitoneum.*

1. The male sex hormones are ___ANDROGEN___, and the female sex hormones are ___ESTROGENS___.

2. Hypofunction of the adrenal cortex in humans is called ___ADDISON'S___ disease.

3. The steroids secreted by the adrenal cortex fall into the following three main categories: ___MINERALO CORTICOIDS___, ___GLUCOCORTICOIDS___, and ___SEX HORMONES___.

4. ___MINERALO CORTICOIN___ regulate electrolyte metabolism.

5. The principal mineralocorticoid is ___ALDOSTERONE___.

6. ___GLUCOCORTICOIDS___ play a principal role in carbohydrate metabolism.

7. The primary glucocorticoids are ___CORTISONE___ and ___HYDRO CORTISONE___.

8. Adrenal tumors in women can promote secondary ___MASCULINE___ characteristics.

9. The adrenal cortex is controlled by ___ADRENO CORTICOTROPIC___ hormone (ACTH) from the pituitary.

10. Epinephrine and norepinephrine are amines, sometimes referred to as ___CATECHOLAMINE___, that elevate the blood pressure. *adrenaline / noradrenaline*

## SONOGRAPHIC EVALUATION

**Exercise 6**

*Fill in the blank(s) with the word(s) that best completes the statements, or provide a short answer about the sonographic evaluation of the retroperitoneum.*

1. Describe the sonographic findings for the paraaortic lymph nodes.

_____

_____

_____

2. Explain how to distinguish enlarged lymph nodes from bowel.

LYMPH NODES · NO PERISTALSIS, NOT COMPRESSIBLE/DISPLACABLE

_____

_____

3. Adrenal hemorrhages are more common in neonates who experienced a traumatic delivery that included

_____, _____, and _____.

4. The clinical symptoms of pheochromocytoma include intermittent _____, severe

_____, heart _____, and excess perspiration.

5. A _____ is a walled-off collection of extravasated urine that develops spontaneously after trauma, surgery, or a subacute or chronic urinary obstruction.

## PATHOLOGY

### Exercise 7

*Provide a short answer for each question after evaluating the images.*

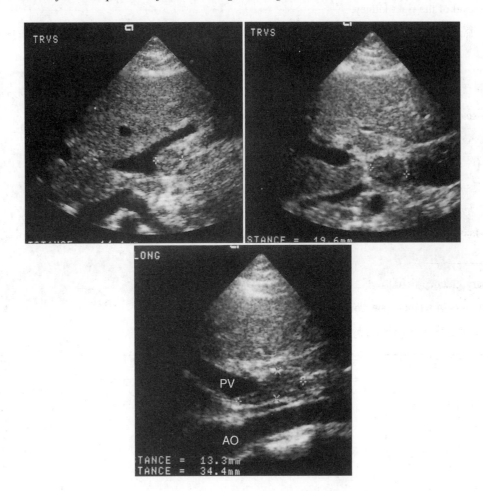

1. A 32-year-old female with a history of lymphoma came in for an abdominal ultrasound exam. Describe the sonographic findings.

_____

_____

2. What structure is the arrow pointing to on this transverse image in this patient with abdominal tenderness?

_____

_____

3. What is the abnormality on this right upper quadrant sonogram?

_____

_____

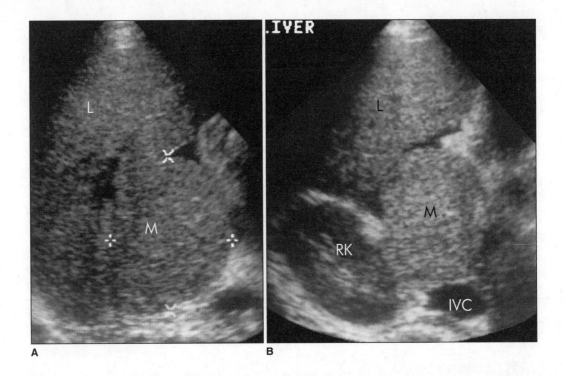

**A**     **B**

4. This patient presents with uncontrollable hypertension. Identify the anomaly shown in the sonograms.

_____

# 17 Abdominal Applications of Ultrasound Contrast Agents

## KEY TERMS

### Exercise 1

*Match the following ultrasound terms to their definitions.*

_____ 1. acoustic emission

_____ 2. contrast-enhanced sonography

_____ 3. tissue-specific ultrasound contrast agent

_____ 4. first-generation agents

_____ 5. gray-scale harmonic imaging

_____ 6. harmonic imaging

_____ 7. induced acoustic emission

_____ 8. intravenous injection

_____ 9. mechanical index

_____ 10. second-generation agents

_____ 11. molecular imaging agents

_____ 12. ultrasound contrast agents

_____ 13. vascular ultrasound contrast agents

A. Index that defines the low acoustic output power that can be used to minimize the destruction of microbubbles by energy in the acoustic field

B. Agents containing room air

C. After the injection of the tissue-specific ultrasound contrast agents (UCA) Sonazoid, the reflectivity of the contrast-containing tissue increases; when the right level of acoustic energy is applied to tissue, the contrast microbubbles eventually rupture, resulting in random Doppler shifts; these shifts appear as a transient mosaic of colors on the color Doppler display; masses that have destroyed or replaced normal Kupffer cells will be displayed as color-free areas

D. Agent used to reduce or eliminate some of the current limitations of ultrasound imaging and Doppler blood flow detection color flow imaging

E. Type of ultrasound contrast agent whose microbubbles are contained in the body's vascular spaces

F. Agents include Optison, Definity, Imagent, Levovist, and SonoVue

G. Allows detection of contrast-enhanced blood flow and organs with gray-scale ultrasound

H. Agents that can be administered intravenously to evaluate blood vessels, blood flow, and solid organs

I. Occurs when an appropriate level of acoustic energy is applied to the tissue; the microbubbles first oscillate and then rupture

J. Hypodermic injection into a vein for the purpose of injecting a contrast medium

K. In this mode, the ultrasound system is configured to receive only echoes at the second harmonic frequency, which is twice the transmit frequency

L. Agents containing heavy gases

M. Type of contrast agent whose microbubbles are removed from the blood and are taken up by specific tissues in the body

## Exercise 2

*Identify the abbreviations related to the use of contrast agents for ultrasound.*

1. AE _____

2. CES _____

3. CFI _____

4. GSHI _____

5. HI _____

6. IAE _____

7. MI _____

8. PDI _____

9. UCA _____

## Exercise 3

*Answer the following review questions regarding ultrasound contrast agents.*

1. Most of the research and development of ultrasound contrast agents has centered on creating agents that can:
   a. enhance the detection of stationary blood.
   b. be administered by intraarterial injection.
   c. be administered intravenously.
   d. enhance the detection of tumors in solid organs.
   e. be used for therapeutic applications.

2. Vascular ultrasound contrast agents enhance Doppler flow signals by:
   a. increasing the velocity of blood flow.
   b. adding more and better acoustic scatterers to the bloodstream.
   c. increasing the number of red blood cells in the vessel being evaluated.
   d. decreasing the speed of sound through tissue.
   e. a and b above.

3. For a vascular ultrasound contrast agent to be clinically useful, it should:
   a. be nontoxic.
   b. have microbubbles that are small enough to traverse the pulmonary capillary beds.
   c. be stable enough to provide multiple recirculations.
   d. be high in viscosity.
   e. a, b, and c above.

4. What type of substance does the microbubble of a "first-generation" ultrasound contrast agent contain?
   a. a heavy gas, such as a perfluorocarbon
   b. a fluid that has low solubility in blood
   c. room air
   d. a fluid that has acoustic properties that are drastically different from human blood
   e. albumin

**138**

5. Depending on the clinical application, vascular ultrasound contrast agents may be administered via:

   a. intravenous bolus injection.

   b. oral ingestion.

   c. intravenous infusion.

   d. all of the above.

   e. a and c above.

6. The microbubbles of tissue-specific ultrasound contrast agents:

   a. are significantly larger than red blood cells.

   b. are significantly larger than liver cells (hepatocytes).

   c. are taken up by or have an affinity toward specific tissue.

   d. are toxic to the targeted tissue.

   e. decrease the echogenicity of targeted tissue.

7. When in harmonic imaging mode, the ultrasound system is configured to receive:

   a. only echoes that are at one half the frequency of the transmitted frequency.

   b. only echoes that are high in amplitude.

   c. only echoes arising from contrast microbubbles.

   d. only echoes at the second harmonic frequency, which is twice the transmit frequency.

   e. only echoes arising from stationary tissue.

8. When insonating microbubble-based ultrasound contrast agents, the energy present within the acoustic field:

   a. has no effect on the microbubbles.

   b. can have a detrimental effect on the contrast microbubbles.

   c. usually increases the microbubble size.

   d. usually results in the creation of more microbubbles.

   e. c and d above.

9. Ultrasound contrast agents have shown the potential to improve the accuracy of hepatic sonography, including:

   a. enhanced detection of hepatic masses.

   b. enhanced characterization of hepatic masses.

   c. improved detection of intrahepatic and extrahepatic blood flow.

   d. a and c above.

   e. a, b, and c above.

10. Vascular ultrasound contrast agents can be useful in the evaluation of patients with suspected renal artery stenosis because they:

    a. increase the ability to visualize blood flow using color flow imaging.

    b. increase the velocity of blood flow to the kidneys.

    c. improve the intensity of spectral Doppler flow signals.

    d. a and c above.

    e. all of the above.

### Exercise 4

*Fill in the blank(s) with the word(s) that best completes the statements, or provide a short answer about the clinical applications of contrast agents in ultrasound.*

1. What are the current limitations of ultrasound imaging and Doppler blood flow detection?

   _____

   _____

   _____

2. What are the limitations of sonographic detection of blood flow?

   _____

   _____

   _____

3. Vascular or blood pool ultrasound contrast agents enhance Doppler (color and spectral) flow signals by adding more and better acoustic _____ to the bloodstream.

4. Some vascular agents also improve gray-scale ultrasound visualization of flowing blood and demonstrate changes to the _____ of tissue.

5. For an agent to be clinically useful, it should have these three qualities:

   _____

   _____

   _____

6. Agents containing room air are commonly referred to as _____ contrast agents, whereas agents containing heavy gases are referred to as _____ agents.

7. Describe how tissue-specific ultrasound contrast agents differ from vascular agents.

   _____

   _____

   _____

8. The rupture of the _____ results in random Doppler shifts appearing as a transient mosaic of colors on a color Doppler display.

9. Currently, tissue-specific agents that are taken up by the _____ system appear to be most useful in the assessment of patients with suspected liver abnormalities.

10. In harmonic imaging mode, the ultrasound system is configured to receive only echoes at the _____ harmonic frequency, which is twice the transmit frequency.

11. When using a microbubble-based ultrasound contrast agent, the microbubbles _____ (that is, they get larger and smaller) when subjected to the acoustic energy present in the ultrasound field with gray-scale ultrasound.

12. In the harmonic imaging mode, the echoes from the oscillating microbubbles have a higher _____ ratio than would be provided by using conventional ultrasound so that regions with microbubbles are more easily appreciated visually.

13. Wideband gray-scale harmonic imaging provides a way to better differentiate areas with and without contrast and has the potential to demonstrate real-time gray-scale blood pool imaging, or _____ imaging.

14. Although ultrasound is usually sensitive for the detection of medium to large hepatic lesions, it is limited in its ability to detect _____, isoechoic, or peripherally located lesions, particularly in obese patients or in patients with diffuse liver disease.

15. Hepatic ultrasound blood flow studies are limited by _____-velocity blood flow.

# 18 Ultrasound-Guided Interventional Techniques

## Exercise 1

*Match the following terms with their definitions.*

_____ 1. freehand technique

_____ 2. coagulopathy

_____ 3. hypovolemia

_____ 4. international normalized ratio

_____ 5. pneumothorax

_____ 6. prostate-specific antigen

_____ 7. hypotension

_____ 8. partial thromboplastin time (PTT)

_____ 9. thoracentesis

_____10. vasovagal

A. Defect in blood-clotting mechanisms

B. Surgical puncture of the chest wall for removal of fluids; usually done by using a large-bore needle

C. Decreased systolic and diastolic blood pressure below normal

D. Laboratory test that can be used to evaluate the effects of heparin, aspirin, and antihistamines on the blood-clotting process by detecting clotting abnormalities of the intrinsic and common pathways

E. Method of performing an ultrasound-guided procedure without the use of a needle guide on the transducer

F. Concerning the action of stimuli from the vagus nerve on blood vessels; vasovagal syncope is a brief loss of consciousness caused by a sudden drop in heart rate and blood pressure, which reduces blood flow to the brain

G. Collection of air or gas in the pleural cavity

H. Diminished blood volume

I. Laboratory test that measures levels of this antigen in the body, elevated levels of which could indicate prostate cancer

J. Method developed to standardize prothrombin time (PT) results among laboratories by accounting for the different thromboplastin reagents used to determine PT

## Exercise 2

*Identify the abbreviations related to ultrasound-guided interventional techniques.*

1. AFP _____

2. FNA _____

3. INR _____

4. PSA _____

5. PT _____

6. PTT _____

**Exercise 3**

*Fill in the blank(s) with the word(s) that best completes the statements, or provide a short answer about the ultrasound-guided procedures.*

1. Discuss the main advantages of using ultrasound for biopsy guidance.

_____

_____

2. List the limitations of ultrasound guidance.

_____

_____

3. The most common indication for a biopsy is to confirm _____ in a mass.

4. Identify the contraindications of a biopsy.

_____

_____

5. Which laboratory test is used to evaluate the effects of heparin, aspirin, and antihistamines on the blood-clotting process?

_____

6. Biopsies are used to confirm if a mass is _____, _____, or _____.

7. A(n) _____ uses an automated spring-loaded device, termed a biopsy gun, to provide a core of tissue for histologic analysis.

8. FNA uses a(n) _____ needle to obtain cells from a mass.

9. One method of ultrasound-guided intervention is called the _____ technique and is performed without the use of a needle guide on the transducer.

10. Identify the benefits of using a needle guide.

_____

_____

11. The patient must be informed of the potential _____, the alternate methods of obtaining the same information, and what the course of the disease would be if the biopsy were not performed and the correct treatment could not be planned.

12. The national patient safety standards (www.jcaho.org) mandate that a "timeout" be performed before beginning any procedure. Explain what a "timeout" is and what its purpose is.

_____

_____

_____

_____

13. Complications from an ultrasound-guided biopsy are usually minor and may include _____,

_____ reactions, and _____.

14. It is important to determine how much the mass moves with _____ and also how well and how long the patient can hold his or her breath.

15. Describe how to see the needle tip in ultrasound.

_____

_____

16. Whenever possible, a(n) _____ approach should be used to prevent the possibility of a pneumothorax or damage to the intercostal arteries.

17. Typically the _____ pole of the kidney is biopsied to prevent possible lacerations of the main renal vessels and ureter.

18. Patients may be marked for a thoracentesis or may have the procedure under sonographic guidance. Patients should be scanned in the _____ position that the procedure will be performed in, which is usually in an upright position, through the back.

# 19 Emergent Ultrasound Procedures

## Exercise 1

*Match the following abdominal ultrasound terms with their definitions.*

_____1. focused assessment with sonography for trauma

_____2. hemoperitoneum

_____3. incarcerated hernia

_____4. intravenous urography

_____5. peritoneal lavage

_____6. pseudodissection

_____7. reducible hernia

_____8. strangulated hernia

A. Collection of bloody fluid in the abdomen or pelvis secondary to trauma or surgical procedure

B. Capable of being replaced in a normal position; the visceral contents can be returned to normal intraabdominal location

C. Invasive procedure that is used to sample the intraperitoneal space for evidence of damage to viscera and blood vessels

D. Limited examination of the abdomen or pelvis to evaluate free fluid or pericardial fluid

E. An incarcerated hernia with vascular compromise

F. Procedure used in radiography wherein contrast is administered intravenously to help the technician visualize the urinary system

G. Condition seen in a patient with aortic dissection

H. Imprisonment or confinement of a part of the bowel; the visceral contents cannot be reduced

## ANATOMY AND PHYSIOLOGY

### Exercise 2

*Label the following illustrations.*

1. The two common sites for peritoneal lavage.

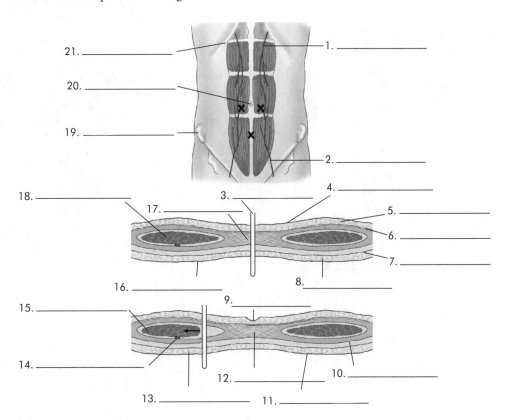

**147**

2. Transverse view of the perihepatic space and Morison's pouch.

10. _____
9. _____
8. _____
7. _____
6. _____
1. _____
2. _____
3. _____
4. _____
5. _____

**A**

15. _____
14. _____
13. _____
12. _____
11. _____
10. _____
1. _____
2. _____
3. _____
4. _____
5. _____
6. _____
7. _____
8. _____
9. _____

**B**

11. _____
Right          Left

Left anterior
(perigastric)

10. _____
9. _____
8. _____
4. _____
7. _____

1. _____
2. _____
3. _____
5. _____
6. _____

**C**                                    **D**

**Exercise 3**

*Fill in the blank(s) with the word(s) that best completes the statements, or provide a short answer about emergent abdominal ultrasound procedures.*

1. This procedure, called _____, is used to sample the intraperitoneal space for evidence of damage to the viscera and blood vessels.

2. Peritoneal lavage is usually used as a diagnostic technique in certain cases of _____ abdominal trauma.

3. Peritoneal lavage carries a risk of organ injury and decreases the specificity of subsequent ultrasonography or CT because of the introduction of _____ fluid and air.

4. The _____ scan in the emergency department is a limited examination of the abdomen or pelvis to evaluate free fluid or pericardial fluid.

5. In the context of traumatic injury, free fluid is usually a result of _____ and contributes to the assessment of the circulation.

6. The FAST scan area of evaluation is widespread, extending from the pericardial sac to the urinary bladder and including the _____ area (including Morison's pouch), the _____ region (including splenorenal recess), and _____ and _____.

7. Accessibility and _____ of performance are critical in the trauma setting.

8. The goal is to scan the _____ quadrants, _____ sac, and cul-de-sac for the presence of free fluid or hemoperitoneum.

9. Hemorrhage in the peritoneal cavity collects in the most _____ area of the abdomen.

10. _____ lacerations or contusions are more easily detected with ultrasound than are any other visceral abdominal injury.

11. A brisk intraparenchymal hemorrhage may be identified as a(n) _____ region within the abnormal parenchyma, whereas a global parenchymal injury may project into the liver as a widespread architectural disruption with absence of the normal vascular pattern.

12. In female patients of reproductive age with trauma, free fluid isolated to the cul-de-sac is likely

    _____.

13. If the patient is female with symptoms of right upper quadrant pain, fever, and leukocytosis, _____ should be ruled out.

14. The most common cause of acute cholecystitis is _____ with a cystic duct obstruction.

15. Midepigastric pain that radiates to the back is characteristic of _____.

16. Sonographic findings in acute pancreatitis show a normal to edematous gland that is somewhat

    _____ to normal texture.

17. Flank pain caused by _____ is a common problem in patients presenting to the emergency department.

18. If the stone completely obstructs the ureter, no _____ will be present.

19. When obstruction occurs, ultrasound is very effective in demonstrating the secondary sign of _____.

20. With the bladder distended, the color Doppler is an excellent tool to image the presence of ureteral jets into

the bladder; the transducer should be angled in a(n) _____ presentation through the distended urinary bladder.

21. The pulse repetition frequency should be _____ to assess the low velocity of the ureteral jet flow.

22. A(n) _____ is a condition in which a propagating intramural hematoma actually dissects along the length of the vessel, stripping away the intima and, in some cases, part of the media.

23. Most aortic dissections will occur at one of three sites:

_____

_____

24. Most aortic dissections are located in the _____ aorta.

25. _____ hypertension is nearly always associated with aortic dissection.

26. The most typical presentation of an aortic dissection is that of a sudden onset of severe, tearing _____ pain radiating to the arms, neck, or back.

27. With appendicitis, the patient will usually have rebound tenderness, "_____ sign," associated with peritoneal irritation.

28. A(n) _____ forms when the abdominal wall muscles are weakened, which allows the viscera to protrude into the weakened abdominal wall.

29. Sonography allows visualization of the _____ movement of the bowel during Valsalva maneuvers and determines the presence or absence of vascular flow within the defect.

30. Most paraumbilical hernias contain _____, _____, and _____.

31. The patient should be instructed to perform a(n) _____ maneuver to determine the site of the wall defect and to confirm the presence of the protruding hernia.

## Exercise 4

*Provide a short answer for each question after evaluating the images.*

1. Identify the abnormality visible in this image of the left upper quadrant.

_____

2. A trauma patient demonstrated fluid in the right upper quadrant in the area of Morison's pouch. Identify the other area(s) where the sonographer should look for fluid.

_____

A                                                                 B

3. After evaluating these images, determine whether this patient has an acute or chronic cholecystitis.

_____

_____

4. Describe what the sonographer should look for in this patient with shortness of breath in the parasternal long-axis view of the heart. What are the arrows pointing to?

_____

5. What structure is seen in this image?

_____

# 20 Sonographic Techniques in the Transplant Patient

## Exercise 1

*Match the following abdominal ultrasound terms with their definitions.*

_____1. Model for End-Stage Liver Disease (MELD)

_____2. Organ Procurement and Transplantation Network (OPTN)

_____3. pediatric end-stage liver

_____4. PTLF

_____5. renal autotransplantation

_____6. SPK

_____7. United Network for Organ Sharing (UNOS)

A. The patient's own kidney is removed from the retroperitoneum and reimplanted into the iliac fossa
B. Maintains a centralized computer networking system for all organ procurement organizations and transplant centers while seeking to be fair and effective in selecting transplant candidates
C. Simultaneous pancreas-kidney transplant
D. Initially used to predict death within 3 months in patients who had a transjugular intrahepatic portosystemic shunt (TIPS) performed. The MELD score is a mathematical calculation based on lab values of bilirubin (measurement of bile pigment), creatinine (kidney function), and international normalized ratio (INR) (blood clotting ability).
E. Organ allocation process
F. For children under 12 years of age
G. Posttransplant lymphoproliferative disorder

## TRANSPLANTATION

## Exercise 2

*Fill in the blank(s) with the word(s) that best completes the statements about transplantation.*

1. _____ is sudden and most commonly caused from a drug-induced injury such as an acetaminophen overdose.

2. The most common reason for transplantation in the United States is cirrhosis due to chronic _____,

   followed by _____ abuse.

3. List other liver diseases that can cause the liver to fail, resulting in the need for transplantation:

   _____

   _____

   _____

4. _____ is the most common primary malignant tumor in the liver

5. The most common cause for requiring a renal transplant is _____ end-stage renal disease or renal failure.

6. List some conditions that can lead to renal failure and a need for transplantation:

   _____

   _____

   _____.

7. High blood _____ can lead to many complications such as amputations, heart disease, stroke, vascular disease, blindness, nerve damage, or kidney damage.

**Exercise 3**

**Evaluation of the Liver Allograft**

*Fill in the blanks with the word(s) that best completes the statements about the evaluation of liver allografts.*

1. As a sonographer, state what you should evaluate in the liver transplant patient.

   _____

   _____

   _____

   _____

   _____

2. Why is Doppler crucial for the transplanted liver patient?

   _____

   _____

   _____

   _____.

3. On gray-scale imaging, the transplanted liver parenchyma should appear smooth and _____, being isoechoic relative to the right renal cortex.

4. The spectral waveform of the portal vein (PV) has _____ flow with minimal respiratory changes.

5. Postoperative edema can create _____ blood flow velocities within the hepatic arteries (HAs) or venous system.

6. The most common cause for liver transplant failure is _____.

7. Intrahepatic _____ are localized fluid collections of necrotic inflammatory tissue that contain purulent material and an infectious organism.

8. Thrombosis and _____ occur most commonly at anastomosis sites due to size discrepancy between the native and transplant vessels or suprahepatic caval kinking.

9. Intraluminal thrombus is identified filling the vessel with _____ color Doppler flow.

10. Thrombosis of the PV occurs in about 3% of liver transplants. List the common causes:

    _____

    _____

    _____

11. With chronic PV thrombosis, _____ can occur with the hepatic artery.

12. The most common cause for hepatic artery stenosis is postoperative _____.

13. The most common vascular complication of liver transplantation is _____ thrombosis.

14. _____ complications taken as a whole are the second most common cause of allograft dysfunction following rejection.

15. The most common biliary complication is _____, which is usually caused from a stricture at the anastomosis but may also be secondary to choledocholithiasis.

16. Hematomas are most common along the _____ spaces and near the vascular and biliary anastomosis sites. _____

17. _____ are clear serous fluid collections that are usually found within the first few days after transplantation.

18. The most common complication of venovenous bypass during liver transplantation is a(n) _____.

19. Bile leaks seep into the peritoneal cavity and may form a contained perihepatic collection, or _____.

20. The most common site of hepatocellular carcinoma (HCC) recurrence is the _____, followed by the liver.

21. Hepatitis _____ virus reinfection occurs in nearly all patients who receive a liver transplant for HCV cirrhosis.

22. Portal venous _____ is a common finding on ultrasound during the early postoperative period following transplantation.

23. One of the most severe complications found in both solid organ and stem cell transplantations is _____.

**Exercise 4**

**Renal Transplant**

*Fill in the blanks with the word(s) that best completes the statements about the evaluation of renal allografts.*

1. Describe what structures the sonographer should evaluate in a renal transplant patient.

   _____

   _____

   _____

2. Why is Doppler critical for the renal transplant evaluation?

   _____

   _____

   _____

3. What is a common indirect Doppler technique to evaluate the arterial and venous flow?

   _____

   _____

   _____

4. A high resistive index (RI) may indicate:

   _____

   _____

   _____

5. For all spectral Doppler, the angle should be _____ with the vessel that is sampled and less than 60 degrees to ensure accurate velocity measurements.

6. List the urgent findings immediately post renal transplant:

_____

_____

_____

_____

7. Postoperative edema can create _____ blood flow velocities within the renal artery (RA) or renal vein (RV), and the arcuate arteries may have an elevated RI and may demonstrate little or no diastolic flow.

8. What is the most common complication of renal biopsy? _____

9. What are the causes for renal graft rejection?

_____

_____

_____

10. More than 80% of renal transplant recipients develop at least one _____ within the first year.

11. Any peritransplant fluid collection should be considered infected in the _____ patient.

12. Focal pyelonephritis can be an isolated area of increased or decreased echogenicity with nonspecific findings. (T or F)

13. The most common site of obstruction is at the site of ureteral implantation into the _____.

14. Renal transplant recipients are at a higher risk for developing urinary _____.

15. Slow flow, extrinsic compression, or a narrowing at the anastomosis may be a precursor to developing

_____.

16. _____ renal vein thrombosis is an urgent finding, and the patient should undergo thrombectomy to avoid allograft loss.

17. Renal artery _____ is one of the most common vascular complications and usually occurs within the first year following transplantation.

18. Segmental infarction within the transplant is a result of:

_____

_____

19. A(n) _____ is a focal disruption of the artery with no direct communication with a vein and can occur in any vessel.

20. The most common peritransplant fluid collection is a(n) _____.

## Exercise 5

### Pancreatic Transplant

*Fill in the blanks with the word(s) that best completes the statements about the evaluation of the pancreatic transplant.*

1. Describe the sonographic evaluation of the pancreatic transplant:

_____

_____

_____

2. The transplanted pancreas will appear different from the native organ; typically, it has a(n) _____ appearance, and the borders can be difficult to visualize at times.

3. Describe the different types of rejection that may occur with a pancreatic transplant:

   a. Hyperacute:

   _____

   _____

   b. Acute:

   _____

   _____

   c. Chronic:

   _____

   _____

4. _____ is the second most common complication following transplantation.

5. _____ thrombosis is the second most common cause of allograft failure and typically is seen within the first 6 weeks following transplantation.

6. Some risk factors of thrombosis include:

   _____

   _____

7. On ultrasound, _____ appears as a round cystic structure that demonstrates disorganized "yin-yang" color flow within.

8. _____ collections are the most common complication following pancreatic transplantation, with the most common being a hematoma.

9. Following pancreatic transplantation, _____ has been reported in as many as 30% of cases.

**Exercise 6**

*Provide a short answer for each question after evaluating the images.*

A                                    B

1. Describe the spectral waveform in the main portal vein.

   _____

   _____

Chapter **20** **Sonographic Techniques in the Transplant Patient**

2. Describe the spectral waveform in the hepatic veins.

_____

_____

3. Describe the spectral waveform in the main hepatic artery.

_____

_____

4. Describe your findings in this post liver transplant patient.

_____

_____

5. Describe your findings in this patient post renal biopsy.

_____

_____

6. Describe your findings in this renal transplant patient.

_____

_____

Chapter **20**  **Sonographic Techniques in the Transplant Patient**

A

B

7. Describe your findings in this renal transplant patient.

_____

_____

A

B

8. Describe your findings in this recent renal transplant patient.

_____

_____

9. Describe your findings in this recent pancreatic transplant patient.

_____

_____

10. Describe your findings in this pancreatic transplant patient.

_____

_____

11. Describe your findings in this pancreatic transplant patient.

_____

_____

# 21 Breast

## Exercise 1

*Match the following anatomy terms with their definitions.*

_____ 1. acinus (acini)

_____ 2. areola

_____ 3. axilla

_____ 4. breast

_____ 5. Cooper's ligaments

_____ 6. mammary layer

_____ 7. retromammary layer

_____ 8. subcutaneous layer

_____ 9. tail of Spence

_____10. terminal ductal lobular unit (TDLU)

A. Connective tissue septa that connect perpendicularly to the breast lobules and extend out to the skin
B. Most superficial of the three layers of the breast identified on breast ultrasound
C. Armpit
D. Glandular (milk-producing) component of the breast lobule
E. Middle layer of the breast tissue that contains the ductal, glandular, and stromal portions of the breast
F. Smallest functional portion of the breast involving the terminal duct and its associated lobule containing at least one acinus
G. Differentiated apocrine sweat gland with a functional purpose of secreting milk during lactation
H. Deepest of the three layers of the breast noted on breast ultrasound
I. The pigmented skin surrounding the breast nipple
J. Normal extension of breast tissue into the axillary region

## Exercise 2

*Match the following breast evaluation terms with their definitions.*

_____ 1. antiradial

_____ 2. asymptomatic

_____ 3. breast imaging reporting and data system

_____ 4. breast self-examination

_____ 5. clinical breast examination

_____ 6. diagnostic breast imaging

_____ 7. fremitus

_____ 8. juxtathoracic

_____ 9. hyperechoic

_____10. palpable

_____11. isoechoic

_____12. radial

_____13. sentinel node

_____14. spiculation

_____15. nonpalpable

A. Plane of imaging on ultrasound of the breast
B. Part of breast cancer screening best done at the end of menses each month
C. Plane of imaging on ultrasound of the breast that is perpendicular to the radial plane of imaging
D. Echo texture that is more echogenic than the surrounding tissue
E. Type of breast imaging examination that is more intensive than routine screening mammography
F. Finger-like extension of a malignant tumor
G. Near the chest wall
H. Part of breast cancer screening done by a health care provider
I. Represents the first lymph node along the axillary node chain
J. Refers to vibrations produced by phonation and felt through the chest wall during palpation
K. Without symptoms
L. Can be felt on clinical examination
M. Trademark system created by the American College of Radiology (ACR) to standardize mammographic reporting terminology, to categorize breast abnormalities according to the level of suspicion for malignancy, and to facilitate outcome monitoring
N. Echo texture that resembles the surrounding tissue

_____16. anechoic

_____17. hypoechoic

_____18. cyst aspiration

_____19. breast cancer screening

O. Having relatively weak echoes
P. Preventive care that includes annual screening mammography (starting at age 40), monthly breast self-examination, and regular clinical breast examination
Q. Cannot be felt on clinical examination
R. Without echoes
S. Common diagnostic and interventional procedure that involves placing a needle through the skin of the breast into a cystic mass and pulling fluid out of the cyst through the needle

## Exercise 3

*Match the following pathology terms with their definitions.*

_____ 1. adenosis

_____ 2. apocrine metaplasia

_____ 3. atypical ductal hyperplasia

_____ 4. atypical hyperplasia

_____ 5. atypical lobular hyperplasia

_____ 6. cyst

_____ 7. epithelial hyperplasia

_____ 8. fibroadenoma

_____ 9. fibrocystic condition

_____10. Paget's disease

_____11. peau d'orange

_____12. infiltrating ductal carcinoma

_____13. infiltrating lobular carcinoma

_____14. isoechoic

_____15. lobular carcinoma in situ (LCIS)

_____16. lobular neoplasia

_____17. multicentric breast cancer

_____18. multifocal breast cancer

_____19. breast cancer

_____20. gynecomastia

A. Descriptive term for skin thickening of a breast that resembles the skin of an orange
B. Abnormal proliferation of cells with atypical features involving the TDLU, with an increased likelihood of evolving into breast cancer
C. Neither considered a true cancer nor treated as such
D. Most common benign solid tumor of the breast, consisting primarily of fibrous and epithelial tissue elements
E. Hypertrophy of residual ductal elements that persist behind the nipple in the male
F. Fluid-filled sac of variable size
G. Overgrowth of the stromal and epithelial elements of the acini within terminal ductal lobular unit (TDLU) of the breast
H. Cancer of the lobular epithelium of the breast, arises at the level of the TDLU
I. Breast cancer occurring in more than one site within the same quadrant of the same ductal system of the breast
J. Condition that represents different, essentially normal, tissue processes within the breast that in some patients become exaggerated to the point of raising concern for breast cancer
K. The pathologist recognizes some, but not all, of the features of ductal carcinoma in situ
L. Breast cancer occurring in different quadrants of the breast at least 5 cm apart
M. Shows some, but not all, of the features of lobular carcinoma in situ
N. Echo texture that resembles the surrounding tissue
O. Form of fibrocystic change in which the epithelial cells of the acini undergo alteration
P. Cancer of the ductal epithelium; most common general category of breast cancer, accounting for approximately 85% of all breast cancers
Q. Proliferation (hyperplasia) of epithelial cells lining the terminal duct-lobular unit
R. Term preferred by many authors to replace LCIS and atypical hyperplasia
S. Surface erosion of the nipple characterized by redness with flaking and crusting caused by direct invasion of the skin of the nipple by underlying breast cancer
T. Involves two main types of cells (ductal and lobular)

**Exercise 4**

*Label the following illustrations.*

1. Breast anatomy.

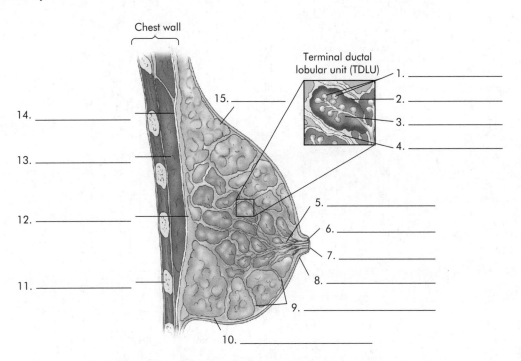

Chest wall

Terminal ductal
lobular unit (TDLU)

1. _____

2. _____

3. _____

4. _____

14. _____

13. _____

12. _____

11. _____

15. _____

5. _____

6. _____

7. _____

8. _____

9. _____

10. _____

2. Lymphatic drainage of the breast.

A

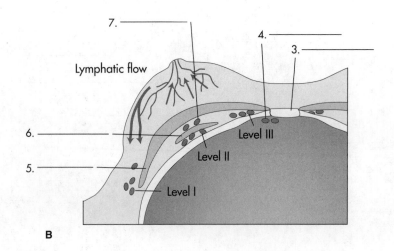

Lymphatic flow

Level III

Level II

Level I

B

Chapter **21**  **Breast**

3. Description of right breast anatomy.

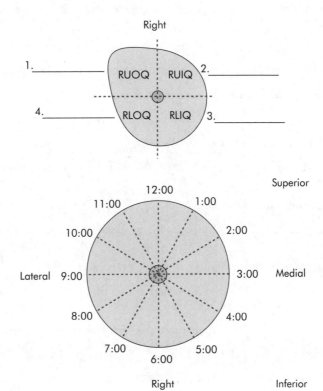

4. Description of left breast anatomy.

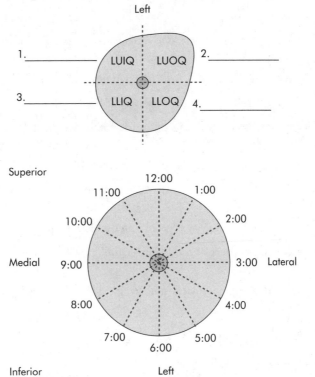

**Exercise 5**

*Fill in the blank(s) with the word(s) that best completes the statements, or provide a short answer about the anatomy and sonographic appearance of the breast.*

1. The breast is a modified _____ gland located in the superficial fascia of the anterior chest wall.

2. Sonographically the breast is divided into three layers located between the skin and the pectoralis major muscle on the anterior chest wall. These layers are the _____ layer, the _____ layer, and the _____ layer.

3. Fat is the least _____ tissue within the breast.

4. The fatty tissue appears _____, whereas the ducts, glands, and supporting ligaments appear echogenic.

5. The _____ quadrant of the breast contains the highest concentration of lobes.

6. Each lobule contains _____ (milk-producing glands) that are clustered on the terminal ends of the ducts like grapes on a vine.

7. The _____ muscle lies posterior to the retromammary layer.

8. The _____ tissue can situate itself in and among the areas of glandular tissue, and in some scanning planes it can mimic isoechoic or hypoechoic masses.

9. Sonographically, cancers can be difficult to differentiate in the fatty breast because most cancers appear _____ and can be difficult to differentiate from the normal breast tissue.

10. The main arterial supply to the breast comes from the internal _____ and the lateral _____ artery.

11. Lymphatic drainage from all parts of the breast generally flows to the _____ lymph nodes.

**Exercise 6**

*Fill in the blank(s) with the word(s) that best completes the statements, or provide a short answer about the physiology of the breast.*

1. The primary function of the breast is _____ transport.

2. The _____ system is critical in the transport of fluids within the breast.

3. An important function during the reproductive years is for the breast to make _____ from nutrients and water taken from the bloodstream.

4. Milk is produced within the _____ and carried to the nipple by the ducts.

5. Breast development begins before _____ and continues until the patient is approximately 16 years old.

6. During this time of development, the ductal system proliferates under the influence of _____.

7. During pregnancy, acinar development is accelerated to enable milk production by estrogen, _____, and prolactin.

8. The hormone produced by the pituitary gland that stimulates the acini to produce and excrete milk is called _____.

9. The expulsion of the placenta after the birth of a baby causes a drop in circulating progesterone, initiating _____ production within the breasts.

10. The physical stimulation of suckling by the baby initiates the release of _____ (produced by the hypothalamus and released by the pituitary gland), which further incites prolactin secretion, stimulating additional milk production.

11. Full maturation of the acini occurs during lactation and is thought to be mildly protective against the development of breast _____.

## SONOGRAPHIC EVALUATION

### Exercise 7

*Fill in the blank(s) with the word(s) that best completes the statements, or provide a short answer about the sonographic evaluation of the breast.*

1. Ultrasound may be used for screening purposes in _____ breasts that are _____ and difficult to penetrate by mammography, to evaluate palpable masses that are not visible on a mammogram, and to image the deep juxtathoracic tissues not normally visible by mammography.

2. Ultrasound is also useful in _____ structures within uniformly dense breast tissue where mammography is limited (e.g., in differentiating solid, round masses from fluid-filled cysts and visualizing tissue adjacent to implants or other structures that limit visualization by mammography).

3. A(n) _____ aspiration can be performed to determine whether a lesion is a complex cyst or truly a solid mass.

4. What basic clinical information must the sonographer have for any patient referred for breast ultrasound?

   _____

   _____

5. Pertinent clinical information that should be provided by the referring physician includes size and location of the lump, when it was noticed, and its relation to the _____.

6. A dominant cyst is frequently _____ or _____ (long axis toward nipple), smooth, soft (some cysts under tension can be firm and are usually very tender), and easily movable.

7. Fibroadenomas are usually similar in shape, but they are often quite firm and rubbery in consistency and _____ on ultrasound.

8. Breast cancer is usually lobular or _____ in shape, uneven in surface contour (sometimes gritty in texture), and fixed or poorly movable.

9. Most breast masses that arise during the adolescent years are _____.

10. A(n) _____ implant rupture occurs when there is a breach of the membrane surrounding an implant, but the silicone that leaks out is still confined within the fibrous scar tissue that forms a "capsule" around the implant.

11. As the implant collapses and the membrane folds inward, a series of discontinuous echogenic lines parallel to the face of the transducer may be seen and are referred to as the "stepladder sign" or "_____ sign."

12. The use of the _____ positions is unique to the breast and can often pick up subtle abnormalities extending toward the nipple along the ductal system from the mass.

13. _____ tend to grow within the ducts and will often follow the ductal system in a radial plane, toward the convergence at the nipple.

14. To be considered a simple cyst, a lesion must meet which three criteria on ultrasound?

   _____

   _____

15. Discuss the disruption of breast architecture with both benign and malignant tumors of the breast.

   _____

   _____

   _____

   _____

16. A rounded or oval shape is usually associated with _____ lesions, whereas sharp, angular

    margins are associated with _____ lesions.

17. The normal tissue planes of the breast are _____ oriented.

18. Benign lesions tend to grow within the normal tissue planes, and their long axis lies _____ to the chest wall.

19. Malignant lesions are able to grow through the connective tissue and may have a(n) _____ orientation when imaging the breast from anterior to posterior.

20. If a mass measures longer in the anteroposterior dimension (_____) than in either transverse

    or sagittal planes (_____), the mass has a vertical orientation that is usually described as being "taller than wide" and is suspicious for malignancy.

21. Malignant masses will often demonstrate increased _____ within the lesion and often have a feeder vessel, which can be identified with careful evaluation.

**PATHOLOGY**

**Exercise 8**

*Fill in the blank(s) with the word(s) that best completes the statements about the abnormalities of the breast.*

1. Lesions more common to younger women are _____ disease and fibroadenomas.

2. Older or postmenopausal women are more likely to have _____ papillomas, duct ectasia, and cancer.

3. Skin dimpling or ulceration and nipple retraction nearly always result from _____.

4. Benign tumors are rubbery, _____, and well delineated (as seen in a fibroadenoma), whereas malignant tumors are often stone hard and irregular with a gritty feel.

5. Clinical signs and symptoms of _____ include the lumps and pain that the patient feels that fluctuate with every monthly cycle. In most cases both breasts are equally involved.

6. The growth of a fibroadenoma is stimulated _____.

7. Sonographically, fat necrosis appears as an irregular, complex mass with low-level echoes, may mimic a(n)

   _____ lesion, and may appear as fat, but it is separate and different from the rest of the breast parenchyma.

8. _____ may result from infection, trauma, mechanical obstruction in the breast ducts, or from other conditions. It often occurs during lactation, beginning in the lactiferous ducts and spreading via the lymphatics or blood.

9. An intraductal papilloma is a small, _____ tumor that grows within the acini of the breast.

10. In _____ tissue, most cancer growth occurs along the borders.

11. _____ and _____ are frequently used as pathways for new tumor development.

12. If the tumor is _____, it continues to grow in one area, compressing and distorting the surrounding architecture.

13. Most cancer originates in the _____ ductal lobular units, whereas a smaller percentage originates in the glandular tissue.

14. _____ refers to breast tumors that arise from the epithelium, in the ductal and glandular tissue, and usually have tentacles.

15. Breast carcinomas are generally categorized by two factors: where the cancer cells originate (_____

or _____) and whether the cancer is prone to spreading (_____ or _____).

16. Carcinomas that do not normally spread outside of the duct or lobule are called noninvasive, noninfiltrating,

or _____ cancers, whereas cancers that spread into nearby tissue are said to be invasive or infiltrating.

**Exercise 9**

*Provide a short answer for each question after evaluating the images.*

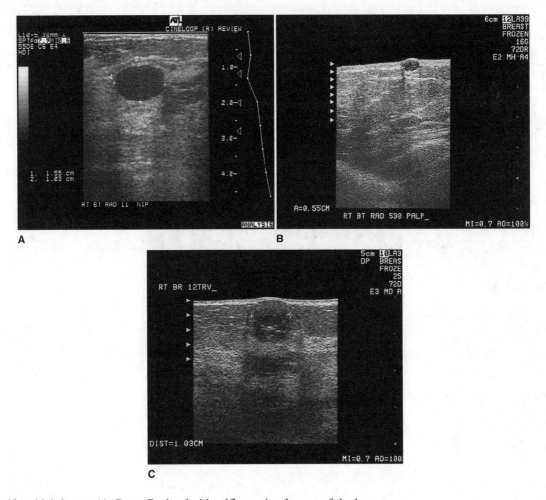

1. Identify which image (*A, B,* or *C*) clearly identifies a simple cyst of the breast.

_____

_____

2. Image A shows the breast lesion without compression, and image B shows the lesion with compression. Would you suspect this breast lesion is benign or malignant? Why?

_____

_____

3. Would you say this breast lesion is benign or malignant? Why?

_____

_____

A

B

C

D

BREAST MASS

4. Describe the following lesions of the breast.

a. _____

b. _____

c. _____

d. _____

# 22 | Thyroid and Parathyroid Glands

## KEY TERMS

### Exercise 1

*Match the following terms related to normal and abnormal anatomy and physiology with their definitions.*

| | | |
|---|---|---|
| C | 1. calcitonin | A. Group of three muscles (sternothyroid, sternohyoid, and omohyoid) that lies anterior to the thyroid |
| I | 2. euthyroid | B. Undersecretion of thyroid hormones |
| L | 3. hyperthyroidism | C. Thyroid hormone important for maintaining a dense, strong bone matrix and regulating the blood calcium level |
| D | 4. hypophosphatasia | D. Low phosphate level associated with hyperparathyroidism |
| B | 5. hypothyroidism | E. Laboratory value that is elevated with hyperparathyroidism |
| J | 6. isthmus | F. Hormone secreted by the pituitary gland that stimulates the thyroid gland to secrete thyroxine and triiodothyronine |
| G | 7. longus colli muscles | G. Wedge-shaped muscle posterior to the thyroid lobes |
| H | 8. parathyroid hormone (PTH) | H. Hormone secreted by parathyroid glands that regulates serum calcium levels |
| M | 9. pyramidal lobe | I. Refers to a normal functioning thyroid gland |
| E | 10. serum calcium | J. Small piece of thyroid tissue that connects the right and left lobes of the gland |
| K | 11. sternocleidomastoid muscles | K. Large muscles anterolateral to the thyroid |
| A | 12. strap muscles | L. Oversecretion of thyroid hormones |
| F | 13. thyroid-stimulating hormone | M. Present in small percentage of patients; extends superiorly from the isthmus |

### Exercise 2

*Match the following terms related to parathology pathology and miscellaneous neck masses with their definitions.*

| | | |
|---|---|---|
| B | 1. brachial cleft cyst | A. Disorder characterized by a localized or generalized enlargement of the lymph nodes or lymph vessels |
| H | 2. fine-needle aspiration | B. Remnant of embryonic development that appears as a cyst in the neck |
| C | 3. hyperparathyroidism | C. Disorder associated with elevated serum calcium level, usually caused by a benign parathyroid adenoma |
| A | 4. lymphadenopathy | D. Oversecretion of parathyroid hormone, usually from a parathyroid adenoma |
| F | 5. parathyroid hyperplasia | E. Congenital anomalies that present in the midline of the neck anterior to the trachea |
| D | 6. primary hyperparathyroidism | F. Enlargement of the multiple parathyroid glands |
| G | 7. secondary hyperparathyroidism | G. Enlargement of parathyroid glands in patients with renal failure or vitamin D deficiency |
| E | 8. thyroglossal duct cysts | H. Use of a fine-gauge needle to obtain cells from a mass |

## Exercise 3

Match the following terms related to thyroid pathology with their definitions.

F 1. adenoma
H 2. anaplastic carcinoma
J 3. follicular carcinoma
K 4. goiter
D 5. Graves' disease
I 6. Hashimoto's thyroiditis
L 7. medullary carcinoma
M 8. microcalcification
E 9. multinodular goiter
A 10. nodular hyperplasia
G 11. papillary carcinoma
C 12. subacute (de Quervain's) thyroiditis
B 13. thyroiditis

A. Degenerative nodules within the thyroid
B. Inflammation of the thyroid
C. Viral infection of the thyroid that causes inflammation
D. Autoimmune disorder characterized by a diffuse toxic goiter, bulging eyes, and cutaneous manifestations
E. Nodular enlargement of the thyroid associated with hyperthyroidism
F. Benign thyroid neoplasm characterized by complete fibrous encapsulation
G. Most common form of thyroid malignancy
H. Rare, undifferentiated carcinoma occurring in middle age
I. Chronic inflammation of the thyroid gland caused by the formation of antibodies against normal thyroid tissue
J. Occurs as a solitary malignant mass within the thyroid gland
K. Enlargement of the thyroid gland that can be focal or diffuse; multiple nodules may be present
L. Neoplastic growth that accounts for 10% of thyroid malignancies
M. Tiny echogenic foci within a nodule that may or may not shadow

## ANATOMY AND PHYSIOLOGY

## Exercise 4

Label the following illustrations.

1. Anterior view of the thyroid and parathyroid glands.

12. SUP THYROID ARTERY
11. SUP THYROID VEIN
10. INTERNAL JUGULAR VEIN
9. MIDDLE THYROID VEIN
8. COMMON CAROTID ART RT
7. INF. THYROID VEIN

1. THYROID CARTILAGE
2. CRICOID CARTILAGE
3. PYRAMIDAL LOBE
4. ISTHMUS (TM)
5. PARATHYROID GLAND
6. TRACHEA

} Thyroid gland

2. Cross section of the thyroid region.

1. _THYROID GLAND_
15. _TRACHEA_
14. _PARATHYROID GLAND_
13. _RECURRENT LARYNGEAL N._
12. _INT JUGULAR V._
11. _COMMON CAROTID A._
10. _INF THYROID A._

2. _STERNOHYOID M._
3. _OMOHYOID M._ } Strap muscles
4. _STERNOTHYROID M._
5. _SCM_
6. _MINOR N-V BUNDLE_
7. _ESOPHAGUS_
8. _LONGUS COLLI M._
9. _VERTEBRAL BODY C5_

## THE THYROID AND PARATHYROID GLANDS

### Exercise 5

*Fill in the blank(s) with the word(s) that best completes the statements about the thyroid and parathyroid glands.*

1. The thyroid straddles the trachea anteriorly, whereas the paired lobes extend on either side bounded laterally by the _COMMON CAROTID_ arteries and _INTERNAL JUGULAR_ veins.

2. Along the anterior surface of the thyroid gland lie the _STRAP_ muscles, including the sternothyroid, omohyoid, sternohyoid, and sternocleidomastoid muscles.

3. The parathyroid glands are normally located on the _POSTERIOR MED_ surface of the thyroid gland.

4. The parathyroid glands are the _Ca++ SENSING_ organs in the body.

5. The parathyroid glands produce _PARATHYROID Hormone_ and monitor the serum calcium feedback mechanism.

6. When the serum calcium level _DECREASES_, the parathyroid glands are stimulated to release PTH.

7. PTH acts on _BONE_, _KIDNEY_, and intestine to enhance calcium absorption.

8. Primary hyperparathyroidism is characterized by _HYPERCALCEMIA_, hypercalciuria, and low serum levels of phosphate.

9. Primary hyperparathyroidism occurs when increased amounts of PTH are produced by a(n) _ADENOMA_, primary hyperplasia, or, rarely, carcinoma located in the parathyroid gland.

10. A chronic hypocalcemia caused by renal failure, vitamin D deficiency (rickets), or malabsorption syndromes is _SECONDARY_ hyperparathyroidism.

### Exercise 6

*Fill in the blank(s) with the word(s) that best completes the statements about the thyroid and parathyroid glands.*

1. The thyroid gland is the part of the endocrine system that maintains body _METABOLISM_, _GROWTH_, and _DEVELOPMENT_ through the synthesis, storage, and secretion of thyroid hormones.

2. These hormones include triiodothyronine (_T3_), thyroxine (_T4_), and _CALCITONIN_.

3. The mechanism for producing thyroid hormones is _IODINE_ metabolism.

4. When the body needs thyroid hormone, it is released into the bloodstream by the action of thyrotropin, or thyroid-stimulating hormone (_TSH_), which is produced by the pituitary gland.

5. The secretion of TSH is regulated by thyrotropin-releasing factor, which is produced by the _HYPOTHALAMUS_

6. The concentration of calcium in the blood is decreased by _CALCITONIN_, which first acts on the bone to inhibit its breakdown.

7. Low intake of iodine (goiter) in the body may cause either _HYPOTHYROIDISM_, or the inability of the thyroid to produce the proper amount of thyroid hormone, or a problem in the pituitary gland that does not control the thyroid production.

8. The metabolic rate is dramatically increased _IN HYPERTHYROIDISM_; clinical signs include weight loss, increased appetite, high degree of nervous energy, tremor, excessive sweating, heat intolerance, and palpitations, and many patients show signs of exophthalmos (protruding eyes).

9. How the thyroid is functioning is evaluated by _NUCLEAR MEDICINE (LAB TESTS?)_

10. An enlargement of the thyroid gland is a(n) _GOITER_, which is often visible on the anterior neck.

※11. One of the most common forms of thyroid disease is _MULTINODULAR_ goiter.

12. _GRAVES'_ disease is characterized by these findings: hypermetabolism, diffuse toxic goiter, exophthalmos (inflammatory infiltration of the orbital tissue resulting in proptosis, or bulging of the eyes), and cutaneous manifestations (thickening of the dermis of the pretibial areas and the dorsum of the feet).

13. A benign thyroid neoplasm characterized by complete fibrous encapsulation is a(n) _ADENOMA_.

14. The most common of the thyroid malignancies is _PAPILLARY CANCER_ of the thyroid and is the preponderant cause of thyroid cancer in children.

15. The normal thyroid gland has a fine _HOMOGENEOUS_ echotexture that is more echogenic than the surrounding muscle structure.

16. A normal lymph node is oval in shape with a(n) _HOMOGENEOUS_ texture with a central core echo complex.

17. The _LONGUS COLLI_ muscle is posterior and lateral to each thyroid lobe and appears as a hypoechoic triangular structure adjacent to the cervical vertebrae.

## PATHOLOGY

### Exercise 7
*Provide a short answer for each question after evaluating the images.*

1. Identify the structure measured by the cross marks.

   _ISTHMUS_

2. A young woman presented with a palpable mass in her neck. Describe the sonographic findings.

MULTINODULAR HETEROGENEOUS ENLARGED TISSUE MASS WITHIN THYROID GLAND
INCREASED VASCULARITY DEMONSTRATED WITH COLOR DOPPLER

3. An asymptomatic female patient appeared with a mass in her neck. Identify the sonographic findings.

WELL-DEFINED ADENOMA WITH A CYSTIC COMPONENT SEEN
- HYPOECHOIC 'HALO' NOTED SURROUNDING THE LESION

**179**

RIGHT THYROID SAG UPPER

4. A 44-year-old female presented with a palpable mass in her neck. Identify the sonographic findings.

SOLID MASS OF THYROID (PAPILLARY CARCINOMA); MICROCALCIFICATIONS SEEN

# 23 Scrotum

## KEY TERMS

### Exercise 1

*Match the following anatomy terms with their definitions.*

____F____ 1. cremasteric muscle

____A____ 2. ejaculatory ducts

____J____ 3. epididymis

____L____ 4. mediastinum testis

____C____ 5. pampiniform plexus

____H____ 6. pudendal artery

____Q____ 7. scrotum

____B____ 8. seminal vesicles

____N____ 9. septa testis

____P____ 10. spermatic cord

____E____ 11. testicle

____K____ 12. testicular artery

____O____ 13. tunica albuginea

____G____ 14. tunica vaginalis

____M____ 15. urethra

____I____ 16. vas deferens

____D____ 17. verumontanum

A. Connect the seminal vesicle and the vas deferens to the urethra at the verumontanum
B. Reservoirs for sperm located posterior to the bladder
C. Plexus of veins in the spermatic cord that drain into the right and left testicular veins
D. Junction of the ejaculatory ducts with the urethra
E. Male gonad that produces hormones that induce masculine features and spermatozoa
F. An extension of the internal oblique muscle that descends to the testis with the spermatic cord
G. Membrane consisting of a visceral layer and a parietal layer lining the inner wall of the scrotum
H. Partially supply the scrotal wall and epididymis and occasionally the lower pole of the testis
I. Tube that connects the epididymis to the seminal vesicle
J. Anatomic structure formed by the network of ducts leaving the mediastinum testis that combine into a single convoluted epididymal tubule
K. Artery arising from the aorta just distal to each renal artery
L. Central linear structure formed by the convergence of multiple thin septations within the testicle, which are invaginations of the tunica albuginea
M. Small membranous canal that extends from the bladder to the end of the penis
N. Multiple septa formed from the tunica albuginea that course toward the mediastinum testis and separate the testicle into lobules
O. Inner fibrous membrane surrounding the testicle
P. Structure made up of vas deferens, testicular artery, cremasteric artery, and pampiniform plexus that suspends the testis in the scrotum
Q. Sac containing the testes and epididymis

### Exercise 2

*Match the following vascular supply terms with their definitions.*

____D____ 1. centripetal artery

____A____ 2. cremasteric artery

____C____ 3. deferential artery

____E____ 4. recurrent rami

____B____ 5. testicular vein

A. Small artery arising from the inferior epigastric artery, which supplies the peritesticular tissue, including the cremasteric muscle
B. Formed by the pampiniform plexus.
C. Arises from the vesicle artery and supplies the vas deferens and epididymis
D. Terminal intratesticular arteries arising from the capsular arteries
E. Terminal ends of the centripetal arteries that curve backward toward the capsule

## Exercise 3

*Match the following pathology terms with their definitions.*

___F___1. cryptorchidism

___B___2. epididymal cyst

___E___3. epididymitis

___I___4. hematocele

___C___5. hydrocele

___G___6. pyocele

___H___7. rete testis

___D___8. spermatocele

___A___9. varicocele

A. Dilated veins in the pampiniform plexus caused by obstruction of the venous return from the testicle
B. Cyst filled with clear serous fluid located in the epididymis
C. Fluid formed between the visceral and parietal layers of the tunica vaginalis
D. Cyst in the vas deferens containing sperm
E. Inflammation of the epididymis
F. Testicles remain within the abdomen or groin and fail to descend into the scrotal sac
G. Pus located between the visceral and parietal layers of the tunica vaginalis
H. Network of the channels formed by the convergence of the straight seminiferous tubules in the mediastinum testis
I. Blood located between the visceral and parietal layers of the tunica vaginalis

## ANATOMY AND PHYSIOLOGY

### Exercise 4

*Fill in the blank(s) with the word(s) that best completes the statements about the anatomy and physiology of the scrotum.*

1. The testes are symmetric, oval-shaped glands residing in the _SCROTAL SAC_.

2. The seminiferous tubules converge at the apex of each lobule and anastomose to form the _RETE TESTIS_ in the mediastinum.

3. The largest part of the epididymis is the _HEAD_, measuring 6 to 15 mm in width.

4. The ductus epididymis becomes the _VAS DEFERENS_ and continues in the spermatic cord.

5. The testis is completely covered by a dense, fibrous tissue termed the _TUNICA ALBUGINEA_

6. The _MEDIASTINUM_ supports the ducts coursing within the testis.

7. The space between the layers of the tunica vaginalis is where _HYDROCELES_ can form.

8. The _VAS DEFERENS_ is a continuation of the ductus _EPIDIDYMIS_.

9. The vas deferens dilates at the terminal portion near _SEMINAL VESICLES_

10. Right and left testicular arteries arise from the _ABD. AORTA_ just below the level of the renal arteries.

11. Venous drainage of the scrotum occurs through the veins of the _PAMPINIFORM_ plexus.

12. Power Doppler is often used as a way to quickly get to a sensitive setting that will demonstrate _SLOW_ flow.

## PATHOLOGY

### Exercise 5

*Fill in the blank(s) with the word(s) that best completes the statements, or provide a short answer about the pathologic conditions of the scrotum.*

1. The most important goal of the ultrasound examination in testicular trauma is to determine if _RUPTURE_ has occurred.

2. An acute hematocele is _ECHOGENIC_ with numerous, highly visible echoes that can be seen to float or move in real time.

3. The most common cause of acute scrotal pain in adults is _____ infection of the epididymis and testis.

4. The normal epididymis shows _____ flow with color Doppler.

5. With epididymitis, Doppler waveforms demonstrate _____ velocities in both systole and diastole. A low resistance waveform pattern is present.

6. Hydroceles are found around the _____ aspect of the testis.

7. _____ of the spermatic cord occurs as a result of abnormal mobility of the testis within the scrotum.

8. The _____ anomaly occurs when the tunica vaginalis completely surrounds the testis, epididymis, and distal spermatic cord, allowing them to move and rotate freely within the scrotum.

9. Torsion is the most common cause of acute scrotal pain in _____.

10. A(n) _____ of perfusion in the symptomatic testis with normal perfusion demonstrated in the asymptomatic side is considered to be diagnostic of torsion.

11. Extratesticular cysts are found in the tunica _____ or epididymis.

12. _____ are usually caused by incompetent venous valves within the spermatic vein.

13. Omental hernias appear _____ because of the omental fat.

14. A(n) _____ contains serous fluid and is the most common cause of painless scrotal swelling.

15. Testicular cancer occurs most frequently between the ages of ___20___ and ___34___ years.

16. Patients with _UNDESCENDED_ testes are 2.5 to 8 times more likely to develop cancer.

17. These masses called _____ are usually benign, whereas _____ masses are more likely to be malignant.

18. The term _CRYPTORCHIDISM_ describes a condition in which the testis has not descended into the scrotum and cannot be brought into the scrotum with external manipulation.

## Exercise 6

*Provide a short answer for each question after evaluating the images.*

1. What anatomic structure does the arrow point to?
   ___MEDIASTINUM TESTIS___

A  B

2. Identify the abnormality in these images of the testes.

RETE TESTIS DILATATION

A  B

3. What is the arrow pointing to?

EPIDIDYMAL CYST (pedunculated cyst/appendix epididymis)

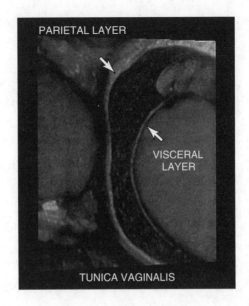

PARIETAL LAYER

VISCERAL
LAYER

TUNICA VAGINALIS

4. Describe the sonographic findings on this image of the tunica vaginalis.

HYDROCELE - develop b/t visceral and parietal layers of tunica vaginalis

UNDESCENDED

CRYPTORCHIDISM

# 24 Musculoskeletal System

## Exercise 1

*Match the following anatomy terms with their definitions.*

___E___ 1. aponeurosis

___H___ 2. bursa

___B___ 3. epineurium

___K___ 4. fasciculi

___E___ 5. ligament

___A___ 6. muscle

___I___ 7. myelin

___L___ 8. pennate

_____ 9. perineurium

___C___ 10. synovial sheath

___G___ 11. tendon

___J___ 12. volar

A. Type of tissue consisting of contractile cells or fibers that affects movement of an organ or part of the body

B. Covering of a nerve that consists of connective tissue

C. Membrane surrounding a joint, tendon, or bursa that secretes a viscous fluid called synovia

D. Connective tissue that surrounds muscle

E. Bandlike flat tendons connecting the process of the scapula

F. Fibrous band of tissue connecting bone or cartilage to bone that aids in stabilizing a joint

G. Fibrous tissue connecting muscle to bone

H. Saclike structure containing thick fluid that surrounds areas subject to friction, such as the interface between bone and tendon

I. Substance forming the sheath of Schwann cells

J. The anterior portion of the body when in the anatomic position

K. Small bundle of muscles, nerves, and tendons

L. A featherlike pattern of muscle growth

## Exercise 2

*Match the following artifact, sonography, and pathology terms with their definitions.*

_____ 1. acromioclavicular joint

_____ 2. anisotropy

_____ 3. nerve

_____ 4. comet tail artifact

_____ 5. dorsiflexion

_____ 6. Guyon's canal or tunnel

_____ 7. plantar flexion

_____ 8. refractile shadowing

_____ 9. seroma

_____ 10. tendinitis

A. Conduit for impulses sent to and from the muscles and the central nervous system

B. Fibrous tunnel that contains the ulnar artery and vein, ulnar nerve, and some fatty tissue

C. Accumulation of serous fluid within tissue

D. The joint found in the shoulder that connects the clavicle to the acromion process of the scapula

E. Pointing of the toes toward the plantar surface of the foot

F. The quality of comprising varying values of a given property when measured in different directions

G. The bending of the sound beam at the edge of a circular structure that results in the absence of posterior echoes

H. Upward movement of the hand and foot

I. Inflammation of the tendon

J. Posterior linear equidistant artifact created when sound reverberates between two strong reflectors, such as air bubbles, metal, and glass

**187**

## Exercise 3

*Label the following illustrations.*

1. Different types of muscle.

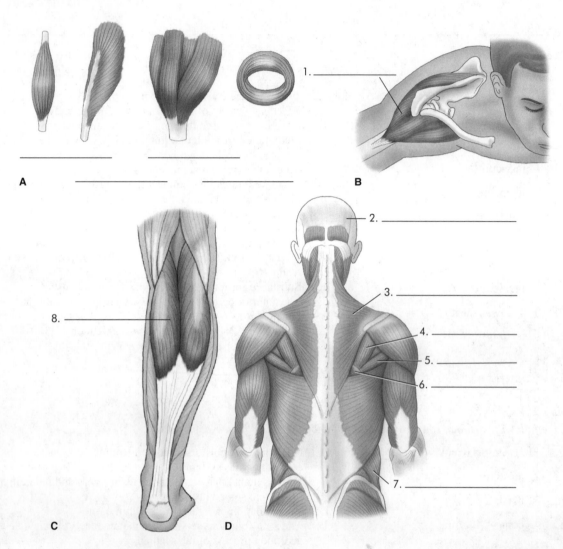

2. The subscapularis, biceps tendon, and the acromioclavicular joint image.

1. _____

2. _____

3. _____

## Exercise 4

*Fill in the blank(s) with the word(s) that best completes the statements about the anatomy of the musculoskeletal system.*

1. Skeletal muscle contains long organized units called muscle _____.

2. The characteristic long fibers are under voluntary control, allowing us to contract a(n) _____ and move a joint.

3. A(n) _____ muscle has a division of several feather-like sections in one muscle, and the

   _____ is the convergence of fibers to a central tendon.

4. The attachment of the muscle that occurs at the proximal and distal portion of the bundle is called a(n)

   _____.

5. Tendons occur with or without a(n) _____ sheath.

6. The sheath surrounding a tendon has two layers. The fluid separates the layers in this part of the body:

   _____, _____, _____, and _____.

7. Short bands of tough fibers that connect bones to other bones are _____.

8. The saclike structure surrounding joints and tendons that contains a viscous fluid is the _____.

9. The knee joint has _____ bursa.

10. A loose areolar connective tissue that fills the fascial compartment of the tendon lacking a synovial sheath is a(n)

    _____.

11. The dense _____ is another layer of connective tissue that closely adjoins the tendon.

12. Interwoven and interconnected collagen fibers found in the tendon run in a(n) _____ path.

13. The proximal portion of the muscle is considered the _____, whereas the _____ is the distal end.

14. The normal nerve has a(n) _____ appearance when compared with muscle, but it is

_____ to tendons.

15. The minute amount of viscous fluid contained within the bursa helps reduce _____ between the moving parts of the joint.

16. A Baker's cyst is an example of a(n) _____ bursa in the medial popliteal fossa.

## SIGNS AND TESTS

### Exercise 5

*Match the following musculoskeletal signs and tests with their definitions.*

_____1. cartilage interface sign

_____2. clapper-in-the-bell sign

_____3. naked tuberosity sign

_____4. Phalen's sign

_____5. Thompson's test

_____6. Tinel's sign

A. Increase in wrist compression caused by hyperflexion of the wrist for 60 seconds; patient is holding the forearms upright and pressing the ventral side of the hands together

B. Pins-and-needles type of tingling felt distally to a percussion site and either a normal or abnormal occurrence (e.g., hitting the elbow creates a tingling in the distal arm)

C. The deltoid muscle is on the humeral head; seen with a full-thickness tear of the rotator cuff

D. Test used to evaluate the integrity of the Achilles tendon that involves plantar flexion with squeezing of the calf

E. Hypoechoic hematoma found at the end of a completely retracted muscle fragment

F. Echogenic line on the anterior surface of the cartilage surrounding the humeral head

## SONOGRAPHIC EVALUATION

### Exercise 6

*Fill in the blank(s) with the word(s) that best completes the statements, or provide a short answer about the sonographic evaluation of the musculoskeletal system.*

1. To begin the examination of the biceps, place the patient with a slight _____ rotation of the shoulder.

2. When facing the patient and imaging the right shoulder, the lateral anatomy displays on the _____ side of the image and the medial anatomy on the _____ side of the screen.

3. The groove located between the greater and lesser tuberosities, coupled with the overlying transverse ligament, maintains the _____ tendon location.

4. Using the biceps tendon as a landmark, angle the transducer _____ to locate the subscapularis tendon.

5. The bandlike tendon that has a medium-level echotexture is the _____ tendon and originates from the greater tuberosity of the humerus.

6. A good landmark to help find the anteriorly located infraspinatus tendon is the posterior _____.

7. Fluid imaged _____ to the infraspinatus tendon indicates bursal fluid, whereas _____ fluid indicates joint effusion.

8. The carpal tunnel is located between the _____ bones and the _____ retinaculum on the palmar side of the wrist.

9. The ulnar artery and veins indicate the medial border of the carpal tunnel, whereas the most lateral structure is the _____ artery and veins.

10. The tendon that connects the gastrocnemius and soleus muscles to the calcaneus is the _____ tendon.

11. The dislocation of the biceps tendon from the bicipital groove may be due to a problem with

_____

_____

12. The _____ thickness tear involves either the bursal or articular cuff surface or the intrasubstance material.

13. The presence of large amounts of fluid in the subacromial-subdeltoid bursa raises the chance of a nonvisualized _____ tear.

14. The normal tendon cannot be compressed; however, the injured tendon _____ as the torn edges move apart.

15. Joint effusion around the biceps tendon combined with subacromial-subdeltoid bursitis results in the _____ sign.

16. Acute tendinitis involves not only the tendon but the surrounding _____ sheath.

17. The normal synovial sheath appears as a hypoechoic _____ around the tendon.

18. The abrupt stretching of the muscle beyond the maximum length results in a(n) _____ tear.

19. External force resulting in a crush injury is considered a(n) _____ tear.

## PATHOLOGY

### Exercise 7

*Provide a short answer for each question after evaluating the images.*

1. The arrow is pointing to which mildly hyperechoic structure in the shoulder?

_____

2. What abnormality does this comparison of the normal with the injured tendon reveal?

_____

A

B

3. De Quervain's tendinitis is identified in this patient. What are the sonographic findings?

_____

_____

4. A soccer player experienced intense pain in his calf after a sudden blow in a championship game. What are the sonographic findings?

_____

_____

5. This sonographic image demonstrates an abnormality that may be seen in carpal tunnel syndrome. What is the abnormality?

_____

_____

# Neonatal and Pediatric Abdomen

---

## KEY TERMS

### Exercise 1

*Match the following key terms with their definitions.*

_____ 1. acholic

_____ 2. appendicolith

_____ 3. atretic

_____ 4. Beckwith-Wiedemann syndrome

_____ 5. biliary atresia

_____ 6. choledochal cyst

_____ 7. hemihypertrophy

_____ 8. hypertrophic pyloric stenosis

_____ 9. intussusception

_____10. neuroblastoma

_____11. projectile vomiting

_____12. pyloric canal

_____13. target (donut) sign

_____14. Wilms' tumor

A. Congenital absence or closure of a normal body opening or tubular structure

B. Excessive development of one side or one half of the body or an organ

C. Frequently associated with sectional areas of the gastrointestinal tract; the muscle is hyperechoic, and the inner core is hypoechoic

D. Congenital cystic malformation of the common bile duct

E. Fecalith or calcification located within the appendix

F. Occurs when bowel prolapses into distal bowel and is propelled in an antegrade fashion

G. Autosomal recessive condition characterized by macroglossia, exophthalmos, and gigantism, often accompanied by visceromegaly and dysplasia of the renal medulla

H. Describes the absence of bile secretion or failure of bile to enter the alimentary tract

I. Located between the stomach and duodenum

J. Thickened muscle in the pylorus that prevents food from entering the duodenum

K. Closure or absence of some or all of the major bile ducts

L. Rapidly developing tumor of the kidney that usually occurs in children

M. Malignant hemorrhagic tumor composed principally of cells resembling neuroblasts that give rise to cells of the sympathetic system

N. Sign of pyloric stenosis in the neonatal period

### Exercise 2

*Label the following illustration.*

1. Diagram of hypertrophic pyloric stenosis.

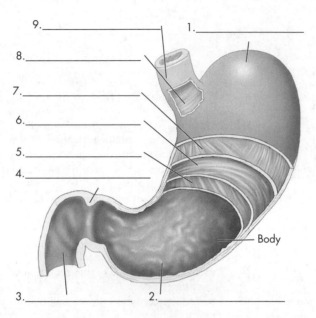

9._____  1._____

8._____

7._____

6._____

5._____

4._____

Body

3._____  2._____

## THE PEDIATRIC ABDOMEN

### Exercise 3

*Fill in the blank(s) with the word(s) that best completes the statements, or provide a short answer about the pediatric abdomen.*

1. The right hepatic lobe should not extend more than _____ cm below the costal margin in the young infant.

2. The common bile duct should measure less than _____ mm in neonates, less than

   _____ mm in infants up to 1 year old, less than _____ mm in older children,

   and less than _____ mm in adolescents and adults.

3. The length of the gallbladder should not exceed the length of the _____.

4. The three most common causes for jaundice in the neonate are _____, _____,

   and _____.

5. Identify the clinical features of biliary atresia in the neonate.

   _____

   _____

   _____

6. An abnormal cystic dilation of the biliary tree that most frequently affects the common bile duct is a(n)

   _____.

7. When a choledochal cyst is present, there is usually _____ of the common bile duct with associated _____ ductal dilation.

8. The most common benign vascular liver tumor of early childhood is infantile hepatic _____.

9. The most common sonographic appearance of hemangioendothelioma is that of multiple _____ lesions and _____.

10. The most common primary malignant disease of the liver is _____ and occurs most frequently in children under 5 years of age.

11. The _____ is located between the stomach and duodenum.

12. _____ occurs most commonly in male infants between 2 and 6 weeks of age.

13. As the pyloric muscle thickens and elongates, the stomach outlet obstruction increases, and vomiting is more constant and _____.

14. A muscle thickness of _____ mm or greater on the long-axis view, a channel length of _____ mm or greater, and pyloric muscle length of _____ or greater are reliable indicators of HPS.

15. In infants and young children, the progression of acute appendicitis to _____ is more rapid than in older children.

16. With ultrasound the acutely inflamed appendix is _____.

17. _____ produced by overlying transducer pressure is an additional finding consistent with appendicitis.

18. The most common acute abdominal disorder in early childhood is _____.

19. The presence of alternating hypoechoic and hyperechoic rings surrounding an echogenic center as seen in a short-axis view of the involved area is known as the _____ sign.

20. Intussusception may be reduced with _____ pressure or by air reduction.

## Exercise 4

*Provide a short answer for each question after evaluating the images.*

1. An 11-year-old child presented with increasing abdominal pain several days after blunt trauma to the abdomen from striking the handlebars on her bike.

_____

_____

Spleen  Long

2. Describe this image obtained from a 17-year-old male with leukemia.

_____

_____

3. A 5-day-old infant with a history of a palpable abdominal mass. What are the sonographic findings?

_____

_____

_____

**199**

Copyright © 2018 Elsevier Inc. All rights reserved.

Chapter **25**  **Neonatal and Pediatric Abdomen**

A

B

C

D

E

F

4. A neonate presented with an abdominal mass. What are the sonographic findings?

_____

_____

5. A child presented with nausea and vomiting, fever, and intense left lower quadrant pain. What is the sonographic finding?

---

6. An infant presented with fever and peritoneal signs. What is the sonographic finding?

---

**201**

7. A 5-week-old male presented with projectile vomiting. What is the sonographic finding?

_____

# 26 Neonatal and Pediatric Adrenal and Urinary System

## Exercise 1

*Match the following terms related to neonatal and pediatric kidneys with their definitions.*

_____ 1. adrenal hemorrhage

_____ 2. arcuate arteries

_____ 3. autosomal dominant polycystic kidney disease (ADPKD)

_____ 4. autosomal recessive polycystic kidney disease (ARPKD)

_____ 5. congenital mesoblastic nephroma

_____ 6. cortex

_____ 7. ectasia

_____ 8. ectopic ureterocele

_____ 9. hydronephrosis

_____ 10. medullary pyramids

_____ 11. multicystic dysplastic kidney (MCDK)

_____ 12. nephroblastomatosis

_____ 13. neuroblastoma

_____ 14. polycystic renal disease

_____ 15. posterior urethral valves

_____ 16. Potter facies

_____ 17. prune-belly syndrome

_____ 18. pulmonary hypoplasia

_____ 19. renal vein thrombosis

_____ 20. ureteropelvic junction obstruction

_____ 21. VACTERL

_____ 22. VATER

_____ 23. Wilms' tumor (nephroblastoma)

A. Malignant adrenal mass seen in pediatric patients; hemorrhaging tumor consisting primarily of cells resembling neuroblasts

B. Dilation of the renal collecting system

C. Large and hypoechoic in the neonate

D. Poorly functioning enlarged kidneys

E. Most common benign renal tumor of the neonate and infant

F. Underdevelopment of the lung tissue that occurs in utero secondary to oligohydramnios

G. Classification of cystic renal disease

H. Abnormal persistence of fetal renal blastoma

I. Most common neonatal obstruction of the urinary tract; results from intrinsic narrowing or extrinsic vascular compression

J. Lie at the base of the medullary pyramids and appear as echogenic structures

K. Congenital polycystic kidney disease that usually presents during middle age; the severity of the disease varies widely

L. Adds cardiac and limb anomalies to the VATER syndrome

M. Most common malignant tumor in the neonate and infant

N. Dilation of any tubular vessel

O. Kidney becomes enlarged and edematous as a result of obstruction of the renal vein

P. Ectopic insertion and cystic dilation of distal ureter of duplicated renal collecting system

Q. Most common cause of bladder outlet obstruction in the male neonate

R. Occurs when the fetus is stressed during a difficult delivery or a hypoxic insult

S. Vertebral, anal, tracheoesophageal fistula and renal anomalies

T. Most common cause of renal cystic disease in the neonate; multiple cystic masses within the kidney; may have contralateral ureteral pelvic junction obstruction

U. Dilation of the fetal abdomen secondary to severe bilateral hydronephrosis and fetal ascites; fetus also has oligohydramnios and pulmonary hypoplasia

V. Outer rim of the kidney; in the neonate it has an echogenicity similar to that of the normal liver parenchyma

W. Rare congenital polycystic renal disease; typically occurs with diffuse enlargement, sacculations, and cystic diverticula of the medullary portions of the kidneys

## Exercise 2

*Fill in the blank(s) with the word(s) that best completes the statements about the neonatal and pediatric kidneys and adrenal glands.*

1. In the second trimester, the kidney develops from small _____ composed of a central large pyramid with a thin peripheral rim of cortex.

2. As the renunculi fuse progressively, their adjoining cortices form a(n) _____.

3. The former renunculi are at that point called _____.

4. The _____ continues to grow throughout childhood, whereas the _____ become smaller in size.

5. The larger amount of cortical _____ is not present in the neonate and pediatric patient, which allows clear distinction of the corticomedullary junction.

6. The _____ are large and hypoechoic and should not be mistaken for dilated calyces or cysts.

7. The surrounding cortex is quite thin, with echogenicity essentially similar to or slightly greater than that of normal _____ parenchyma.

8. The _____ vessels are seen as intense specular echoes at the corticomedullary junction.

9. At the site of the fetal lobulation, a parenchymal triangular defect may be identified in the anterosuperior or inferoposterior aspect of the kidney, known as a(n) _____ defect.

10. Each adrenal gland lies immediately _____ to the upper pole of the kidney.

11. The normal urinary bladder is thin-walled in the distended state and should measure less than _____ mm.

## PATHOLOGY

## Exercise 3

*Fill in the blank(s) with the word(s) that best completes the statements about the pathology of the neonatal and pediatric kidney and adrenal gland.*

1. The dilatation of the urinary collecting system is known as _____.

2. The most common type of obstruction of the upper urinary tract is _____; it most often results from intrinsic narrowing or extrinsic vascular compression at the level of the ureteropelvic junction.

3. The obstruction produces _____ (proximal or distal) dilatation of the collecting system; the ureter is normal in caliber.

4. The most common cause of bladder outlet obstruction in the male neonate is _____ valves.

5. Urinary _____ or a perirenal _____ can result from high-pressure vesicoureteral reflux rupturing a calyceal fornix or tearing the renal parenchyma.

6. The ectopic _____ is seen as a fluid mass within the urinary bladder and is located inferomedially to the ureteral insertion of the lower pole ureter.

7. The triad of hypoplasia, or deficiency, of the abdominal musculature, cryptorchidism, and urinary tract anomalies is known as the _____ syndrome.

8. The most common cause of renal cystic disease presenting in the neonate is _____, and when hydronephrosis is excluded, it is the most common cause of an abdominal mass in the newborn.

9. Sonographically, the classic appearance of MCDK is of a unilateral mass resembling a bunch of grapes, which represents a cluster of discrete _____ cysts, the largest of which are peripheral.

10. The kidneys are hyperechoic and greatly enlarged with a hypoechogenic outer rim, which represents the cortex compressed by the expanded pyramids in _____.

11. The most common intraabdominal malignant renal tumor is _____ in young children.

12. A(n) _____ is a malignant tumor that arises in sympathetic chain ganglia and adrenal medulla; it may be detected on antenatal sonography or at birth.

13. About half of neuroblastoma tumors arise in the medulla of the _____, although tumors have also been found in the neck, mediastinum, retroperitoneum, and pelvis.

14. Sonographically, adrenal _____ results in ovoid enlargement of the gland or a portion of the gland.

## Exercise 4

*Provide a short answer for each question after evaluating the images.*

1. Describe the findings in this 28-day-old infant.

_____

_____

2. What anatomic structure are the arrows pointing to?

_____

3. Identify whether this obstruction to the kidney is minor or major.

_____

4. Identify the abnormality demonstrated in these views of the neonatal pelvis.

_____

_____

5. Does this neonate show sonographic evidence of hydronephrosis or of multicystic dysplastic kidney disease?

_____

_____

Chapter **26** **Neonatal and Pediatric Adrenal and Urinary System**

A B

6. This neonate had abdominal distention at 1 day after birth. Describe the appearance of the kidneys.

_____

_____

_____

7. A 2-year-old with a palpable abdominal mass, nausea and vomiting, and appetite loss was imaged with ultrasound. Describe the sonographic findings.

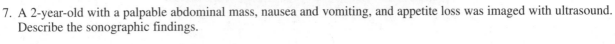

Chapter **26** **Neonatal and Pediatric Adrenal and Urinary System**

8. A 2-week-old male neonate with a history of neonatal infections, increased bilirubin, and an abdominal mass had an ultrasound. Describe the sonographic findings.

_____

_____

_____

# 27 Neonatal and Infant Head

## KEY TERMS

### Exercise 1

*Match the following embryology and anatomy terms with their definitions.*

_____ 1. neonate

_____ 2. atrium (trigone) of the lateral ventricles

_____ 3. brain stem

_____ 4. caudate nucleus

_____ 5. cavum septum pellucidum

_____ 6. cerebellum

_____ 7. cerebrum

_____ 8. choroid plexus

_____ 9. cistern

_____ 10. corpus callosum

_____ 11. falx cerebri

_____ 12. fontanelle

_____ 13. germinal matrix

_____ 14. meninges

_____ 15. sulcus

_____ 16. tentorium cerebelli

_____ 17. thalamic-caudate groove

_____ 18. thalamus

A. Echogenic cluster of cells important in the production of cerebrospinal fluid that lies along the atrium of the lateral ventricles

B. Three membranes enclosing the brain and spinal cord

C. Echogenic fibrous structure that separates the cerebral hemispheres

D. Part of the brain connecting the forebrain and spinal cord; consists of the midbrain, pons, and medulla oblongata

E. Prominent structure best seen in the midline filled with cerebrospinal fluid in the premature infant

F. The region at which the thalamus and caudate nucleus join

G. Largest part of the brain consisting of two equal hemispheres

H. Prominent group of nerve fibers that connect the right and left sides of the brain

I. Infant during the early newborn period

J. Fragile periventricular tissue that bleeds easily in the premature infant; includes the caudate nucleus

K. Area of the brain that forms the lateral borders of the anterior horns, anterior to the thalamus

L. Echogenic V-shaped "tent" structure in the posterior fossa that separates the cerebellum from the cerebrum

M. Area of the brain that lies posterior to the brain stem below the tentorium

N. Two ovoid brain structures located midbrain, situated on either side of the third ventricle superior to the brain stem

O. The ventricle is measured at this site on the axial view; anterior, occipital, and temporal horn junction

P. Groove on the surface of the brain that separates the gyri

Q. Soft space between the bones

R. Reservoir for cerebrospinal fluid

## Exercise 2

*Match the following terms related to pathology and sonographic evaluation with their definitions.*

_____ 1. aqueductal stenosis

_____ 2. asphyxia

_____ 3. axial plane

_____ 4. Chiari malformation

_____ 5. coronal plane

_____ 6. Dandy-Walker malformation

_____ 7. extracorporeal membrane oxygenation

_____ 8. holoprosencephaly

_____ 9. hydrocephalus

_____10. hypoxia

_____11. periventricular leukomalacia

_____12. sagittal plane

_____13. subependyma

_____14. subependymal cyst

_____15. ventriculitis

A. Transducer is placed above the ear (above the canthomeatal line)

B. Ventriculomegaly in the neonate resulting in compression and often destruction of brain tissue

C. Abnormal development of the fourth ventricle; often accompanied by hydrocephalus

D. Severe case of inadequate oxygenation

E. Echogenic white matter necrosis best seen in the posterior aspect of the brain or adjacent to the ventricular structures

F. Congenital defect characterized by abnormal single ventricular cavity with some form of thalami fusion

G. Congenital blockage of the aqueduct connecting the third and fourth ventricles causing dilation of the third and fourth ventricles

H. Treatment for infants with severe respiratory failure who have not responded to conventional ventilatory support

I. Perpendicular to the coronal plane with the transducer in the anterior fontanelle

J. Transducer is perpendicular to the anterior fontanelle in the coronal axis of the head

K. Site of hemorrhage for the germinal matrix; fragile area beneath the ependyma that is subject to bleeding in the premature neonate

L. Congenital defect in which the cerebellum and brain stem are pulled toward the spinal cord (banana sign)

M. Decreased oxygen in the body

N. Inflammation/infection of the ventricles, which appears as echogenic linear structures along the gyri

O. Cyst that occurs at the site of a previous bleed in the germinal matrix

## ANATOMY AND PHYSIOLOGY

### Exercise 3

*Label the following illustrations.*

1. Neonatal skull showing the sutures and open anterior fontanelle.

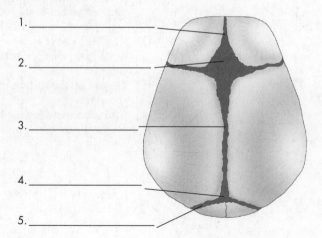

1._____

2._____

3._____

4._____

5._____

2. Sagittal view of the ventricular system.

1._____

8._____

7._____

6._____

5._____

2._____

3._____

4._____

3. Sagittal view of choroid plexus and cisterns of the ventricular system.

9._____

8._____

7._____

6._____

1._____

2._____

3._____

4._____

5._____

4. Sagittal view of cerebral cortex.

20. _____
19. _____
18. _____
17. _____
16. _____
15. _____
14. _____
13. _____
12. _____
11. _____
10. _____
9. _____

1. _____
2. _____
3. _____
4. _____
5. _____
6. _____
7. _____
8. _____

5. Coronal view of cerebral lobes, corpus callosum, and sylvian fissure.

5. _____
4. _____

1. _____
2. _____
3. _____

6. Lateral and axial view of the basal ganglia.

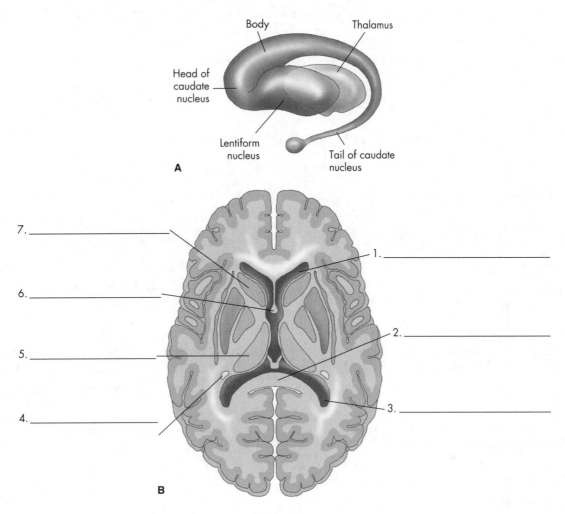

**Exercise 4**

*Fill in the blank(s) with the word(s) that best completes the statements about the anatomy of the neural axis.*

1. The _____ forms from the cavity of the hindbrain and contains choroid plexus like the lateral and third ventricles.

2. The spaces between the bones of the skull are called _____.

3. The _____ fontanelle is located at the top of the neonatal head and may be easily felt as the "soft spot."

4. A double-layered outer membrane that forms the toughest barrier is the _____.

5. A V-shaped echogenic structure known as the _____ separates the cerebrum and the cerebellum; it is an extension of the falx cerebri.

6. The _____ ventricles communicate with the third ventricle through the interventricular foramen of Monro.

7. The cavum septum pellucidum forms the medial wall, and the _____ forms the roof.

8. The _____ touches the inferior lateral ventricular wall, and the body of the caudate

   _____ borders the superior wall.

9. The third and fourth ventricles are connected by the _____.

10. The lateral angles of the fourth ventricle form the foramen of _____.

11. The mass of special cells that regulate the intraventricular pressure by secretion or absorption of cerebral spinal fluid is the _____.

12. The _____ is located along the lateral-most aspect of the brain and is the area where the middle cerebral artery is located.

13. The _____ borders the third ventricle and connects through the middle of the third ventricle by the massa intermedia.

14. The _____ extends from the pons to the foramen magnum, where it continues as the spinal cord.

15. Three pairs of nerve tracts, the _____, connect the cerebellum to the brain stem.

## SONOGRAPHIC EVALUATION

### Exercise 5

*Fill in the blank(s) with the word(s) that best completes the statements about neonatal encephalography.*

1. Technically a(n) _____ view is 90 degrees to Reid's baseline.

2. When the transducer is angled _____, the frontal horns of the lateral ventricles appear as slitlike hypoechoic to cystic formations.

3. As the transducer is angled _____, the ventricles acquire a commalike shape.

4. Sonography depicts the choroid plexus as a very _____ structure inside the ventricular cavities surrounding the thalamic nuclei.

5. In premature infants, the caudate nuclei may have _____ echogenicity than the rest of the brain parenchyma.

6. The _____ ventricle appears in the midline as a small anechoic space approximately 2 to 3 mm wide, located anteriorly to the vermis.

## PATHOLOGY

### Exercise 6

*Fill in the blank(s) with the word(s), or provide a short answer that best completes the statements about the pathology of the neonatal head.*

1. A congenital anomaly associated with spina bifida is a(n) _____ malformation in which the cerebellum and brain stem are pulled toward the spinal cord and secondary hydrocephalus develops.

2. Chiari malformation is frequently associated with myelomeningocele, _____, dilation of the third ventricle, and absence of the septum pellucidum.

3. _____ is characterized by a grossly abnormal brain in which there is a common large central ventricle.

4. Dandy-Walker syndrome is a congenital anomaly in which a huge _____ ventricle cyst occupies the area where the cerebellum usually lies, with secondary dilation of the third and lateral ventricles.

5. A Dandy-Walker variant is present when there is an enlarged _____ communicating with the fourth ventricle in the presence of a normal or hypoplastic cerebellar vermis.

6. Complete absence of the _____ is distinguished by narrow frontal horns, as well as marked separation of the anterior horns and bodies of the lateral ventricles associated with widening of the occipital horns and the third ventricle.

7. Any condition in which enlargement of the ventricular system is caused by an imbalance between production and reabsorption of cerebrospinal fluid (CSF) is referred to as _____.

8. The CSF pathways are open within the ventricular system in _____ hydrocephalus, but there is decreased absorption of CSF.

9. The most common cause of congenital hydrocephalus is _____.

10. The most common hemorrhagic lesions in preterm newborn infants are _____ hemorrhages.

11. Subependymal hemorrhages are caused by capillary bleeding in the _____.

12. Studies from the anterior fontanelle may not detect small intraventricular hemorrhage (IVHs), because intraventricular blood tends to "settle out" in the _____ horns.

13. Intraparenchymal hemorrhages appear as very _____ zones in the white matter adjacent to the lateral ventricles.

14. _____ can result from a variety of insults including respiratory failure, congenital heart disease, and sepsis.

15. White matter ischemia leads to white matter volume loss or _____ leukomalacia.

16. The chronic stage of white matter necrosis (WMN) is identified with ultrasound when _____ develop in the echogenic white matter.

17. A common complication of purulent meningitis in newborn infants is _____.

18. _____ occurs when the ependyma becomes thickened and hyperechoic as a result of irritation from hemorrhage within the ventricle.

## Exercise 7

*Provide a short answer for each question after evaluating the images.*

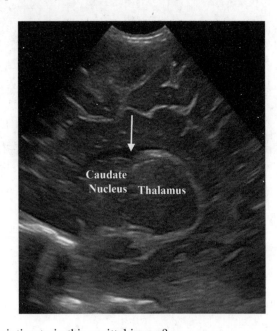

1. What structure is the arrow pointing to in this sagittal image?

_____

2. Identify the following structures:

   1)_____

   2)_____

   3)_____

   4)_____

3. Identify the following structures:

   6)_____

   15)_____

   30)_____

4. A 4-month-old infant was evaluated. What are the sonographic findings?

_____

_____

A                                           B

5. These sonographic images are typical of what abnormality of the premature neonatal head?

_____

_____

_____

A

B

C

6. An 8-day-old premature infant with an acute drop in hematocrit was referred for a head ultrasound. What are your findings?

_____

_____

Chapter **27**   **Neonatal and Infant Head**

7. A head ultrasound was performed on an 11-day-old full-term infant. What are your sonographic findings?

_____

_____

_____

# 28 | Infant and Pediatric Hip

### Exercise 1

*Match the following anatomy terms with their definitions.*

_____1. fascia lata

_____2. femoral triangle

_____3. hip joint

_____4. pelvic girdle

_____5. saphenous opening

_____6. sciatic nerve

A. Formed by the articulation of the head of the femur with the acetabulum of the hip bone
B. Deep fascia of the thigh
C. Largest nerve in the upper thigh
D. Formation of the hip bones by the ilium, ischium, and pubis
E. Description of a region at the front of the upper thigh, just below the inguinal ligament
F. Gap in the fascia lata, which is found 4 cm inferior and lateral to the pubic tubercle

### Exercise 2

*Match the following sonographic evaluation and pathology terms with their definitions.*

_____1. Barlow maneuver

_____2. developmental displacement of the hip (DDH)

_____3. frank dislocation

_____4. Galeazzi sign

_____5. Ortolani maneuver

_____6. subluxation

A. The hip is laterally and posteriorly displaced to the extent that the femoral head has no contact with the acetabulum and the normal "U" configuration cannot be obtained on ultrasound.
B. The patient lies in the supine position. The examiner's hand is placed around the hip to be examined with the fingers over the femoral head. The hip is flexed 90 degrees, and the thigh is abducted.
C. On physical exam, the knee is lower in position on the affected side of the neonate with DDH when the patient is supine and the knees are flexed.
D. The patient lies in the supine position with the hip flexed 90 degrees and adducted. Downward and outward pressure is applied. If the hip is dislocated, the examiner will feel the femoral head move out of the acetabulum.
E. This occurs when the femoral head moves posteriorly and remains in contact with the posterior aspect of the acetabulum.
F. This abnormal condition of the hip results in congenital hip dysplasia; includes dysplastic, subluxated, dislocatable, and dislocated hips.

**Exercise 3**

*Label the following illustrations.*

1. Coronal section of the right hip joint and articular surfaces of the right hip joint.

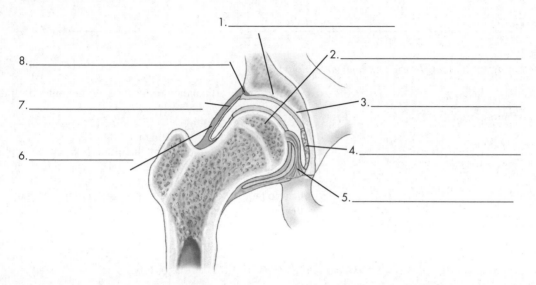

2. Coronal section of the right hip joint and arterial supply of the head of the femur.

**Exercise 4**

*Fill in the blank(s) with the word(s) that best completes the statements about the anatomy of the neonatal hip.*

1. The _____ joints unite the two hip bones with the sacral part of the vertebral column.

2. The hip bones are the fusion of three separate bones, the _____, the _____, and the _____, which together form the pelvic girdle.

3. The bone of the upper thigh is the _____.

4. The femoral artery branches into the _____ artery, which is the main artery supply for the thigh muscles.

5. The largest nerve in the upper thigh is the _____ nerve.

6. The deep fascia of the thigh, the _____, forms a tough connective tissue surrounding the muscles.

7. The _____ is formed by the inguinal ligament, the adductor longus (medially), and the sartorius (laterally).

8. The contents of the femoral triangle include the femoral _____, the femoral _____ and _____, and the femoral _____.

9. The femoral vein and artery and the femoral canal are enclosed in a connective tissue sleeve called the femoral _____.

10. The contents of the femoral triangle are separated from the more deeply lying hip joint by muscles; the _____ is medial, and the _____ is lateral.

11. The articulation of the head of the femur with the acetabulum of the hip bone forms the _____.

12. The gluteus _____ muscle is the immediate cover for the upper part of the hip joint, whereas the obturator externus is found winding below it from front to back.

13. The _____ muscle is immediately posterior to the joint, and the obturator internus and the gemelli and quadratus femoris are lower down.

14. The rounded shape of the femur and the cup shape of the _____ form the "ball and socket" hip joint.

15. One of the strongest ligaments in the body is the _____; it is very important for standing and maintaining correct upright balance.


## MOVEMENTS OF THE HIP

**Exercise 5**

*Match the following terms regarding movements of the hip with their definitions.*

_____1. flexion

_____2. extension

_____3. abduction

_____4. adduction

_____5. medial rotation

_____6. lateral rotation

A. To move away from the body
B. Turning inward
C. Bending forward
D. Turning outward
E. Bending backward
F. To move toward the body

## Exercise 6

*Fill in the blank(s) with the word(s) that best completes the statements about the movement of the hip.*

1. The primary flexors of the hip are the _____ major, the _____, and the _____ femoris.

2. When the trochanter moves forward, the femur rotates _____, and when the trochanter moves backward, the femur rotates _____.

3. The medial rotators are the anterior fibers of gluteus _____ and _____.

4. The lateral rotators are the small muscles at the back of the joint: _____, _____, and _____ femoris, with assistance of the gluteus _____.

## SONOGRAPHIC EVALUATION

### Exercise 7

*Fill in the blank(s) with the word(s) that best completes the statements, or provide a short answer about the sonographic evaluation of the neonatal hip.*

1. Ossification of the femoral head begins between _____ and _____ months of age, occurs earlier in girls than boys, and is often complete by 1 year.

2. Sonography of the neonatal hip is performed with a(n) _____ transducer.

3. Sonographically, the femoral head is _____ because it is cartilaginous and contains a focal echogenic ossification nucleus.

4. The femoral head sits within the acetabulum, which is _____ and has a deep concave configuration.

5. Two thirds of the head should be covered by the _____.

6. The basic hip anatomy is imaged in four different views:

   _____

   _____

7. The _____ view is performed with the infant in the supine position from the lateral aspect of the hip joint with the plane of the transducer oriented coronally with respect to the hip joint.

8. The transducer is maintained in the lateral position while the hip is moved into a 90-degree angle of flexion in the _____ view. During this assessment, the transducer is moved in an anteroposterior direction with respect to the body to allow visualization of the entire hip.

9. A normal hip gives the appearance of a "ball on a spoon" in the midacetabulum. The _____ is the ball, the _____ forms the spoon, and the iliac line is the handle.

10. The transverse plane is rotated 90 degrees and moved posteriorly into a posterolateral position over the hip joint in the _____ view.

11. From the transverse or flexion view, the leg is brought down into a neutral position to the _____ view.

### Exercise 8

*Fill in the blank(s) with the word(s) that best completes the statements, or provide a short answer about the pathology of the neonatal hip.*

1. _____ causes of hip dislocation can be traumatic or nontraumatic (i.e., neuromuscular diseases).

2. _____ dislocations occur in utero and are associated with neuromuscular disorders.

3. _____ of the hip includes dysplastic, subluxated, dislocatable, and dislocated hips.

4. Describe the multiple risk factors that may contribute to the developmental displacement of the hip.

   _____

   _____

   _____

   _____

5. Name the two basic maneuvers that help in diagnosing DDH.

   _____

   _____

### Exercise 9

*Provide a short answer for each question after evaluating the images.*

1. What is the arrow pointing to in this 4-month-old infant?

   _____

   _____

2. Name the normal "_____" appearance seen in this coronal/flexion view.

_____

_____

3. This transverse view without any added stress is the normal "_____" shape.

_____

RIGHT ADD STRESS _

4cm

4. With stress added in the transverse view, this demonstrates the "_____" shape.

_____

_____

5. This image demonstrates what abnormality?

_____

_____

6. The abnormality demonstrated in these images is:

_____

_____

# 29 Neonatal and Infant Spine

**Exercise 1**

*Match the following neonatal spine anatomy and pathology terms with their definitions.*

_____ 1. cauda equine

_____ 2. conus medullaris

_____ 3. diastematomyelia

_____ 4. dysraphic

_____ 5. filum terminale

_____ 6. hydromyelia

_____ 7. lipoma

_____ 8. meningocele

_____ 9. myelomeningocele

_____ 10. myeloschisis

_____ 11. spina bifida aperta

_____ 12. spina bifida occulta

_____ 13. tethered spinal cord

A. Protrusion of the meninges through the gap in the spine, the skin covering being vestigial

B. Bundle of nerve roots from the lumbar, sacral, and coccygeal spinal nerves that descend nearly vertically from the spinal cord until they reach their respective openings in the vertebral column

C. Slender tapering terminal section of the spinal cord

D. Caudal end of the spinal cord

E. Fixed spinal cord that is in an abnormal position

F. Congenital fissure of the spinal cord, frequently associated with spina bifida cystica

G. Open (non-skin-covered lesions) neural tube defects, such as myelomeningocele and meningocele

H. Dilation of the central canal of the spinal cord

I. Describes anomalies associated with incomplete embryologic development

J. Closed (skin-covered lesions) neural tube defects, such as spinal lipoma and tethered cord

K. Cleft spinal cord resulting from failure of the neural tube to close

L. Spinal cord and nerve roots are exposed, often adhering to the fine membrane that overlies them

M. Common benign tumor composed of fat cells

## Exercise 2

*Label the following illustrations.*

1. Basic features of the vertebrae.

2. Longitudinal section of the sacrum.

3. Joints in the cervical, thoracic, and lumbar regions of the vertebral column.

1. _____

2. _____

3. _____

4. _____

5. _____

6. _____

4. Section through the thoracic part of the spinal cord.

1. _____

2. _____

3. _____

4. _____

5. _____

6. _____

7. _____

8. _____

## ANATOMY AND PATHOLOGY

### Exercise 3

*Fill in the blank(s) with the word(s) that best completes the statements about the anatomy and pathology of the neonatal spine.*

1. One of the clinical signs of a spinal problem in an infant is a(n) _____ on the posterior surface of the body along the spinal canal.

2. Other suspicious findings that an abnormality may be present include a(n) _____, a raised midline area, a(n) _____ patch, or even a tail-like projection from the lower spine.

3. A dimple is suspicious if it is of greater than _____ from the anus.

4. Spinal _____ includes disorders of the spine involving absent or incomplete closure of the neural tube.

5. The defects of the spinal canal occur in the first _____ weeks of life as the fetal nervous system develops.

6. The bony spine, meninges, and muscle form the _____.

7. Incomplete separation of the neural tube from the ectoderm may result in cord tethering, _____, or a dermal sinus.

8. If the neural tube fails to fold and fuse in the midline, defects, such as _____, occur.

9. Within the vertebral cavity lie the spinal cord, the roots of the spinal nerves, and the covering _____, which provide protection for the vertebral column.

**Exercise 4**

*Fill in the blank(s) with the word(s) that best completes the statements about the anatomy of the vertebral column and spinal cord.*

1. Each vertebra consists of a rounded body _____ and a vertebral arch _____.

2. The vertebrae enclose a space called the vertebral _____, through which run the spinal cord and its coverings.

3. The vertebral arch consists of a pair of cylindrical pedicles, which form the sides of the arch, and a pair of flattened _____, which complete the arch posteriorly.

4. Laterally the sacrum articulates with the two iliac bones to form the _____ joints.

5. The laminae of the fifth sacral vertebra (and sometimes those of the fourth) fail to meet in the midline, forming the sacral _____.

6. The _____ disks are responsible for one fourth of the length of the vertebral column.

7. Each disk consists of a peripheral part, the *annulus* _____, and a central part, the *nucleus* _____.

8. The spinal cord begins above at the foramen magnum, where it is continuous with the medulla oblongata of the brain. In the younger child, it is relatively longer and ends at the upper border of the _____ lumbar vertebra.

9. Inferiorly the cord tapers off into the conus _____, from the apex of which a prolongation of the pia mater, the filum _____, descends to be attached to the back of the coccyx.

10. The cord has a deep longitudinal fissure in the midline anteriorly called the anterior _____ fissure, and a shallow furrow on the posterior surface called the posterior median sulcus.

11. The lower nerve roots together are called the _____.

12. The spinal cord is surrounded by three meninges: the _____ mater, the _____ mater, and the _____ mater.

13. The most external membrane is the _____ mater and is a dense, strong, fibrous sheet that encloses the spinal cord and cauda equina.

14. The _____ mater is a delicate, impermeable membrane covering the spinal cord and lying between the pia mater internally and the dura mater externally.

15. The vascular membrane that closely covers the spinal cord is the _____ mater; below, it fuses with the filum terminale.

**Exercise 5**

*Fill in the blank(s) with the word(s) that best completes the statements about the anatomy and pathology of the spinal cord.*

1. The spinal cord is _____ with slightly echogenic borders and an echogenic line extending longitudinally along its midline.

2. This central echo complex represents or is close to the cord's central _____.

3. The spinal cord and roots of the cauda equina are normally observed to _____ with the frequency of the heartbeat, and there is also a superimposed motion that occurs with respirations.

4. The _____ spinal cord is a pathologic fixation of the spinal cord in an abnormal caudal location so that the cord suffers mechanical stretching, distortion, and ischemia with daily activities, growth, and development.

5. In addition to being in a more caudal location, the tethered spinal cord is often fixed _____ within the canal.

6. Lipomas are usually _____ and may present as a small or large mass.

7. A(n) _____ shows a flat nontubulated cord (neural placode) with nerve roots extending into the defect.

8. In contrast, a(n) _____ shows nothing but fluid within the sac.

9. _____ seem to have a high association with tethered spinal cord.

**Exercise 6**

*Provide a short answer for each question after evaluating the images.*

1. Identify the structure the arrows are pointing to on this image.

_____

_____

_____

Chapter **29** Neonatal and Infant Spine

2. Identify the structures lettered on this sagittal image.

_____

_____

_____

3. A neonate presented with a fatty mass near the lower back with increased areas of pigmentation. Describe the sonographic finding.

_____

_____

_____

4. What abnormality of the neonatal spine is demonstrated in this image?

_____

_____

_____

# 30 Anatomic and Physiologic Relationships within the Thoracic Cavity

## KEY TERMS

### Exercise 1

*Match the following heart and cardiac cycle terms with their definitions.*

_____1. atrioventricular valves

_____2. endocardium

_____3. epicardium

_____4. myocardium

_____5. pericardium

_____6. semilunar valves

A. Outer layer of the heart wall
B. Inner layer of the heart wall
C. Sac surrounding the heart, reflecting off the great arteries
D. Valves located between the atria and ventricles
E. Thick, contractile middle layer of the heart
F. Valves located in the aortic or pulmonic artery

### Exercise 2

*Match the following electrical conduction system and auscultation terms with their definitions.*

_____1. continuous murmur

_____2. depolarization

_____3. diastolic murmur

_____4. electrocardiography

_____5. frequency

_____6. intensity

_____7. murmur

_____8. repolarization

_____9. systolic murmur

A. The predominant frequency band of the murmur, which varies from high to low as determined by auscultation
B. Method of recording the electrical activity generated by the heart muscle
C. Heart murmur that begins with or after the time of the first heart sound and ends at or before the time of the second heart sound
D. Describes the electrical activity that triggers contraction of the heart muscle
E. A relatively prolonged series of auditory vibrations of varying intensity (loudness), frequency (pitch), quality, configuration, and duration; produced by structural changes and/or hemodynamic events in the heart or blood vessels
F. Heart murmur that begins with or after the time of the second heart sound and ends at or before the time of the first heart sound
G. Describes electrical activity just before the relaxation phase of cardiac muscle activity
H. Heart murmur that begins in systole and continues without interruption through the time of the second heart sound into all or part of diastole
I. A grading scale of 1 to 6 describes this aspect of systolic and diastolic murmurs

**Exercise 3**

*Label the following illustrations.*

1. Anterior view of the right ventricle.

12. _____
11. _____
10. _____
9. _____
8. _____

1. _____
2. _____
3. _____
4. _____
5. _____
6. _____
7. _____

2. Right atrium viewed from the right side.

12. _____
11. _____
10. _____
9. _____
8. _____
7. _____
6. _____

1. _____
2. _____
3. _____
4. _____
5. _____

3. Tricuspid valve.

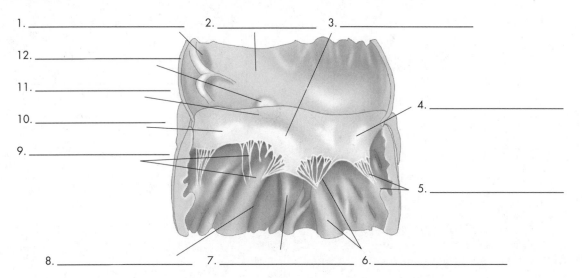

1. _____    2. _____    3. _____

12. _____

11. _____

10. _____                                    4. _____

9. _____

                                                               5. _____

8. _____    7. _____    6. _____

4. Posterolateral view of the left atrium and ventricle.

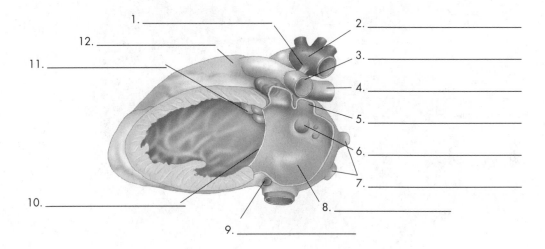

1. _____                                    2. _____

12. _____                                   3. _____

11. _____                                   4. _____

                                                              5. _____

                                                              6. _____

                                                              7. _____

10. _____                                   8. _____

9. _____

5. Mitral valve.

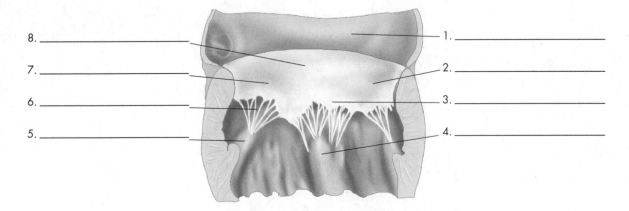

8. _____

7. _____

6. _____

5. _____

1. _____

2. _____

3. _____

4. _____

6. Posterolateral view of the left ventricle.

23. _____

22. _____

21. _____

20. _____

19. _____

18. _____

17. _____

16. _____

15. _____

14. _____

13. _____

1. _____

2. _____

3. _____

4. _____

5. _____

6. _____

7. _____

8. _____

9. _____

10. _____

11. _____

12. _____

7. Aortic valve.

1. _____    2. _____

10. _____

9. _____

8. _____

3. _____

4. _____

5. _____

6. _____

7. _____

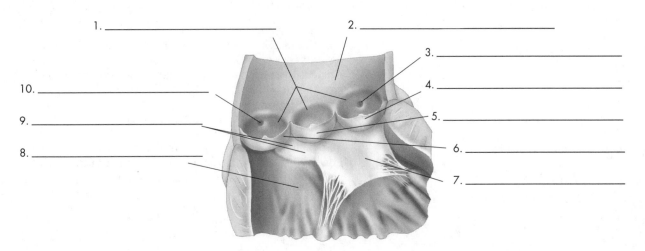

8. Aortic arch and branches.

13. _____

12. _____

11. _____

10. _____

9. _____

8. _____

1. _____

2. _____

3. _____

4. _____

5. _____

6. _____

7. _____

Chapter **30** **Anatomic and Physiologic Relationships within the Thoracic Cavity**

**Exercise 4**

*Match the following landmarks of the thorax with their locations.*

_____1. midaxillary line

_____2. sternal angle

_____3. costal margin

_____4. midsternal line

_____5. xiphoid

_____6. suprasternal notch

_____7. midclavicular line

_____8. xiphisternal joint

A.   Lies in the median plane over the sternum
B.   Superior margin of the manubrium sterni; lies opposite the lower border of the body of the second thoracic vertebra
C.   Angle between the manubrium and the body of the sternum; also known as the angle of Louis
D.   Junction between the xiphoid and the sternum
E.   Runs vertically from a point midway between the anterior and posterior axillary folds
F.   Vertical line from the midpoint of the clavicle
G.   Lower boundary of the thorax, formed by the cartilages of the seventh through tenth ribs and the ends of the eleventh and twelfth cartilages
H.   Lowest point of the sternum

**Exercise 5**

*Fill in the blank(s) with the word(s) that best completes the statements about the anatomy of the cardiovascular system.*

1. The cardiovascular system delivers _____ blood to tissues in the body and removes

   _____ products from these tissues.

2. The thoracic cavity lies within the thorax and is separated from the abdominal cavity by the

   _____.

3. The junction between the manubrium and the body of the sternum is a prominent ridge called the

   _____.

4. The greater part of the thoracic cavity is occupied by two lungs that are enclosed by the _____.

5. The pleural reflection between the costal and diaphragmatic portions of the parietal pleura is known as the

   _____.

6. The heart lies obliquely in the chest, posterior to the sternum, with the greater portion of its muscular mass lying

   slightly to the _____ of midline.

7. The right heart is located more _____ than its left-side chambers.

8. The right atrium is _____ to the left atrium and lies to the _____ of the sternum.

9. The left atrium becomes the most _____ chamber to the left of the sternum.

10. The _____ layer lines the fibrous pericardium and is reflected around the roots of the great vessels to become continuous with the visceral layer of serous pericardium.

11. The slit between the parietal and visceral layers is the _____.

12. The intimal lining of the heart is the _____ and is continuous with the intima of the vessels connecting to it.

13. The muscular part of the heart is the _____.

14. The primary purpose of the atrium is to act as a _____ chamber that drives the blood into the relaxed ventricular cavity.

15. The left ventricle has the greatest muscle mass because it must pump blood to _____, whereas

   the right ventricle needs only enough pressure to pump the blood to the _____.

16. The _____ enters the upper posterior border, and the _____ enters the lower posterolateral border of the right atrium.

17. The medial wall of the right atrium is formed by the _____ septum.

18. The _____ part of the membranous septum separates the right atrium and the left ventricle.

19. The inferior vena cava is guarded by a fold of tissue called the _____ valve, and the coronary sinus is guarded by the _____ valve.

20. The _____ drains the blood supply from the heart wall.

21. The valve that separates the right atrium from the right ventricle is the _____ valve.

22. The base of the right ventricle lies on the diaphragm, and the roof is occupied by the crista _____, which lies between the tricuspid and pulmonary orifices.

23. The outflow portion of the right ventricle, or _____, is smooth walled and contains few trabeculae.

24. The valve that separates the left atrium from the left ventricle is the _____ valve.

25. The functions of the _____ are to prevent the opposing borders of the leaflets from inverting into the atrial cavity, to act as mainstays of the valves, and to form bands or foldlike structures that may contain muscle.

26. The smaller end of the ventricle represents the _____ of the heart, and the larger end, near the orifice of the mitral valve, is near the _____ of the heart.

27. The ventricular septum is formed of _____, _____, _____, and _____ parts.

28. The _____ septum is located just inferior to the aortic root in the area of the left ventricular outflow tract.

29. The _____ arise from the right and left coronary cusps.


**Exercise 6**

*Fill in the blank(s) with the word(s) that best completes the statements about the cardiac cycle and conduction system of the heart.*

1. The heart beats in sinus rhythm at _____ beats per minute.

2. Forceful contraction of the cardiac chambers is _____, and the relaxed phase of the cycle is

   _____.

3. During diastole, venous blood enters the _____ from the superior and inferior venae cavae.

4. Oxygenated blood returns from the lungs through the _____ to enter the left atrium.

5. The _____ pressure in the ventricular cavity closes the atrioventricular valves.

6. The blood fills the sinuses of _____ and forces the cusps to close.

7. The conducting system of the heart consists of specialized cardiac muscle in the _____ node,

   _____ node, _____ bundle, and _____ fibers.

8. The _____ node initiates the normal cardiac impulse and is often called the pacemaker of the heart.

9. The _____ node is located in the right posterior portion of the interatrial septum.

10. Atrial contraction follows the _____ wave on an ECG and generates the atrial systolic activity.

Chapter **30** Anatomic and Physiologic Relationships within the Thoracic Cavity

11. The impulse spreads via the Purkinje fibers to activate the ventricles, generating the _____ waves of the ECG.

12. The _____ interval is measured from the beginning of the P wave to the beginning of the QRS complex.

13. The _____ wave represents ventricular repolarization.

14. The _____ law of the heart states that the output of the heart increases in proportion to the degree of diastolic stretch of the muscle fibers.

15. The longer the initial resting length of the cardiac muscle, called _____, the greater the strength of the contraction of the following beat.

16. The shortening velocity of cardiac muscle is inversely related to the _____.

**Exercise 7**

*Fill in the blank(s) with the word(s) that best completes the statements about cardiac physiology.*

1. When the blood moves in smooth layers that slide against each other, this is known as _____ flow.

2. When blood cells move in different directions with varying velocities, this is known as _____ flow.

3. The flow dynamics depend on the fluid _____ and the _____ of molecules in the fluid.

4. The _____ profile is such that as fluid moves through a tube, fluid layers in the center have a higher velocity than those on outer surfaces.

5. The _____ profile states that as flow accelerates and converges, more fluid travels at velocities closer to peak velocity than layers in the center.

6. In _____, the ventricles eject blood into the aorta and pulmonary artery.

7. In _____, the ventricles fill with blood from the atria that flows to the body organs.

8. Blood flow through a constriction creates a _____ pressure upstream from the constriction.

9. High fluid pressure forces blood through the constriction in the form of laminar _____ velocity jet.

10. The normal left ventricular ejection fraction is _____%.

11. Myocardial ischemia may occur in situations in which blood pressure is acutely _____.

# 31 Understanding Hemodynamics

## KEY TERMS

### Exercise 1

*Match the following heart and cardiac cycle terms with their definitions.*

_____ 1. afterload

_____ 2. Bernoulli equation

_____ 3. blood flow velocity profiles

_____ 4. cardiac output

_____ 5. color Doppler

_____ 6. continuous wave Doppler

_____ 7. continuity principle

_____ 8. Doppler effect

_____ 9. frequency shift

_____10. hemodynamics

_____11. preload

_____12. pressure

_____13. pulsed wave Doppler

_____14. stroke volume

_____15. velocity

_____16. volume

A. The product of stroke volume and heart rate

B. Refers to a change in the frequency of waves (through sound, light etc.) that occurs as the source and observer change in motion relative to each other (away or toward)

C. Measures the pressure gradient across the orifice using blood flow velocities. Three components are present: convective acceleration, flow acceleration, and viscous friction

D. The exertion of force upon a surface by an object, fluid, etc., it is in contact with, or the force per unit area

E. Displays intracavitary blood flow in shades of red, blue, yellow, or green depending on the velocity, direction, and extent of turbulence

F. Refers to the aortic arterial pressure and vascular resistance the ventricle must overcome to eject blood, or any resistance against which the ventricles must pump to eject its volume

G. Transducers send and receive ultrasound pulses at timed intervals so that the location of where the sample volume is positioned can be known

H. Depends on many factors including the shape and size of the vessel or chamber it's traveling through, wall characteristics, the timing within the cardiac cycle, flow rate, and the viscosity of the blood

I. Refers to the change or shift in received sound waves from the initial transmitted sound waves or pulse

J. Transducer delivers continuous pulses out and back; it constantly transmits and receives, with no specific pulse duration or sample volume area

K. The amount of space occupied by a three-dimensional object as measured in cubic units such as $cm^3$ or mL

L. Derived from one of the fundamental laws of physics, the conservation of energy, which states that energy cannot be created or destroyed, only transferred from one form to another

M. The speed with which something moves in a given direction

N. The study of the forces involved with blood flow and circulation

O. The volume of blood ejected by the ventricles with each contraction

P. The degree that the muscle fiber stretches prior to contraction (end-diastole)

## Exercise 2

*Fill in the blank(s) with the word(s) that best completes the statements or answers questions about hemodynamics.*

1. What is hemodynamics?

   _____

   _____

2.

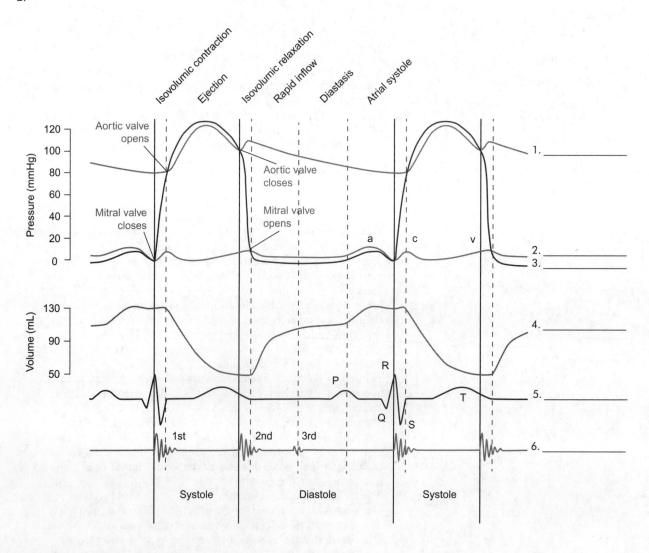

3. Fill in the correct mmHg for each structure in the box:

| Right atrium (RA) _____ mmHg | Left atrium (LA) _____ mmHg |
|---|---|
| Right ventricle (RV): | Left ventricle (LV): |
| _____ mmHg in systole | _____ mmHg in systole |
| _____ mmHg in diastole | _____ mmHg in diastole |
| Pulmonary artery (PA) | Aorta (Ao) |
| _____ mmHg in systole | _____ mmHg in systole |
| _____ mmHg in diastole | _____ mmHg in diastole |

4. The average CO for adults is _____ liters per minute.

5. Cardiac output has a direct effect on blood pressure; as the cardiac output _____, so does the blood pressure.

6. _____ can also be considered the diastolic filling or ventricular end-diastolic volume and pressure.

7. The flow velocities will be _____ toward the middle of the vessel or area and slowest along the walls or edges of the surface it travels through.

8. When the flow is moving away from the transducer or source, the velocity will be _____, displaying a negative shift with lower frequencies.

9. As flow moves toward the transducer or source, the velocity is _____, displaying a positive shift.

10. If flow is _____ to the transducer, it will exhibit no change in frequency, giving no frequency shift.

11. One of the limitations of pulsed wave Doppler is that higher velocities will exceed the Nyquist limit, and _____ of the spectral trace will occur.

12. The _____ pressure is estimated by ultrasound from the size and collapsibility of the inferior vena cava.

## Exercise 3

*Identify and answer the questions for the following images:*

1. Which valve is demonstrated in this image? Is the Doppler waveform pulsed or continuous?

_____

_____

Chapter **31** **Understanding Hemodynamics**

2. Describe this Doppler artifact.

_____

_____

3. Is this image captured in systole or diastole?

_____

_____

# 32 Introduction to Echocardiographic Techniques, Termniology and Tips

## KEY TERMS

### Exercise 1

*Match the following echocardiography terms with their definitions.*

_____1. color flow mapping

_____2. continuous wave probe

_____3. diastole

_____4. Doppler frequency

_____5. pulsed wave transducer

_____6. spectral analysis waveform

_____7. systole

A. Name for the change in frequency when red blood cells move from a lower-frequency sound source at rest toward a higher-frequency sound source

B. Part of the cardiac cycle in which the ventricles are filling with blood; the tricuspid and mitral valves are open during this time

C. Sound is continuously emitted from one transducer and is continuously received by a second transducer

D. Graphic display of flow velocity over time

E. Ability to display blood flow in multiple colors, depending on the velocity, direction of flow, and extent of turbulence

F. Part of the cardiac cycle in which the ventricles are pumping blood through the outflow tract into the pulmonary artery or the aorta

G. Single crystal that sends and receives sound intermittently; a pulse of sound is emitted from the transducer, which also receives the returning signal

## ECHOCARDIOGRAPHY EXAMINATION

### Exercise 2

*Match the following terms for imaging planes and transducer locations with their definitions.*

_____1. apical

_____2. four chamber

_____3. long axis

_____4. parasternal

_____5. short axis

_____6. subcostal

_____7. suprasternal

A. Transducer placed over the area bounded superiorly by the left clavicle, medially by the sternum, and inferiorly by the apical region

B. Transects the heart perpendicular to the dorsal and ventral surfaces of the body and parallel to the long axis of the heart

C. Transducer placed in the suprasternal notch

D. Transects the heart approximately parallel to the dorsal and ventral surfaces of the body

E. Transducer located near the body midline and beneath the costal margin

F. Transects the heart perpendicular to the dorsal and ventral surfaces of the body and perpendicular to the long axis of the heart

G. Transducer located over the cardiac apex (at the point of maximal impulse)

**Exercise 3**

*Fill in the blank(s) with the word(s) that best completes the statements about the echocardiography examination.*

1. The cardiac window is found between the _____ and _____ intercostal spaces, slightly to the left of the sternal border. The cardiac window may be considered that area on the anterior chest where the heart is just beneath the skin surface, free of lung interference.

2. Doppler echocardiography has emerged as a valuable noninvasive tool in clinical cardiology to provide

   _____ information about the function of the cardiac valves and chambers of the heart.

3. The best-quality Doppler signals are obtained when the sample volume is _____ to the direction of flow.

4. Blood flow toward the transducer is displayed by a time velocity waveform _____ the baseline at

   point zero, or a _____ deflection.

5. The maximum frequency shift that can be measured by a pulsed Doppler system is called the _____ limit and is one half of the pulsed repetition frequency.

6. The _____ waveform allows the operator to print a graphic display of what the audio signal is recording as it provides a representation of blood flow velocities over time.

7. The Doppler equation is based on the principle that the velocity of blood flow is _____ proportional to the Doppler frequency shift and the speed of sound in tissue and is inversely related to twice the frequency of transmitted ultrasound and the cosine of the angle of incidence between the ultrasound beam and the direction of blood flow.

**Exercise 4**

1. Identify the echocardiographic view demonstrated in this image.

_____

2. Identify the echocardiographic view demonstrated in this image.

_____

3. What is demonstrated in each M-mode tracing?

_____

Chapter **32**  **Introduction to Echocardiographic Techniques, Termniology and Tips**

4. What is measured in this image?

_____

5. What pathology is demonstrated in these images?

_____

6. Identify the echocardiographic view demonstrated in this image.

_____

7. Identify the echocardiographic view demonstrated in this image.

_____

8. Identify the echocardiographic view demonstrated in this image.

_____

9. Identify the echocardiographic view demonstrated in this image.

10. Identify the echocardiographic view demonstrated in this image.

11. Identify the echocardiographic view demonstrated in this image.

_____

# 33 Introduction to Clinical Echocardiography: Left-Sided Valvular Heart Disease

## KEY TERMS

### Exercise 1

_____ 1. Aortic stenosis

_____ 2. Bicuspid aortic valve

_____ 3. Pressure half-time (PHT)

_____ 4. Pseudoaneurysm

_____ 5. PISA

_____ 6. Mitral regurgitation

A. Time it takes for the transmitral pressure gradient to decrease by half
B. May lead to aortic stenosis and/or insufficiency
C. Proximal isovelocity surface area (PISA) method
D. Congenital abnormality that causes two of the three aortic leaflets to fuse together, resulting in a two-leaflet valve instead of the normal three leaflets
E. Well-defined collection of blood and connective tissue outside the vessel wall; typically results from a contained rupture of the aortic wall
F. Occurs when the mitral leaflet is thickened and deformed and unable to close properly, allowing blood to leak from the left ventricle into the left atrium during systole

### Exercise 2

_Fill in the blank(s) with the word(s) that best completes the statements regarding valvular heart disease._

1. The anterior and posterior leaflets are pliable with _____ attached to the tips of the leaflets.

2. The chordae tendineae are attached to the _____ papillary muscles.

3. The leaflets open in _____ and close in _____.

4. Mitral regurgitation is defined as the systolic retrograde flow from the left _____ into the left

   _____.

5. What echocardiographic parameters should the sonographer assess for mitral regurgitation?

   a. _____

   b. _____

   c. _____

   d. _____

6. The vena contracta width should be measured in the parasternal _____ axis view at the narrowest portion of the regurgitant jet, just after the orifice.

7. Analysis of the pulmonary vein flow into the left atrium with posterior wall (PW) Doppler may show systolic flow

   _____ due to the mitral regurgitation (MR) jet and elevated left atrium (LA) pressure.

8. The two common causes of mitral stenosis are _____ and degenerative mitral stenosis.

9. Degenerative mitral stenosis is secondary to _____, which is associated with advanced age, hypertension, atherosclerosis, and renal disease/dialysis.

10. The normal mitral valve area is _____ $cm^2$.

11. The reduced valve area in mitral stenosis leads to _____ diastolic flow into the left ventricle, causing _____ of the left atrial pressure and pulmonary venous pressure, which leads to pulmonary edema and right-sided heart failure.

12. List the distinct features of mitral stenosis on echocardiography.

_____

_____

_____

_____

13. List four of the causes of aortic regurgitation.

_____

_____

_____

_____

14. With _____ aortic regurgitation, there is a sudden large regurgitant volume in the left ventricle, causing early closure of the mitral valve.

15. Describe what effect the aortic regurgitation has on the anterior leaflet of the mitral valve.

_____

_____

16. The vena contracta is measured in the parasternal long-axis view with the beam _____ to the jet of regurgitation at the smallest neck of the flow region at the level of the aortic valve immediately below the flow convergence region.

17. Aortic regurgitation may show flow reversal in the _____ aorta as imaged from the suprasternal notch view.

18. The _____ aortic stenosis occurs inferior to the aortic leaflets in the left ventricular outflow tract.

19. What is the most common congenital valvular aortic stenosis? _____

20. The most common cause of adult aortic stenosis is _____ and senile or degenerative disease.

21. Name the Doppler measurements that are useful in determining the severity of aortic stenosis.

_____

_____

_____

22. It is important to note that any misalignment of the transducer to the jet direction leads to _____.

23. List the transducer positions and locations necessary to obtain the maximum velocity flow signal from the aortic valve.

_____

_____

_____

24. The high flow rate (hyperdynamic status secondary to aortic insufficiency) may lead to _____ of the severity of aortic stenosis, while the low flow rate (left ventricular dysfunction or mitral regurgitation) may lead to _____ of the severity of aortic stenosis.

## Exercise 3

*Fill in the blank(s) with the word(s) that best completes the statements regarding aortic abnormalities.*

1. The _____ view will image the aortic sinuses of Valsalva and the sinotubular junction; with medial angulation, the right parasternal view shows the midascending aorta.

2. The aortic arch is seen from the _____ notch, the descending thoracic aorta is imaged from the apical _____ chamber view, and the subcostal long-axis view demonstrates the distal thoracic and _____ aorta.

3. The definition of an aneurysm implies there has been _____ expansion of all three layers of the vessel wall in diameter.

4. The risk of rupture is greatest when the aneurysm exceeds _____ cm or when the aneurysm is rapidly expanding.

5. A _____ is the loss of integrity of the aortic wall with a blood collection outside the aorta.

6. The aortic _____ is a tear in the aortic intima that leads to a false lumen with blood between the intima and media and/or adventitia.

7. The true lumen expands with _____ and shows normal laminar flow with color Doppler. The false lumen may be crescent shaped, usually _____ than the true lumen, with thrombosis within the lumen.

8. This aneurysm occurs at the base of the aorta in the area of the sinus of Valsalva and is called _____.

## Exercise 4

*Provide an answer to the question regarding each of the following images.*

A        B

1. Which image shows "tenting" of the mitral valve?

_____

2. What structure are the arrows pointing to in this image?

_____

3. What measurement is this used for?

_____

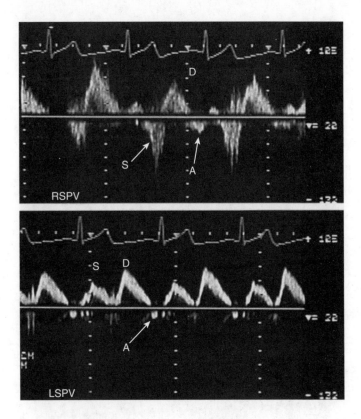

4. Describe what is happening to the systolic flow in the pulmonary vein analysis.

_____

5. What does this parasternal long-axis image represent?

_____

6. Describe what is happening with the anterior leaflet of the mitral valve.

_____

7. What is this arrow pointing to in the ascending aorta?

_____

8. What type of aortic valve is shown?

_____

9. This is a patient with aortic valve disease. What is the aortic gradient?

_____

10. The patient presented in the ED hypertensive with acute onset of chest pain. What do you see on the TEE image of the ascending aorta?

_____

# Introduction to Clinical Echocardiography: Pericardial Disease, Cardiomyopathies, and Tumors

## KEY TERMS

### Exercise 1

*Match the word with the definition.*

_____ 1. cardiac tamponade

_____ 2. constrictive pericarditis

_____ 3. dilated cardiomyopathy

_____ 4. exudative

_____ 5. fibrous pericardium

_____ 6. hypertrophic cardiomyopathy

_____ 7. lipomatous hypertrophy

_____ 8. malignant primary cardiac tumors

_____ 9. myxoma

_____ 10. papillary fibroelastoma

_____ 11. rhabdomyoma

_____ 12. serous pericardium

_____ 13. takotsubo cardiomyopathy

_____ 14. transudative

A. In chronic pericardial disease the pericardium may become thickened and inelastic, which in turn limits the ventricular filling, leading to chronic biventricular diastolic dysfunction, right-sided heart failure, and low systemic output

B. Tumors include angiosarcoma, rhabdomyosarcoma, mesothelioma, fibrosarcoma, and synovial fibrosarcoma

C. Accumulative fluid in a cavity

D. Benign cardiac tumor is the most common tumor in children with tuberous sclerosis

E. Common benign tumor of the heart

F. Outer sac of the pericardium

G. Inner sac of the pericardium with two layers: visceral and parietal

H. Hypertrophied, nondilated left ventricle in the absence of another cardiac or systemic disease capable of producing hypertrophy

I. Thickening that is seen along the superior/inferior interatrial septum

J. Arises on the aortic or mitral valve tissue and is usually quite small

K. Acute cardiac syndrome that is characterized by transient left ventricular regional wall motion abnormalities, chest pain and/or dyspnea, ST segment elevations, and minor elevations in cardiac enzymes

L. This condition occurs when the intrapericardial pressure increases to the point of compromising systemic venous return to the right atrium

M. Fluid that passes through a membrane

N. Characterized by the dilation and reduced contractility of the left ventricle or both the left and right ventricles

Chapter **34** **Introduction to Clinical Echocardiography: Pericardial Disease, Cardiomyopathies, and Tumors**

**Exercise 2**

*Fill in the blank(s) with the word(s) that best completes the statements regarding pericardial disease.*

1. The inner layer of the pericardium is further divided into the _____ (epicardium) that is continuous with the pericardial surface and covers the heart and proximal great vessels and the fibrous parietal layer.

2. The visceral layer is reflected to form the _____.

3. List the functions of the pericardium.

   _____

   _____

   _____

4. The effusions first accumulate _____ to the heart and, as the size increases, extend laterally and then circumferentially.

5. The pericardial effusion always is found _____ to the descending aorta, while the pleural effusion

   is _____ to the descending aorta.

6. Describe the echocardiographic features of cardiac tamponade.

   _____

   _____

   _____

**Exercise 3**

*Fill in the blank(s) with the word(s) that best completes the statements regarding cardiomyopathies.*

1. The _____ cardiomyopathy is characterized by the dilation and reduced contractility of the left ventricle or both the left and right ventricles.

2. _____ of the left ventricle implies that the myocardial wall segments are extremely thick (>2 mm), with peaks and valleys.

3. The _____ properties of the left ventricle may be determined by the E/A ratio, dispersion of the E-wave velocity, color Doppler M-mode velocity of propagation, deceleration time, pulmonary vein flow, and annular Doppler tissue imaging.

4. Describe the characteristics of restrictive cardiomyopathy.

   _____

   _____

   _____

5. The acute cardiac syndrome that is characterized by transient left ventricular regional wall motion abnormalities, chest pain and/or dyspnea, ST segment elevations, and minor elevations in cardiac enzymes is called

   _____ cardiomyopathy.

6. The predominant anatomic features of _____ cardiomyopathy include a narrowed left ventricular outflow tract (LVOT) secondary to the asymmetric septal hypertrophy.

7. The sonographer should evaluate the presence of a(n) _____ of the mitral leaflet to see if further flow velocity is obstructed in the LVOT.

## Exercise 4

*Fill in the blank(s) with the word(s) that best completes the statements regarding cardiac masses.*

1. _____ of the kidney may travel through the renal vein into the inferior vena cava and into the right atrium.

2. _____ malignancy affects the right side of the heart, causing severe tricuspid regurgitation.

3. The more common benign tumor of the heart is a(n) _____.

4. This benign tumor, _____, has a stippled edge with a shimmer or vibration at the tumor-blood interface that is always found downstream of the flow.

5. _____ hypertrophy is a thickening that is seen along the superior/inferior interatrial septum.

6. Predisposing conditions for left ventricular _____ include blood stasis with low-velocity flow, ventricular aneurysm, dilated cardiomyopathy with "swirling" blood flow, or pseudoaneurysm.

7. Contrast injected into the heart will clearly demonstrate a(n) _____ anechoic area if thrombus is present.

8. Patients are usually very symptomatic with _____, presenting with fever, chills, and perhaps a new cardiac murmur.

## Exercise 5

*Complete the following.*

1. Does this image show a pleural effusion or pericardial effusion?

   _____

   _____

2. Describe the size of the pericardial effusion.

   _____

   _____

Chapter **34**  **Introduction to Clinical Echocardiography: Pericardial Disease, Cardiomyopathies, and Tumors**

3. This M mode through the mitral valve is suggestive of what abnormality?

_____

_____

4. What are the areas pointing to in this left ventricle with contrast?

_____

_____

5. What does this apical four-chamber view reveal about the left ventricle?

_____

_____

6. What does this M-mode tracing reveal about the ventricle?

_____

_____

Chapter **34** **Introduction to Clinical Echocardiography: Pericardial Disease, Cardiomyopathies, and Tumors**

7. What does this parasternal long-axis view of the heart reveal?

_____

_____

8. What are the arrows pointing to in this M-mode image?

_____

_____

9. This TEE image of the interatrial septum reveals what abnormality?

_____

_____

10. This adult had a history of tuberous sclerosis. What do you see?

_____

_____

Chapter **34** **Introduction to Clinical Echocardiography: Pericardial Disease, Cardiomyopathies, and Tumors**

# 35 Fetal Echocardiography: Beyond the Four Chambers

## KEY TERMS

### Exercise 1

*Match the following embryology of the cardiovascular system terms with their definitions.*

_____1. atrioventricular node

_____2. bulbus cordis

_____3. foramen ovale

_____4. left and right atria

_____5. left and right ventricles

_____6. septum primum

_____7. septum secundum

_____8. sinoatrial node

A. Filling chambers of the heart
B. First part of the atrial septum to grow from the dorsal wall of the primitive atrium; fuses with the endocardial cushions
C. Primitive chamber that forms the right ventricle
D. Pumping chambers of the heart
E. Area of cardiac muscle that receives and conducts the cardiac impulse
F. Forms in the wall of the sinus venosus near its opening into the right atrium
G. Also termed *fossa ovale*; opening between the free edge of the septum secundum and the dorsal wall of the atrium
H. Grows into the atrium to the right of the septum primum

### Exercise 2

*Match the following fetal circulation terms with their definitions.*

_____ 1. bicuspid aortic valve

_____ 2. ductus arteriosus

_____ 3. fossa ovale

_____ 4. inferior vena cava

_____ 5. main pulmonary artery

_____ 6. mitral valve

_____ 7. patent ductus arteriosus

_____ 8. pulmonary veins

_____ 9. right ventricle

_____10. superior vena cava

_____11. tricuspid valve

A. Vessel receiving venous return from the head and upper extremities into the upper posterior medial wall of the right atrium
B. Four veins that bring blood from the lungs back into the posterior wall of the left atrium
C. Pumping chamber of the heart that sends blood into the pulmonary artery
D. Also termed *foramen ovale*; opening between the free edge of the septum secundum and the dorsal wall of the atrium
E. Atrioventricular valve between the left atrium and the left ventricle
F. Two leaflets instead of the normal three leaflets with asymmetrical cusps
G. Atrioventricular valve found between the right atrium and the right ventricle
H. Venous return into the right atrium of the heart along the posterior lateral wall
I. Open communication between the pulmonary artery and the descending aorta that does not constrict after birth
J. Communication between the pulmonary artery and the descending aorta that closes after birth
K. Main artery that carries blood from the right ventricle to the lungs

### Exercise 3

*Label the following illustrations.*

1. The heart during the fourth week of development.

1._____

2._____

3._____

4._____

11._____

5._____

10._____

6._____

7._____

8._____

9._____

2. Partitioning of the primitive atrioventricular canal, atrium, and ventricle in the developing heart.

1._____
2._____
3._____
4._____
5._____
6._____
7._____
8._____
9._____
15._____
14._____
13._____
12._____
11._____
10._____
16._____
17._____
18._____
19._____
20._____

3. Fetal circulation.

16._____
15._____
14._____
13._____
12._____
11._____
10._____
9._____
8._____
1._____
2._____
3._____
4._____
5._____
6._____
7._____

Chapter **35** **Fetal Echocardiography: Beyond the Four Chambers**

**Exercise 4**

*Fill in the blank(s) with the word(s) that best completes the statements about the embryology and physiology of the fetal heart.*

1. The cardiovascular system is the first organ system to reach a functional state; by the end of the _____ week, circulation of blood has begun, and the heart begins to beat in the _____ week.

2. The vascular system begins during the third week in the wall of the _____, the connecting stalk, and the chorion.

3. The _____ veins return blood from the embryo, and the _____ veins return blood from the yolk sac.

4. The _____ veins return oxygenated blood from the placenta; only one umbilical vein persists.

5. _____ develop in the atrioventricular region of the heart.

6. The _____ grows from the dorsal wall of the primitive atrium and fuses with the endocardial cushions.

7. As the foramen secundum develops, another membranous fold, the _____, grows into the atrium to the right of the septum primum.

8. There is also an opening between the free edge of the septum secundum and the dorsal wall of the atrium, the _____.

9. The right ventricle is formed from the _____.

10. Communication is open between the right and left sides of the heart through the _____ and between the aorta and the pulmonary artery via the _____.

11. A small amount of oxygenated blood from the inferior vena cava is diverted by the _____ and remains in the right atrium to mix with deoxygenated blood from the superior vena cava and the coronary sinus.

12. Some of the blood from the inferior vena cava is directed by the lower border of the _____ (the crista dividens) through the foramen ovale into the left atrium.

13. The blood in the right atrium flows through the three-leaflet _____ into the _____ and leaves the right ventricle through the _____.

14. Most of this blood from the right heart passes through the connection of the _____ into the descending aorta; only a very small amount goes to the lungs.

15. The pulmonary veins enter the _____ of the left atrium.

16. The blood then flows from the left atrium into the _____ through the bicuspid _____ and leaves the heart through the _____.

17. The septum primum forms the _____ of the fossa ovalis.

18. The _____ usually constricts shortly after birth (usually within 24 to 48 hours), once left-sided pressures exceed right-sided pressures.

19. The normal fetal heart rate is between _____ beats per minute.

20. If the heart rate is too slow (less than 60 beats per minute), it is called _____; a heart rate faster than 200 beats per minute is termed _____.

**Exercise 5**

*Fill in the blank(s) with the word(s) that best completes the statements about the anatomy and sonographic evaluation of the fetal heart.*

1. The fetal heart lies in a(n) _____ position within the thorax, and the apex of the heart (the left ventricle) is directed toward the left hip.

2. The right heart is slightly _____ in utero than the left heart.

3. The right and left sides may be identified by the opening flap of the patent foramen ovale; in utero the foramen opens _____ the left atrium.

4. The _____ stretches horizontally across the right ventricle near the apex.

5. Normally the tricuspid valve is located just slightly _____ to the mitral valve.

6. The right and left ventricular width measurements are performed in the four-chamber view at the level of the _____ annulus.

7. The pulmonary artery normally is _____ and to the _____ of the aorta.

8. The _____ membranous septum is best seen on the apical four-chamber view at the level of the atrioventricular valves, whereas the _____ may be seen on the long-axis view.

9. On the long-axis view, the continuity of the right side of the _____ with the _____ wall of the aortic root is important to rule out the presence of a membranous ventricular septal defect (VSD), conal truncal abnormality (such as truncus arteriosus), endocardial cushion defect, or tetralogy of Fallot.

10. Normally the three cusps open in _____ to the full extent of the aortic root and close in midposition in _____.

11. On the short-axis view, normally the right ventricular outflow tract and the pulmonary artery "drape" _____ to the circular aorta.

12. The sonographer may find the fetal spine in the sagittal plane and may angle slightly inward toward the left chest to search for the _____.

13. The three head and neck branch arteries (_____, _____, and _____) may be seen to arise from the perfect curve of the aortic arch as they ascend into the fetal head.

14. A second "arch-type" pattern (which appears as large as the aorta) is shown as the transducer is angled inferiorly from the aortic arch. This represents the _____, a communication between the pulmonary artery and the aorta.

## Exercise 6

*Provide a short answer for each question after evaluating the images.*

1. Which pulmonary vein is not shown?

_____

2. The left ventricle should be measured at the level of which structure?

_____

3. This image shows the mitral valve in which stage of the cardiac cycle?

_____

4. What important relationship does this image show?

_____

Ascending to

Arch

Descending to

5. Does this image show the ductus arteriosus or the aortic arch?

_____

6. What anatomic structure does this image show?

_____

# 36 Fetal Echocardiography: Congenital Heart Disease

## KEY TERMS

**Exercise 1**

*Match the terms related to cardiac malposition, cardiac enlargement, and septal defects with their definitions.*

_____ 1. atrial septal defect

_____ 2. atrioventricular septal defect (AVSD)

_____ 3. bicuspid aortic valve

_____ 4. cardiomyopathy

_____ 5. dextrocardia

_____ 6. dextroposition

_____ 7. levocardia

_____ 8. levoposition

_____ 9. mesocardia

_____ 10. myocarditis

_____ 11. partial anomalous pulmonary venous return

_____ 12. pericardial effusion

_____ 13. ventricular septal defect

A. Disease of the myocardial muscle layer of the heart that causes the heart to dilate secondary to regurgitation; also affects cardiac function

B. The heart is in the right chest with the apex pointed to the right of the thorax

C. Atypical location of the heart in the middle of the chest with the cardiac apex pointing toward the midline of the chest

D. Condition in which the pulmonary veins do not all enter the left atrial cavity

E. Normal position of the heart in the left chest with the cardiac apex pointed to the left

F. Congenital abnormality that causes two of the three aortic leaflets to fuse together, resulting in a two-leaflet valve instead of the normal three-leaflet valve; usually the cusps are asymmetrical in size and position; may be the cause of adult aortic stenosis and/or insufficiency

G. Cardiac disease process of necrosis and destruction of myocardial cells that involves an inflammatory infiltrate

H. Condition in which the heart is located in the right side of the chest with the cardiac apex pointing medially or to the left

I. Condition in which the heart is displaced farther toward the left chest, usually in association with a space-occupying lesion

J. Defect that provides communication between the left atrium and the right atrium that continues after birth

K. Defect in the ventricular septum that provides communication between the right and left chambers of the heart; most common congenital lesion in the heart

L. Abnormal collection of fluid surrounding the epicardial layer of the heart

M. Failure of the endocardial cushion to fuse; this defect of the central heart provides communication between the ventricles, between the atria, or between the atria and ventricles

**Exercise 2**

*Match the terms related to right and left ventricular inflow and outflow disturbances with their definitions.*

_____ 1. aortic stenosis

_____ 2. Ebstein's anomaly of the tricuspid valve

_____ 3. hypoplastic left heart syndrome

_____ 4. hypoplastic right heart syndrome

_____ 5. tetralogy of Fallot

_____ 6. mitral atresia

_____ 7. mitral regurgitation

_____ 8. pulmonary stenosis

_____ 9. subpulmonic stenosis

_____ 10. supravalvular pulmonic stenosis

_____ 11. tricuspid atresia

A. Most common form of cyanotic heart disease characterized by a high, membranous ventricular septal defect; large, anteriorly placed aorta; pulmonary stenosis; and right ventricular hypertrophy

B. Abnormal pulmonary valve characterized by thickened, domed leaflets that restrict the amount of blood flowing from the right ventricle to the pulmonary artery to the lungs

C. Abnormal development of the mitral leaflet (valve between the left atrium and the left ventricle); may lead to development of hypoplastic left ventricle; also called congenital mitral stenosis

D. Abnormal narrowing in the main pulmonary artery superior to the valve opening

E. Abnormal displacement of the septal leaflet of the tricuspid valve toward the apex of the right ventricle; the right ventricle above this leaflet becomes the "atrialized" chamber

F. Underdevelopment of the tricuspid valve; usually associated with hypoplasia of the right ventricle and pulmonary stenosis

G. Underdevelopment of the right ventricular outflow tract secondary to pulmonary stenosis; tricuspid atresia is often found

H. Abnormal development of the cusps of the aortic valve, which results in thickened and domed leaflets

I. Underdevelopment of the left ventricle with aortic and/or mitral atresia; left ventricle is extremely thickened compared with the right ventricle

J. Occurs when the mitral leaflet is deformed and is unable to close properly, allowing blood to leak from the left ventricle into the left atrium during systole

K. Occurs when a membrane or muscle bundle obstructs the outflow tract into the pulmonary artery

**Exercise 3**

*Match the following terms related to great vessel abnormalities, complex cardiac abnormalities, and dysrhythmias with their definitions.*

_____ 1. atrioventricular block

_____ 2. coarctation of the aorta

_____ 3. corrected transposition of the great arteries

_____ 4. cor triatriatum

_____ 5. ductal constriction

_____ 6. premature atrial contractions (PACs) and premature ventricular contractions (PVCs)

_____ 7. single ventricle

_____ 8. supraventricular tachyarrhythmias

_____ 9. total anomalous pulmonary venous return

_____ 10. transposition of the great arteries

_____ 11. truncus arteriosus

A. Benign condition that arises from the electrical impulses generated outside the cardiac pacemaker (sinus node); immature development of the electrical pacing system causes irregular heartbeats scattered throughout the cardiac cycle

B. Right atrium and left atrium are connected to the morphologic left and right ventricles, respectively, and the great arteries are transposed

C. Congenital heart lesion in which only one great artery arises from the base of the heart; the pulmonary trunk, systemic arteries, and coronary arteries arise from this single great artery

D. Congenital anomaly in which there are two atria but only one ventricular chamber, which receives both mitral and tricuspid valves

E. Block of the transmission of electrical impulses from the atria to the ventricles

F. Condition in which the pulmonary veins do not return at all into the left atrial cavity; the veins may return into the right atrial cavity or into a chamber posterior to the left atrial cavity

G. Occurs when flow is diverted from the ductus secondary to tricuspid or pulmonary atresia or secondary to maternal medications given to stop early contractions

H. Occurs when the left atrial cavity is partitioned into two compartments; pulmonary veins drain into an accessory left atrial chamber proximal to the true left atrium

I. Abnormal condition that exists when the aorta is connected to the right ventricle and the pulmonary artery is connected to the left ventricle; the atrioventricular valves are normally attached and related

J. Abnormal cardiac rhythm above 200 beats per minute with a conduction rate of 1:1

K. Narrowing of the aortic arch (discrete, long segment, or tubular); occurs most commonly as a shelflike protrusion in the isthmus of the arch or at the site of the ductal insertion near the left subclavian artery

## CONGENITAL HEART DISEASE

**Exercise 4**

*Fill in the blank(s) with the word(s) that best completes the statements about congenital heart disease.*

1. The most common type of congenital heart disease is the _____, followed by atrial septal defects and then pulmonary stenosis.

2. _____ is usually found when extrinsic factors, such as a space-occupying large diaphragmatic hernia, or hypoplasia of the right lung is present.

3. In the four-chamber view, a hypoechoic area in the peripheral part of the epicardial and/or pericardial interface of

   _____ or less is considered within normal limits and does not represent a pericardial effusion.

4. The _____ defect is the defect in the central atrial septum near the foramen ovale; it is the most difficult to see in utero because the flap of the foramen ovale is mobile at this period of development.

5. The _____ defect is usually associated with the chromosome abnormality of trisomy 21; it often will consist of a cleft mitral valve and abnormalities of the atrioventricular septum.

6. The flap of the foramen ovale should not be so large as to touch the lateral wall of the atrium; when this redundancy of the foramen occurs, the sinoatrial node may become agitated in the right atrium and cause fetal

   _____.

7. The (perimembranous) ventricular septal defect may be classified as _____,

   _____, or _____.

8. Ventricular septal defects may close with the formation of _____ tissue that is commonly found along the right side of the septal defect.

9. Failure of the endocardial cushion to fuse is termed _____ atrioventricular septal defect.

10. The most primitive form of endocardial cushion defect is called _____ atrioventricular septal defect. This defect has a single, undivided, free-floating leaflet stretching across both ventricles.

11. Findings in tricuspid atresia include a large dilated _____ ventricular cavity with a small,

    underdeveloped _____ ventricular cavity.

12. The portion of the right ventricle underlying the adherent tricuspid valvular tissue is quite thin and functions as a

    receiving chamber analogous to the right atrium. This is referred to as the _____ chamber.

13. The right heart is underdeveloped because of obstruction of the right ventricular outflow tract secondary to

    _____.

14. A large septal defect with mild to moderate pulmonary stenosis is classified as _____ disease,

    and a large septal defect with severe pulmonary stenosis is considered _____ disease ("blue baby" at birth).

15. If the override is greater than 50%, the condition is called a(n) _____ ventricle. (Both great vessels arise from the right heart.)

16. In pulmonic stenosis, the abnormal pulmonic cusps become thickened and _____ during diastole.

17. In a(n) _____, the raphe between cusp tissues has not separated; thus the leaflet opens asymmetrically and may show "doming" on the parasternal long-axis view.

18. _____ occurs when a membrane covers the left ventricular outflow tract.

19. _____ is characterized by a small, hypertrophied left ventricle with aortic and/or mitral dysplasia or atresia.

20. _____ is an abnormal condition that exists when the aorta is connected to the right ventricle and the pulmonary artery is connected to the left ventricle. The atrioventricular valves are normally attached and related.

21. _____ shows an abnormal, large, single great vessel arising from the ventricles. Usually an infundibular ventricular septal defect is present. Significant septal override occurs.

22. In the normal fetus, the ductus arteriosus transmits about 55% to 60% of combined ventricular output from the

    _____ to the aorta.

23. _____ tumors tend to be multiple and involve the septum. These tumors are associated with tuberous sclerosis (50% to 86%).

24. _____ occurs when the left atrial cavity is partitioned into two compartments. This anomaly is characterized by drainage of the pulmonary veins into an accessory left atrial chamber that lies proximal to the true left atrium.

25. An enlarged _____ system can serve an important function as a conveyor of inferior vena caval blood to the right atrium even though the inferior vena cava itself communicates with the left atrium.

26. In _____, the venous return may occur totally into the right atrium or into a "common chamber" posterior to the left atrium, into the superior or inferior vena cava, or into the left subclavian vein, azygos vein, or portal vein.

## FETAL CARDIAC RHYTHM

### Exercise 5

*Fill in the blank(s) with the word(s) that best completes the statements about fetal cardiac rhythm.*

1. _____ contractions arise from electrical impulses generated outside the cardiac pacemaker (sinus node).

2. To adequately assess fetal rhythm, ventricular and atrial rates must be analyzed _____.

3. The aortic leaflets may signify the ventricular _____ event, whereas the atrial wall signifies the

   _____ event.

4. _____ include abnormal rhythms above 200 beats per minute with a conduction rate of 1:1.

5. In atrial flutter, the _____ rate is recorded at 300 to 460 beats per minute with a normal ventricular rate.

6. _____ shows the atria to have a rate of more than 400 beats per minute with a ventricular rate of 120 to 200 beats per minute.

7. With supraventricular tachycardia, the fetus develops _____ filling of the ventricles, decreased cardiac output, and right ventricular volume overload leading to subsequent congestive heart failure.

8. When transmission of the electrical impulse from the atria to the ventricles is blocked, the condition is called

   _____.

9. In _____ heart block, atrial and ventricular rates are independent of each other, and the atrial rate is slower.

## Exercise 6

*Provide a short answer for each question after evaluating the images.*

1. From this image identify and answer the following questions:

    a. Where is the fetal spine? (Use a clock identification.)

    b. Describe the left ventricle.

    c. What is the ratio of the cardiac circumference to the thoracic circumference?

    d. What would you expect the contractility to be?

a. _____

b. _____

c. _____

d. _____

2. What fetal defect does this four-chamber view demonstrate?

_____

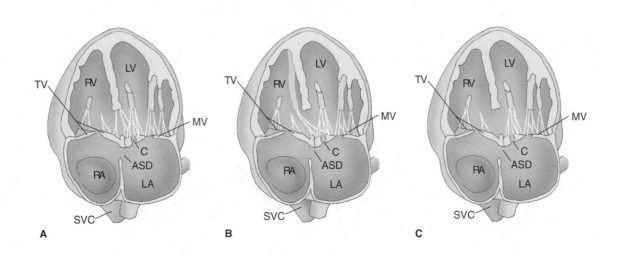

A                                      B                                      C

3. Describe the differences among illustrations *A* through *C*.

_____

_____

_____

4. Identify the fetal cardiac anomaly in this image.

_____

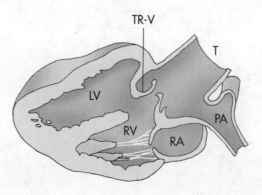

5. Describe the fetal cardiac anomaly in this fetus.

_____

_____

_____

6. Identify the fetal cardiac anomaly in this image.

_____

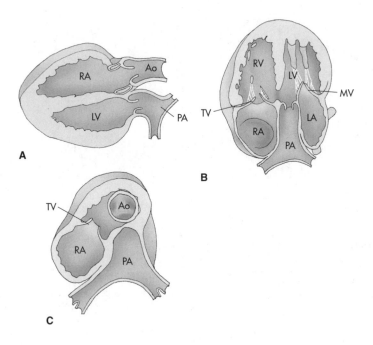

**A**

**B**

**C**

7. Describe the cardiac anomaly represented by this illustration.

_____
_____
_____
_____

Chapter **36**    **Fetal Echocardiography: Congenital Heart Disease**

8. Identify the anomaly that is demonstrated in this fetal heart.

_____

_____

# 37 Extracranial Cerebrovascular Evaluation

## Exercise 1

*Match the following extracranial terms with their definitions.*

___I___ 1. amaurosis fugax

___M___ 2. aphasia

___E___ 3. ataxia

___C___ 4. bruit

___L___ 5. collateral pathway

___B___ 6. common carotid artery (CCA)

___N___ 7. cerebrovascular accident

___Q___ 8. diplopia

___A___ 9. dysarthria

___D___ 10. dysphagia

___O___ 11. external carotid artery (ECA)

___K___ 12. hemiparesis

___G___ 13. internal carotid artery (ICA)

___J___ 14. reversible ischemic neurologic deficit

___P___ 15. transient ischemic attack

___H___ 16. vertebral artery

___F___ 17. vertigo

A. Difficulty with speech caused by impairment of the tongue or muscles essential to speech
B. Arises from the aortic arch on the left side and from the innominate artery on the right side
C. Noise caused by tissue vibration produced by turbulence that causes flow disturbance
D. Inability to swallow or difficulty in swallowing
E. Impaired ability to coordinate movement, especially disturbances in gait
F. Sensation of having objects move about the person or sensation of moving around in space
G. Larger of the two terminal branches that arise from the common carotid artery
H. Large branches of the subclavian artery that merge to form the basilar artery
I. Transient partial or complete loss of vision in one eye
J. Cerebral infarct that lasts longer than 24 hours but less than 72 hours
K. Unilateral partial or complete paralysis
L. Develops because of vessel obstruction; smaller side branches of the vessel provide alternative flow pathways
M. Inability to communicate by speech or writing
N. Abnormal condition of the brain characterized by occlusion by an embolus, thrombus, cerebrovascular hemorrhage, or vasospasm that results in ischemia of brain tissues normally perfused by the damaged vessels
O. Smaller of the two terminal branches of the common carotid artery
P. Episode of cerebrovascular insufficiency, usually associated with partial occlusion of a cerebral artery by an atherosclerotic plaque or an embolus
Q. Double vision

## Exercise 2

*Label the following illustration.*

1. Anatomy of the extracranial carotid system.

1. SUPERFICIAL TEMPORAL A
15. POST AURICULAR A
14. OCCIPITAL A
13. EXT CAROTID A
12. INT CAROTID A
11. CAROTID BULB
10. VERTEBRAL A
9. RT SUBCLAVIAN A

2. MAXILLARY A
3. ASC. PHARYNGEAL A
4. FACIAL A
5. LINGUAL A.
6. SUP THYROID. A
7. RT CCA
8. BRACHIOCEPHALIC TRUNK

## Exercise 3

*Fill in the blank(s) with the word(s) that best completes the statements, or provide a short answer about the anatomy of extracranial cerebrovascular imaging.*

1. The ascending aorta originates from the ___LEFT___ ventricle of the heart.

2. Three main arteries arise from the superior convexity of the arch in its normal configuration: the ___BRACHIOCEPHALIC___ trunk (innominate artery) is the first branch; the ___LEFT___ common carotid artery the second; and the left ___SUBCLAVIAN___ artery the third branch in approximately 70% of cases.

3. The right CCA and the right subclavian artery are divided by the ___INNOMINATE___ artery, which gives rise to the right vertebral artery.

4. Each CCA ascends through the superior mediastinum anterolaterally in the neck and lies ___MEDIAL___ to the jugular vein.

5. The left common carotid is usually ___LONGER___ than the right, because it originates from the aortic arch.

6. The termination of the CCA is the carotid ___BIFURCATION___, which is the origin of the ICA and the ECA.

7. The ECA originates at the midcervical level and is usually the ___SMALLER___ of the two terminal branches of the CCA.

8. The larger of the CCA terminal branches is usually the ___INTERNAL (ICA)___

9. Identify the four main segments into which the ICA can be divided: ___CERVICAL___, ___PETROUS___, ___CAVERNOUS___, and ___CEREBRAL___.

10. In most individuals, the ICA lies ___POSTEROLATERA___ to the ECA and courses medially as it ascends in the neck.

11. The vertebral arteries are large branches of the ___SUBCLAVIAN___ arteries.

12. The ___EXTRAVERTEBRAL___ segment of the vertebral artery courses superiorly and medially from its subclavicular origin to enter the transverse foramen of the sixth cervical vertebra.

## STROKE

**Exercise 4**

*Fill in the blank(s) with the word(s) that best completes the statements, or provide a short answer about stroke risk factors, warning signs, and symptoms.*

1. A stroke or "brain attack" is caused by a(n) _____ of blood flow to the brain (ischemic stroke) or by a ruptured intracranial blood vessel (intracranial hemorrhage).

2. Approximately 80% of all known strokes are _____, and the remaining 20% are hemorrhagic.

3. Nonmodifiable risk factors for stroke include _____, _____, and

    _____.

4. List the modifiable, or controllable, risk factors of stroke.

    _____

    _____

    _____

5. Symptoms of weakness or numbness of a leg or arm on one side of the body indicate disease in the _____ carotid system.

6. Other cerebrovascular symptoms are _____ (transient partial or complete loss of vision in one eye); (unilateral partial or complete paralysis); _____ (difficulty with speech caused by impairment of the tongue or muscles essential to speech); _____ (inability to communicate by speech or writing); _____ (inability or difficulty in swallowing); _____ (gait disturbances); (double vision); and _____ (sensation of having objects move about the person or sensation of moving around in space).

## Exercise 5

*Fill in the blank(s) with the word(s) that best completes the statements about the technical aspects of carotid duplex imaging.*

1. Arm pressures are recorded, and a difference of _____ mmHg pressure between arms suggests a proximal stenosis and/or occlusion of the subclavian or innominate artery on the side of the lower pressure.

2. In the normal setting, the CCA spectral waveform will demonstrate a(n) _____ resistance pattern (end diastole above the zero baseline) because blood travels from the CCA to the brain via the ICA.

3. The CCA Doppler signal will display a _____ Doppler shift throughout the cardiac cycle.

4. The ICA demonstrates blood flow velocity that is _____ and _____ the zero baseline throughout the cardiac cycle.

5. The normal color pattern of the ICA will have _____ color throughout the cardiac cycle because the ICA has diastolic blood flow caused by the low peripheral resistance of the brain.

6. The ECA demonstrates a more _____ Doppler signal (minimum diastolic flow) because it supplies blood to the skin and the muscular bed of the scalp and face.

7. The ECA usually has a(n) _____ slope to peak systole and blood flow velocity at or very close to zero in late diastole.

8. The vertebral arteries are located by angling the transducer slightly _____ from a longitudinal view of the middle or proximal CCA.

## Exercise 6

*Fill in the blank(s) with the word(s) that best completes the statements, or provide a short answer about the interpretation of carotid duplex imaging.*

1. The _____ velocity obtained from an ICA stenosis is used to classify the degree of narrowing.

2. A(n) _____ is present if reversal of vertebral artery blood flow direction occurs secondary to a significant obstruction proximal to the origin of the vertebral artery in the ipsilateral subclavian or innominate artery.

3. Evaluation of normal subclavian arteries produces _____ high-resistance Doppler signals.

4. Identify the important information that should be included in the interpretation of a carotid duplex imaging examination.

   _____

   _____

5. Carotid duplex imaging performed after carotid endarterectomy may reveal _____ or

   _____ stenosis in the ipsilateral ICA and disease progression in the contralateral ICA.

## PATHOLOGY

## Exercise 7

*Fill in the blank(s) with the word(s) that best completes the statements, or provide a short answer about the pathology of the extracranial vessels.*

1. The echogenicity of plaque is usually described as _____ if it demonstrates a uniform level of

   echogenicity and texture throughout the plaque, and as _____ if the plaque has mixed areas of echogenicity and textures.

2. A(n) _____ plaque is usually visualized with an accompanying acoustic shadow that obscures imaging information deep to it.

3. When describing whether the ICA is occluded, the color PRF should be _____ to document the presence of any slow-moving blood flow, and the color gain should be _____ to enhance any blood flow that may be present.

4. The ICA should be sampled at _____ sites with Doppler.

5. A nonatherosclerotic disease that usually affects the media of the arterial wall is _____.

**Exercise 8**

*Provide a short answer for each question after evaluating the images.*

1. How can the sonographer be certain the vessel is the external carotid artery?

_____

2. Does this vertebral artery demonstrate high resistance or low resistance?

_____

3. What does this image of the carotid artery demonstrate?

_____

_____

4. What does this image show of the carotid artery in a 39-year-old patient with strokelike symptoms?

_____

_____

_____

# 38 Intracranial Cerebrovascular Evaluation

## KEY TERMS

### Exercise 1

*Match the following intracranial anatomic terms with their definitions.*

_____1. anterior cerebral artery (ACA)

_____2. anterior communicating artery (ACoA)

_____3. basilar artery (BA)

_____4. circle of Willis

_____5. internal carotid artery (ICA)

_____6. middle cerebral artery (MCA)

_____7. posterior cerebral artery (PCA)

_____8. posterior communicating artery (PCoA)

_____9. vertebral artery

A. A polygon vascular ring at the base of the brain
B. A short vessel that connects the anterior cerebral arteries at the interhemispheric fissure
C. Courses posteriorly and medially from the internal carotid artery to join the posterior cerebral artery
D. Branch of the subclavian artery
E. Smaller of the two terminal branches of the internal carotid artery
F. Originates from the terminal basilar artery and courses anteriorly and laterally
G. Formed by the union of the two vertebral arteries
H. Arises from the common carotid artery to supply the anterior brain and meninges
I. Large terminal branch of the internal carotid artery

### Exercise 2

*Match the following intracranial terms with their definition.*

_____1. cerebral vasospasm

_____2. mean velocity

_____3. ophthalmic artery

_____4. subclavian steal syndrome

_____5. submandibular window

_____6. suboccipital window

_____7. transorbital window

_____8. transtemporal window

A. Characterized by symptoms of brain stem ischemia associated with stenosis or occlusion of the left subclavian, innominate, or right subclavian artery proximal to the origin of the vertebral artery
B. Transducer is placed on the posterior aspect of the neck inferior to the nuchal crest
C. First branch of the internal carotid artery
D. Transducer is placed on the temporal bone cephalad to the zygomatic arch anterior to the ear
E. Vasoconstriction of the arteries
F. Transducer is placed at the angle of the mandible and is angled slightly medially and cephalad toward the carotid canal
G. Transducer is placed on the closed eyelid
H. Based on the time average of the outline velocity (maximum velocity envelope)

### Exercise 3

*Label the following illustrations.*

1. The arteries of the circle of Willis.

1. _____

2. _____

3. _____

4. _____

5. _____

6. _____

7. _____

2. Identify the pathway of blood in the subclavian steal.

1. _____

7. _____

2. _____

6. _____

5. _____

3. _____

4. _____

Chapter **38**  **Intracranial Cerebrovascular Evaluation**

**Exercise 4**

*Fill in the blank(s) with the word(s) that best completes the statements about the anatomy of the intracranial cerebrovascular system.*

1. Blood supply to the brain is provided by the _____ (anterior) and _____ (posterior) arteries.

2. The first branch of the ICA is the _____ artery, which courses anterior laterally and slightly downward through the optic foramen to supply the globe, orbit, and adjacent structures.

3. The artery that courses posteriorly and medially from the ICA to join the posterior cerebral artery is the

   _____ artery.

4. The larger terminal branch of the ICA is the _____ artery.

5. The terminal branches of the MCA anastomose with terminal branches of the _____ cerebral and

   _____ cerebral arteries.

6. The smaller of the two terminal branches of the ICA is the _____ artery.

7. A short vessel that connects the ACAs at the interhemispheric fissure is the _____ artery.

8. The large branches of the subclavian arteries are the _____ arteries.

9. The artery that is formed by the union of the two vertebral arteries and is evaluated during TCD imaging is the

   _____ artery.

10. The arteries that originate from the terminal basilar artery and course anteriorly and laterally are the

    _____ arteries.

11. A polygon vascular ring at the base of the brain that permits communication between the right and left cerebral hemispheres (via the ACoA) and between the anterior and posterior systems (via the PCoAs) is the

    _____.

**Exercise 5**

*Fill in the blank(s) with the word(s) that best completes the statements about the hemodynamics of the intracranial cerebrovascular system.*

1. The percentage of red blood cells by volume in whole blood and a major determinant of blood viscosity is

   _____.

2. Blood viscosity is an important factor influencing intracranial arterial blood _____ velocity.

3. A deficiency of $CO_2$ in the blood, known as hypocapnia or _____, causes a decrease in the MCA mean velocity and an increase in the PI.

4. An excess of $CO_2$ in the blood, referred to as hypercapnia or _____, causes an increase in MCA mean velocity and a decrease in the PI.

## SONOGRAPHIC EVALUATION

### Exercise 6

*Fill in the blank(s) with the word(s) that best completes the statements about the sonographic evaluation of intracranial evaluation.*

1. The approach that is performed with the patient in the supine position with the head aligned straight with the body

   is the _____ window.

2. When the vertebrobasilar system is evaluated, the best results are obtained with the patient lying on his or her side

   with the head bowed slightly toward the chest. This is called the _____ window.

3. The large, circular, anechoic area seen from the suboccipital window is the _____, and the bright,

   echogenic reflection is from the _____ bone.

4. The _____ window evaluation provides information about the ophthalmic artery and the carotid
   siphon.

5. To evaluate the extracranial distal ICA, the transducer is placed at the angle of the mandible and is angled slightly

   medially and cephalad toward the carotid canal with the _____ window.

## PATHOLOGY

### Exercise 7

*Fill in the blank(s) with the word(s) that best completes the statements about the pathology of the intracranial cerebrovascular system.*

1. The most common cause of subarachnoid hemorrhage (SAH) is leakage of blood from intracranial cerebral

   aneurysms into the _____ space.

2. The hemodynamic effect of vasospasm produces a(n) _____ in blood flow velocity coupled with a
   pressure drop distal to the narrowed segment.

3. When intracranial pressure is increased or the vasomotor reserve has been exhausted, cerebral blood flow can be

   reduced to critical levels, resulting in _____ or _____.

4. Intracranial arterial _____ cause characteristic alterations in the Doppler signal (audio and spectral
   waveform), including focal increases in velocity, local turbulence, and a poststenotic drop in velocity.

5. An artery providing collateral circulation usually demonstrates a(n) _____ blood flow velocity.

6. Brain stem ischemia associated with stenosis or occlusion of the left subclavian, innominate, or right subclavian

   artery proximal to the origin of the vertebral artery is a symptom of _____ syndrome.

7. The "stealing" of blood from the _____ artery, via retrograde vertebral artery flow, causes the
   patient to experience neurologic symptoms of brain stem ischemia.

8. Blood flow is normally _____ from the transducer (suboccipital approach) in the vertebrobasilar

   system. If flow is _____ the transducer in a vertebral artery and the basilar artery, there is
   evidence of a steal.

## Exercise 8

*Provide a short answer after evaluating the image.*

1. Describe the abnormality demonstrated on this transcranial image.

   _____

   _____

   _____

# 39 Peripheral Arterial Evaluation

## KEY TERMS

**Exercise 1**

*Match the following peripheral artery terms with their definitions.*

_____ 1. anterior tibial artery

_____ 2. corpus cavernosum

_____ 3. axillary artery

_____ 4. brachial artery

_____ 5. claudication

_____ 6. dorsalis pedis artery

_____ 7. innominate artery

_____ 8. ischemic rest pain

_____ 9. Raynaud's phenomenon

_____10. popliteal artery

_____11. profunda femoris artery

_____12. pseudoaneurysm

_____13. radial artery

_____14. reactive hyperemia

_____15. subclavian artery

_____16. femoral artery

_____17. thoracic outlet syndrome

_____18. tibial-peroneal trunk

_____19. ulnar artery

A. Continuation of the anterior tibial artery on the top of the foot
B. Perivascular collection (hematoma) that communicates with an artery or a graft; pulsating blood is entering the collection
C. Continuation of the axillary artery
D. Posterior and lateral to the superficial femoral artery
E. Changes in arterial blood flow to the arms may be related to intermittent compression of the proximal arteries (or neural and venous structures)
F. Arterial branch that exits after the anterior tibial artery and bifurcates into the posterior tibial artery and the peroneal artery
G. Supplies the corpus cavernosum with blood
H. Begins at the opening of the adductor magnus muscle and travels behind the knee in the popliteal fossa
I. Originates at the inner border of the scalenus anterior and travels beneath the clavicle to the outer border of the first rib to become the axillary artery
J. Branch of the brachial artery that runs parallel to the radial artery in the forearm
K. Walking-induced muscular discomfort of the calf, thigh, hip, or buttock caused by ischemia
L. First branch artery from the aortic arch
M. Branch of the brachial artery that runs parallel to the ulnar artery in the forearm
N. Begins at the popliteal artery and travels down the lateral calf in the anterior compartment to the level of the ankle
O. Courses the length of the thigh through Hunter's canal and terminates at the opening of the adductor magnus muscle
P. Intermittent digital ischemia in response to cold or emotional stress (primary) or caused by vascular occlusion or stenosis to the digits (secondary)
Q. Alternative method to stress the peripheral arterial circulation
R. Continuation of the subclavian artery
S. Symptom of critical ischemia of the distal limb when the patient is at rest

## Exercise 2

*Label the following illustrations.*

1. The arteries of the lower extremity.

1._____

2._____

3._____

4._____

5._____

6._____

7._____

8._____

9._____

10._____

11._____

12._____

13._____

2. The arteries of the upper extremity.

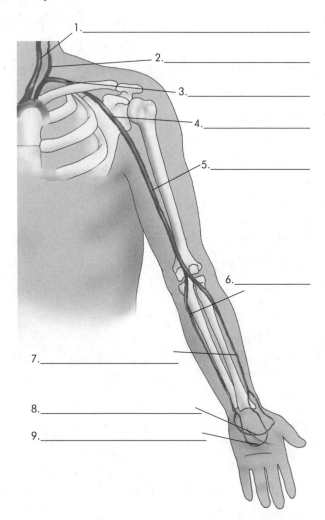

1._____

2._____

3._____

4._____

5._____

6._____

7._____

8._____

9._____

## Exercise 3

*Fill in the blank(s) with the word(s) that best completes the statements about peripheral arterial anatomy.*

1. The descending aorta is divided into a(n)_____ section and a(n) _____ section.

2. The abdominal aorta terminates in the _____ of the right and left common iliac arteries (approximately at the level of the fourth lumbar vertebra).

3. The external iliac artery terminates at the inguinal ligament, where it becomes the _____ artery.

4. The common femoral artery originates beneath the inguinal ligament and terminates by dividing into the femoral artery and the _____ artery.

5. The popliteal artery begins at the opening of the adductor magnus muscle and travels behind the knee in the _____ fossa.

6. The popliteal artery terminates distally into the _____ tibial artery and the tibial _____ trunk.

7. A continuation of the anterior tibial artery on the top of the foot is the _____ artery.

8. The artery that is located deep within the calf and travels near the medial aspect of the fibula is the _____ artery.

9. The artery that originates at the inner border of the scalenus anterior and travels beneath the clavicle to the outer border of the first rib is the _____ artery.

10. The brachial artery is a continuation of the _____ artery.

11. The radial artery begins at the _____ artery bifurcation.

## Exercise 4

*Fill in the blank(s) with the word(s) that best completes the statements, or provide a short answer about the risk factors and symptoms of peripheral arterial disease.*

1. List the risk factors associated with peripheral occlusive arterial disease.

   _____

   _____

   _____

   _____

2. Symptoms of lower extremity occlusive arterial disease are _____ and _____ pain.

3. Ischemic rest pain implies critical ischemia of the _____ limb when the patient is at rest.

## INDIRECT ARTERIAL TESTING

## Exercise 5

*Fill in the blank(s) with the word(s) that best completes the statements about indirect arterial testing.*

1. Before beginning the examination, there should be a(n) _____ minute rest period to allow the patient's blood pressure to stabilize and the legs to recover from walking to the examination room.

2. Segmental pressures are obtained with the patient in the _____ position; the legs should be at the same level as the _____ because this position prevents hydrostatic pressure artifact.

3. To obtain pressures comparable with direct intra-arterial measurements, the blood pressure cuff must have a width _____ greater than the diameter of the limb.

4. Pressures may be falsely _____ in obese patients, and a proximal thigh pressure may be _____ in extremely thin patients.

5. Pulse volume recordings measure changes in _____ limb volume with each cardiac cycle.

**Exercise 6**

*Fill in the blank(s) with the word(s) that best completes the statements or provide a short answer about arterial stress testing.*

1. In a healthy individual without occlusive arterial disease, blood flow will _____ with exercise

   because of a(n) _____ in peripheral vascular resistance.

2. Identify the contraindications to lower extremity arterial stress testing.

   _____

   _____

   _____

3. Indirect arterial testing is helpful in predicting the likelihood of the _____ of skin lesions.

## ARTERIAL DUPLEX IMAGING

**Exercise 7**

*Fill in the blank(s) with the word(s) that best completes the statements, or provide a short answer about arterial duplex imaging.*

1. Arterial duplex imaging provides direct anatomic and physiologic information, but it does not provide information

   regarding overall limb _____.

2. Duplex imaging distinguishes between a stenosis and a(n) _____, determines the length of

   the disease segment and _____ of the distal vessels, evaluates the results of intervention

   (angioplasty, stent placement), aids in diagnoses of aneurysms and _____, and monitors patients'
   postoperative course with continuing bypass graft surveillance.

3. If a(n) _____-degree angle cannot be maintained, documentation of the angle used during the
   examination is important, especially in following the patient over time.

4. In normal vessels, the arterial Doppler signal is _____ from the abdominal aorta to the tibial
   arteries at the ankle.

5. The characteristic aortic waveform has a high-velocity _____ flow component during systole

   (ventricular contraction), followed by a brief _____ of flow in early diastole (because of
   peripheral resistance) and a final low-velocity forward flow phase in late diastole (elastic recoil of the vessel
   wall).

6. Peak systolic velocity gradually _____ from the proximal to the distal arteries.

7. List three major changes in the spectral Doppler arterial waveform that occur because of a significant stenosis.

   a. _____

   b. _____

   c. _____

8. A pseudoaneurysm may be unilocular or multilocular and may partially contain _____.

9. Identification of the _____ of the pseudoaneurysm is important when ultrasound-guided
   compression therapy is attempted and color Doppler imaging permits identification of the vessel of origin, which
   is important when surgical interventions are planned.

10. During _____, blood flows from the native artery into the pseudoaneurysm, and during

    _____, blood flow returns to the native artery.

## Exercise 8

*Provide a short answer for each question after evaluating the images.*

1. Describe the flow pattern in this femoral artery tracing.

_____

_____

_____

2. This patient presented with claudication. A 40-mmHg drop in pressure was noted from the upper to the lower thigh. The Doppler signal is proximal to the narrowed segment. What does this image show?

_____

_____

_____

3. Describe what this waveform tells about flow in the bypass graft.

_____

_____

_____

4. This image was taken along the cephalic vein and brachial artery. What vascular abnormality does it demonstrate?

_____

_____

_____

Chapter **39** Peripheral Arterial Evaluation

# 40 Peripheral Venous Evaluation

## Exercise 1

*Match the following anatomy terms with their definitions.*

_____ 1. anterior tibial veins

_____ 2. axillary vein

_____ 3. cephalic vein

_____ 4. common iliac vein

_____ 5. gastrocnemius veins

_____ 6. innominate veins

_____ 7. perforating veins

_____ 8. popliteal vein

_____ 9. posterior tibial veins

_____ 10. respiratory phasicity

_____ 11. subclavian vein

_____ 12. valves

_____ 13. internal iliac vein

_____ 14. external iliac vein

A. Paired veins that lie in the medial and lateral gastrocnemius muscles; terminate into the popliteal vein

B. Blood flow velocity changes with respiration

C. Connect the superficial and deep venous systems

D. Begins where the basilic vein joins the brachial vein in the upper arm and terminates beneath the clavicle at the outer border of the first rib

E. Originate from the plantar veins of the foot and drain blood from the posterior compartment of the lower leg

F. Begins on the thumb side of the dorsum of the hand and joins the axillary vein just below the clavicle

G. Folds of the intima that temporarily close to permit blood flow in one direction only

H. Right vein: courses vertically downward to join the left innominate vein below the first rib to form the superior vena cava; left vein: longer than right, courses from left chest to the right beneath the sternum to join the right vein

I. Continuation of the axillary vein joins the internal jugular vein to form the innominate vein

J. Drain blood from the dorsum of the foot and the anterior compartment of the calf

K. Originates from the confluence of the anterior tibial vein with the posterior and peroneal veins

L. Formed by the confluence of the internal and external iliac veins

M. Single vein that travels with the artery beginning at the level of the inguinal ligament

N. Single vein that travels with the iliac artery; drains the pelvis

## Exercise 2

*Match the following peripheral venous terms with their definitions.*

_____ 1. augmentation

_____ 2. basilic vein

_____ 3. common femoral vein

_____ 4. deep femoral vein

_____ 5. greater saphenous vein

_____ 6. lesser saphenous vein

_____ 7. peroneal veins

_____ 8. posterior arch vein

_____ 9. pulmonary embolism

A. Formed by the confluence of the profunda femoris and the femoral vein; also receives the greater saphenous vein

B. Originates at the hiatus of the adductor magnus muscle in the distal thigh and ascends through the adductor (Hunter's) canal

C. Main tributary of the greater saphenous vein

D. Travels with the profunda femoris artery to unite with the superficial femoral vein to form the common femoral vein

E. Blockage of the pulmonary circulation by foreign matter

F. Blood flow velocity increases with distal limb compression or with the release of proximal limb compression

G. Dilated, elongated, tortuous superficial veins

H. Originates on the dorsum of the foot and ascends posterior to the lateral malleolus and runs along the midline of the posterior calf; terminates as it joins the popliteal vein

_____10. soleal sinuses

_____11. femoral vein

_____12. varicose veins

_____13. Baker cyst

I. Large venous reservoirs that lie in the soleus muscle and empty into the posterior tibial or peroneal veins
J. Fluid collection that can be found in the popliteal fossa or upper posterior calf; associated with synovial fluid drainage
K. Originates on the small finger side of the dorsum of the hand and enters the brachial veins in the upper arm
L. Drain blood from the lateral compartment of the lower leg
M. Originates on the dorsum of the foot and ascends anterior to the medial malleolus and along the anteromedial side of the calf and thigh; joins the common femoral vein in the proximal thigh

## ANATOMY

### Exercise 3

*Label the following illustrations.*

1. The deep veins of the lower extremity.

1._____

2._____

3._____

4._____

5._____

6._____

7._____

8._____

9._____

10._____

11._____

12._____

2. The greater saphenous vein.

1._____

2._____

3._____

4._____

5._____

**315**

3. The lesser saphenous vein.

1._____

2._____

3._____

4._____

5._____

4. The deep veins of the upper extremity.

1._____

11._____

10._____

9._____

8._____

2._____

3._____

4._____

5._____

6._____

7._____

5. The superficial veins of the upper extremity.

1._____

2._____

3._____

4._____

5._____

6._____

## PERIPHERAL VENOUS EVALUATION

### Exercise 4

*Fill in the blank(s) with the word(s) that best completes the statements about the risk factors and symptoms of vascular disease.*

1. A potentially lethal complication of acute deep vein thrombosis (DVT) is _____.

2. The chronic process, _____ syndrome, is a complication that may follow DVT.

3. List three factors associated with thrombus formation (Virchow's triad):

   a. _____

   b. _____

   c. _____

4. Varicose veins are dilated, elongated, tortuous _____ veins.

5. The venous systems of the lower and upper extremities consist of _____, _____, and perforating (_____) veins.

6. Perforating veins provide a channel between the _____ and _____ veins.

7. Venous blood flow is normally from the _____ veins to the _____ veins.

8. Venous valves are important in maintaining _____ blood flow from the peripheral veins to the central veins.

## Exercise 5

*Fill in the blank(s) with the word(s) that best completes the statements about the technical aspects of venous duplex imaging.*

1. If the patient is symptomatic, it helps to locate the _____ of pain and to measure any limb

   swelling at the _____ level.

2. The bed or table should be placed in reverse Trendelenburg (head elevated) position, which promotes venous

   _____ and optimizes visualization of the veins.

3. The leg being evaluated is _____ rotated and the knee slightly _____.

4. In general, compared with the common femoral artery, the common femoral vein will _____ with

   light to moderate transducer pressure on the skin and usually will _____ in size with respiration.

5. If superficial thrombophlebitis is suspected, the _____ vein should be followed along its entire length.

6. If the saphenous vein is not visualized, _____ the pressure on the transducer to make sure that the vein is not being compressed inadvertently.

7. The popliteal vein is evaluated from a(n) _____ approach with the patient's knee rotated externally,

   with the patient in the _____ position, or with the patient in the _____ position with the foot elevated on a pillow to eliminate extrinsic compression of the vein.

8. The popliteal vein usually lies _____ to the popliteal artery.

## Exercise 6

*Fill in the blank(s) with the word(s) that best completes the statements, or provide a short answer about the peripheral venous examination.*

1. On what three components are the interpretation criteria for venous duplex imaging based?

   a. _____

   b. _____

   c. _____

2. The most significant diagnostic criterion during venous imaging is how the vein responds to transducer

   _____.

3. If the vein still does not _____, remember that visualization of the thrombus is variable.

4. At times the thrombus is very _____ and may blend into the surrounding tissue; at other times the

   clot is _____.

5. The purpose of superficial vein mapping is to determine the vein's suitability for use as a(n) _____ and to identify its anatomic route.

6. The purpose of venous reflux testing is to identify the presence and the location of _____ venous valves.

7. The term _____ femoral vein is often used to describe the deep venous system in the thigh in venous duplex imaging reports. It is advisable to use the term *femoral vein* in venous duplex imaging reports when describing the deep venous system in the thigh.

*Provide a short answer for each question after evaluating the images.*

1. Which image (right or left) was made with transducer pressure?

   _____

   _____

Left CFV GSV DNC

2. This image over the popliteal vein is made with transducer pressure. Describe the sonographic findings. Does this patient have a thrombus?

   _____

   _____

   _____

RT subclvian vein

3. Is this flow pattern normal for the subclavian vein?

_____

_____

_____

4. This patient presented with tenderness and swelling of the upper thigh. Describe the sonographic findings.

_____

_____

_____

# 41 Normal Anatomy and Physiology of the Female Pelvis

**KEY TERMS**

## Exercise 1

*Match the following female pelvis anatomy terms with their definitions.*

D ___ 1. coccygeus muscles

I ___ 2. false pelvis

A ___ 3. iliacus muscle

G ___ 4. iliopectineal line

C ___ 5. levator ani

J ___ 6. obturator internus muscle

E ___ 7. piriformis muscle

H ___ 8. psoas major muscle

F ___ 9. striations

B ___ 10. true pelvis

A. Paired triangular, flat muscles that cover the inner curved surface of the iliac fossae; arise from the iliac fossae and join the psoas major muscles to form the lateral walls of the pelvis

B. Pelvic cavity found below the brim of the pelvis

C. One of two muscles of the pelvic diaphragm that stretch across the floor of the pelvic cavity like a hammock, supporting the pelvic organs and surrounding the urethra, vagina, and rectum; a broad, thin muscle that consists of the pubococcygeus, iliococcygeus, and puborectalis muscles

D. One of two muscles in the pelvic diaphragm; located on the posterior pelvic floor, where it supports the coccyx

E. A flat, pyramidal muscle arising from the anterior sacrum, passing through the greater sciatic notch to insert into the superior aspect of the greater trochanter of the femur; serves to rotate and abduct the thigh

F. Parallel longitudinal lines commonly seen in muscle tissue when imaged sonographically; appear as hyperechoic parallel lines running in the long axis of the hypoechoic muscle tissue

G. A bony ridge on the inner surface of the ilium and pubic bones that divides the true and false pelves

H. Paired muscle that originates at the transverse process of the lumbar vertebrae and extends inferiorly through the false pelvis on the pelvic sidewall, where it unites with the iliacus muscle to form the iliopsoas muscle before inserting into the lesser trochanter of the femur; serves to flex the thigh toward the pelvis

I. Portion of the pelvis found above the brim; that portion of the abdominal cavity cradled by the iliac fossae

J. A triangular sheet of muscle that arises from the anterolateral pelvic wall and surrounds the obturator foramen; passes through the lesser sciatic foramen and inserts into the medial aspect of the greater trochanter of the femur; serves to rotate and abduct the thigh

## Exercise 2

*Match the following terms related to female pelvic anatomy and uterine positions with their definitions.*

___N___ 1. anteverted

___F___ 2. anteflexed

___I___ 3. broad ligament

___D___ 4. cardinal ligament

___B___ 5. estrogen

___J___ 6. mesosalpinx

___E___ 7. mesovarium

___R___ 8. ovarian ligament

___C___ 9. ovum

___L___ 10. perimetrium

___Q___ 11. progesterone

___H___ 12. rectouterine recess (pouch)

___O___ 13. retroflexed

___A___ 14. retroverted

___P___ 15. round ligament

___M___ 16. space of Retzius

___G___ 17. suspensory ligament

___S___ 18. uterosacral ligament

___K___ 19. vesicouterine recess (pouch)

___T___ 20. corpus luteum

A. Position of the uterus when the entire uterus is tipped posteriorly so that the angle formed between the cervix and the vaginal canal is greater than 90 degrees

B. Steroidal hormone secreted by the theca interna and granulosa cells of the ovarian follicle that stimulates the development of female reproductive structures and secondary sexual characteristics; promotes the growth of endometrial tissue during the proliferative phase of the menstrual cycle

C. Female egg; secondary oocyte released from the ovary at ovulation

D. Wide bands of fibromuscular tissue arising from the lateral aspects of the cervix and inserting along the lateral pelvic floor; a continuation of the broad ligament that provides rigid support for the cervix

E. Posterior portion of the broad ligament that is drawn out to enclose and hold the ovary in place

F. Position of the uterus when the uterine fundus bends forward toward the cervix

G. Paired ligaments that extend from the infundibulum of the fallopian tube and the lateral aspect of the ovary to the lateral pelvic wall

H. Area in the pelvic cavity between the rectum and the uterus that is likely to accumulate free fluid

I. Broad fold of peritoneum draped over the fallopian tubes, uterus, and ovaries; extends from the sides of the uterus to the sidewalls of the pelvis, dividing the pelvis from side to side and creating the vesicouterine pouch anterior to the uterus and the rectouterine pouch posteriorly; it is divided into mesometrium, mesosalpinx, and mesovarium

J. Upper portion of the broad ligament that encloses the fallopian tubes

K. Area in the pelvic cavity between the urinary bladder and the uterus

L. Serous membrane enveloping the uterus

M. Located between the anterior bladder wall and the pubic symphysis; contains extraperitoneal fat

N. Position of the uterus when the uterus is tipped slightly forward so that the cervix forms a 90-degree angle or less with the vaginal canal; most common uterine position

O. Position of the uterus when the uterine fundus bends posteriorly upon the cervix

P. Paired ligaments that originate at the uterine cornua, anterior to the fallopian tubes, and course anterolaterally within the broad ligament to insert into the fascia of the labia majora; hold the uterus forward in its anteverted position

Q. Steroidal hormone produced by the corpus luteum that helps prepare and maintain the endometrium for arrival and implantation of an embryo

R. Paired ligament that extends from the inferior and/or medial pole of the ovary to the uterine cornua

S. Posterior portion of the cardinal ligament that extends from the cervix to the sacrum

T. Anatomic structure on the surface of the ovary, consisting of a spheroid of yellowish tissue that grows within the ruptured ovarian follicle after ovulation; acts as a short-lived endocrine organ that secretes progesterone to maintain the decidual layer of the endometrium should conception occur

## Exercise 3

*Match the following terms related to follicular development, ovulation, and menstruation with their definitions.*

__D__ 1. amenorrhea

__G__ 2. dysmenorrhea

__B__ 3. follicle-stimulating hormone

__I__ 4. gonadotropin

__A__ 5. gonadotropin-releasing hormone

__L__ 6. luteinizing hormone

__H__ 7. menarche

__E__ 8. menopause

__J__ 9. menses

__C__ 10. menorrhagia

__F__ 11. oligomenorrhea

__K__ 12. premenarche

A. Hormone secreted by the hypothalamus that stimulates the release of follicle-stimulating hormone and luteinizing hormone by the anterior pituitary gland

B. Hormone secreted by the anterior pituitary gland that stimulates the growth and maturation of graafian follicles in the ovary

C. Abnormally heavy or long menstrual periods

D. Absence of menstruation

E. Refers to cessation of menstruation

F. Abnormally light menstrual periods

G. Pain associated with menstruation

H. Refers to the onset of menstruation and the commencement of cyclic menstrual function; usually occurs between 11 and 13 years of age

I. Hormonal substance that stimulates the function of the testes and the ovaries

J. Periodic flow of blood and cellular debris that occurs during menstruation

K. Time period in young girls before the onset of menstruation

L. Hormone secreted by the anterior pituitary gland that stimulates ovulation and then induces luteinization of the ruptured follicle to form the corpus luteum

## ANATOMY AND PHYSIOLOGY

### Exercise 4

*Label the following illustrations.*

1. Pelvic cavity viewed from above.

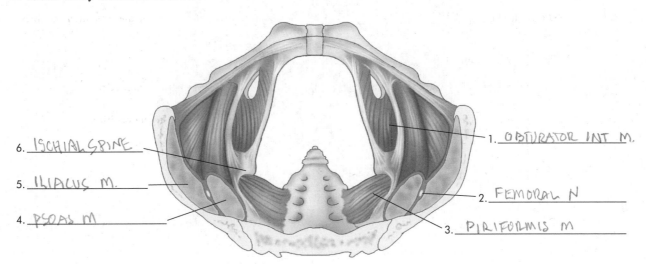

6. ISCHIAL SPINE

5. ILIACUS M.

4. PSOAS M

1. OBTURATOR INT M.

2. FEMORAL N

3. PIRIFORMIS M

2. The floor of the pelvis.

9. URETHRA

8. VAGINA

7. RECTUM

6. ISCHIAL SPINE

1. SYMPHYSIS PUBIS

2. OBTURATOR INT M.

Pubococcygeus
Puborectalis
Iliococcygeus
3. LEVATOR ANI

4. COCCYGEUS M

5. PIRIFORMIS M

Sacrum

3. Lateral view of the pelvis.

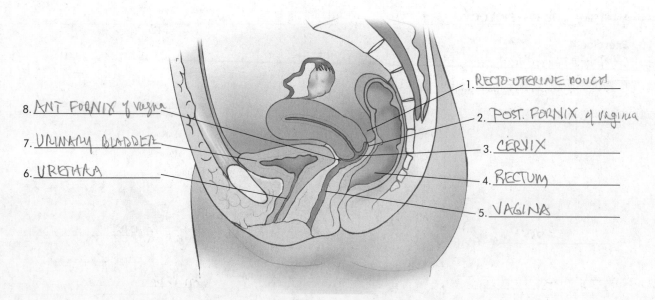

8. ANT FORNIX of vagina

7. URINARY BLADDER

6. URETHRA

1. RECTO-UTERINE POUCH

2. POST. FORNIX of vagina

3. CERVIX

4. RECTUM

5. VAGINA

4. Coronal view of the vagina, cervix, and uterus.

1. OVARY
15. FALLOPIAN TUBE
14. UTERINE A
13. CARDINAL LIG
12. OBTURATOR INT M
11. LEVATOR ANI M.
10. DEEP TRANSVERSE PERINEAL M

2. BODY of UTERUS
3. ROUND LIG
4. ISTHMUS of uterus
5. INTERNAL OS
6. LAT. FORNIX
7. CERVIXAL OS
8. EXTERNAL OS
9. VAGINA

5. Normal female pelvic anatomy.

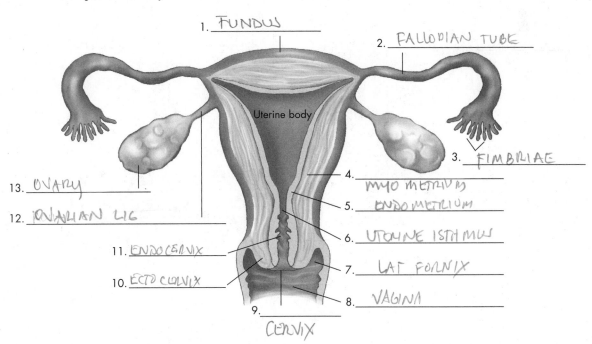

1. FUNDUS
2. FALLOPIAN TUBE
Uterine body
3. FIMBRIAE
13. OVARY
12. OVARIAN LIG
11. ENDOCERVIX
10. ECTO CERVIX
4. MYO METRIUM
5. ENDOMETRIUM
6. UTERINE ISTHMUS
7. LAT FORNIX
8. VAGINA
9. CERVIX

Chapter **41** **Normal Anatomy and Physiology of the Female Pelvis**

6. Identify the uterine positions.

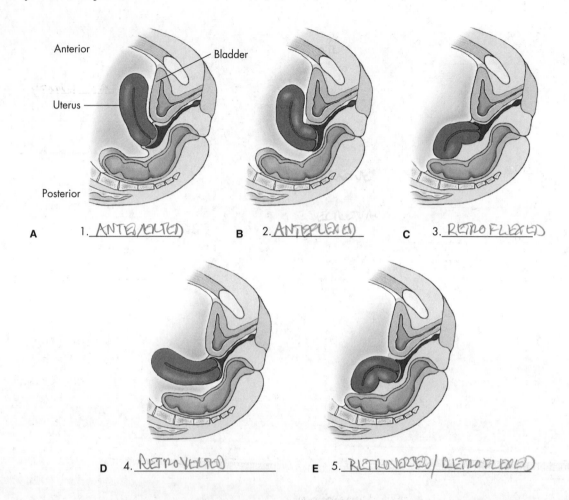

Anterior

Bladder

Uterus

Posterior

A    1. ANTEVERTED

B    2. ANTEFLEXED

C    3. RETROFLEXED

D    4. RETROVERTED

E    5. RETROVERTED/RETROFLEXED

7. Diagram of the fallopian tube.

1. AMPULLA

2. ISTHMUS

3. INTERSTITIAL PORTION

7. MESOSALPINX

6. INFUNDIBULUM

5. FIMBRIAE

4. OVARIAN LIG

8. Blood is supplied to the uterus and the vagina by the uterine and vaginal arteries.

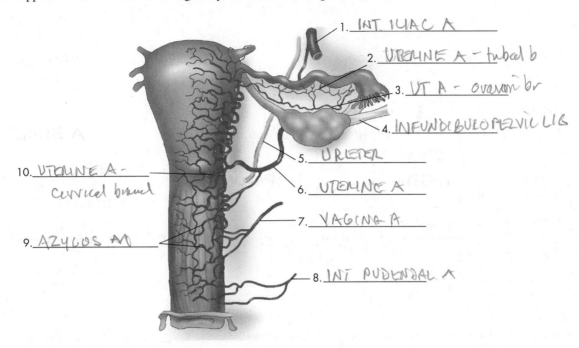

1. INT. ILIAC A

2. UTERINE A - tubal b

3. UT A - ovarian br

4. INFUNDIBULOPELVIC LIG

5. URETER

6. UTERINE A

7. VAGINA A

8. INT PUDENDAL A

9. AZYGOS AN

10. UTERINE A - cervical branch

## Exercise 5

*Fill in the blank(s) with the word(s) that best completes the statements about rectouterine spaces.*

1. The anterior cul-de-sac, or ___VESICO UTERINE___ pouch, is located anterior to the fundus of the uterus between the urinary bladder and the uterus.

2. The posterior cul-de-sac, or ___RECTO UTERINE___ pouch, is located posterior to the uterus between the uterus and the rectum.

3. The rectouterine pouch is often referred to as the pouch of ___DOUGLAS___ and is normally the most inferior and most posterior region of the peritoneal cavity.

4. An additional sonographically significant area is the retropubic space, which is also called the space of
___RETZIUS___.

5. The retropubic space normally can be identified between the ___ANTERIOR___ bladder wall and the pubic symphysis.

6. The retropubic space normally contains subcutaneous fat, but a hematoma or abscess in this location may displace the urinary bladder ___POSTERIORLY___.

7. The greatest quantity of free fluid in the cul-de-sac normally occurs immediately following ___OVULATION___, when the mature follicle ruptures.

## Exercise 6

*Fill in the blank(s) with the word(s) that best completes the statements about the physiology of the menstrual cycle.*

1. The average menstrual cycle is approximately ___28___ days in length, beginning with the first day of menstrual bleeding.

2. The menstrual cycle is regulated by the ___HYPOTHALAMUS___ and is dependent upon the cyclic release of estrogen and progesterone from the ovaries.

3. During the menarchal years, a(n) ___OVUM___ is released once a month by one of the two ovaries in a process known as ovulation.

Chapter **41** **Normal Anatomy and Physiology of the Female Pelvis**

4. Ovulation normally occurs midcycle on about day ___14___ of a 28-day cycle.

5. Secretion of the ___FSH___ by the anterior pituitary gland causes the ovarian follicles to develop during the first half of the menstrual cycle.

6. This phase of the ovulatory cycle, known as the ___FOLLICULAR___ phase, begins with the first day of menstrual bleeding and continues until ovulation on day 14.

7. The ___LUTEINIZING___ hormone level will typically increase rapidly 24 to 36 hours before ovulation in a process known as the LH surge.

8. Cells in the lining of the ruptured ovarian follicle begin to multiply and create the corpus luteum, or yellow body, during the ___LUTEAL___ phase.

9. The phase of endometrial regeneration is called the ___PROLIFERATIVE___ phase and will last until luteinization of the graafian follicle around ovulation.

10. The endometrial phase after ovulation is referred to as the ___SECRETORY___ phase and extends from approximately day 15 to the onset of menses (day 28). The secretory phase of the endometrial cycle corresponds to the luteal phase of the ovarian cycle.

## SONOGRAPHIC EVALUATION

### Exercise 7

*Fill in the blank(s) with the word(s) that best completes the statements about the anatomy and sonographic evaluation of the female pelvis.*

1. The approach that requires a full urinary bladder for use as an "acoustic window" and typically necessitates the use of a 3.5- to 5-MHz transducer for adequate penetration is the ___TA___ approach.

2. A(n) ___TV___ examination is performed with an empty bladder and allows the use of a higher-frequency transducer, typically 7.5 to 10 MHz.

3. The transabdominal scan offers a(n) ___WIDER___ field of view for a general screening of the pelvic anatomy.

4. When a transabdominal scanning technique is used, a(n) ___FULL/DISTENDED___ urinary bladder is essential.

5. The ___LABIA___ are folds of skin at the opening of the vagina; the labia ___MAJORA___ is the thicker external folds, and the ___MINORA___ consists of thin folds of skin between the labia majora.

6. The ___INNOMINATE___ bones make up the anterior and lateral margins of the bony pelvis; the ___SACRUM___ and ___COCCYX___ form the posterior wall.

7. The margins of the posterolateral wall of the true pelvis are formed by the ___PIRIFORMIS___ and ___COCCYGEUS___ muscles.

8. The anterolateral walls of the pelvic cavity are formed by the hip bones and the ___OBTURATOR INT.___ muscles that rim the ischium and pubis.

9. The lower margin of the pelvic cavity, the pelvic floor, is formed by the ___LEVATOR ANI___ and ___COCCYGEUS___ muscles and is known as the pelvic diaphragm.

10. The area below the pelvic floor is the ___PERINEUM___.

11. The muscles of the false pelvis include the ___PSOAS___ major and ___ILIACUS___ muscles.

12. The muscles that arise from the lower part of the pubic symphysis and surround the lower part of the rectum, forming a sling, are the ___PUBORECTALIS___ muscles.

13. A collapsed muscular tube that extends from the external genitalia to the cervix of the uterus is the
_VAGINA_.

14. The cervix lies _POSTERIOR_ to the urinary bladder and urethra and _ANTERIOR_ to the rectum and anus.

15. The largest organ in the normal female pelvis when the urinary bladder is empty is the _UTERUS_.

16. At the lateral borders of the uterine fundus are the _CORNUA_, where the fallopian tubes enter the uterine cavity.

17. The cervix is constricted at its upper end by the _INTERNAL_ os and at its lower end by the _EXTERNAL_ os.

18. The point where the uterus bends anteriorly (anteversion) or posteriorly (retroversion) with an empty bladder is the _ISTHMUS_.

19. The uterine wall consists of three histologic layers: the _PERI-_, the _MYO-_, and the _ENDO-METRIUM_.

20. The endometrium consists primarily of two layers: the superficial functional layer (zona _FUNCTIONALIS_) and the deep basal layer (zona _BASALIS_).

21. The uterus is supported in its midline position by paired _BROAD_ ligaments, _ROUND_ ligaments, _CARDINAL_ ligaments, and _UTEROSACRAL_ ligaments.

22. The average uterine position is considered to be _ANTEVERTED_ and _ANTEFLEXED_.

23. The _FALLOPIAN TUBES_ are contained in the upper margin of the broad ligament and extend from the uterine cornua of the uterus laterally where they curve over the ovary.

24. The fallopian tubes are divided into four anatomic portions: the _INFUNDIBULUM_ (lateral segment), _AMPULLA_ (middle segment), _ISTHMUS_ (medial segment), and _INTERSTITIUM_ portions (segment that passes through the uterine cornua).

25. The _INFUNDIBULUM_ is often referred to as the fimbriated end of the fallopian tube because it contains fringelike extensions, called fimbriae, which move over the ovary, directing the ovum into the fallopian tube after ovulation.

26. The ovaries are usually located _MEDIAL_ to the external iliac vessels and _ANTERIOR_ to the internal iliac vessels and ureter.

27. The cortex of the ovary consists primarily of follicles in varying stages of development and is covered by a layer of dense connective tissue, the _TUNICA ALBUGINEA_.

28. The central _MEDULLA_ is composed of connective tissue containing blood, nerves, lymphatic vessels, and some smooth muscle at the region of the hilum.

29. The ovaries produce the reproductive cell, the _ovum_, and two known hormones: _ESTROGEN_, secreted by the follicles, and _PROGESTERONE_, secreted by the corpus luteum.

30. The common _ILIAC_ arteries course anteriorly and medially to the psoas muscles, providing blood to the pelvic cavity and lower extremities.

31. The _INTERNAL_ iliac arteries extend into the pelvic cavity along the posterior wall and provide multiple branches that perfuse the pelvic structures to include the urinary bladder, uterus, vagina, and rectum.

32. The _RADIAL_ arteries extend through the myometrium to the base of the endometrium, where straight and spiral arteries branch off the radial arteries to supply the zona basalis of the endometrium.

33. The _SPIRAL_ arteries will lengthen during regeneration of the endometrium after menses to traverse the endometrium and supply the zona functionalis.

**331**

# 42 Sonographic and Doppler Evaluation of the Female Pelvis

## KEY TERMS

### Exercise 1

*Match the following patient history and sonographic technique terms with their definitions.*

B ___ 1. adnexa
O ___ 2. anteverted
F ___ 3. coronal plane
D ___ 4. endometrium
L ___ 5. introitus
A ___ 6. menarche
N ___ 7. menopause
J ___ 8. myometrium
C ___ 9. parity
M ___ 10. premenarche
G ___ 11. retroverted
K ___ 12. sagittal plane
E ___ 13. translabial
I ___ 14. transperineal
H ___ 15. cornu

A. State after reaching puberty in which menses occurs normally every 21 to 28 days
B. Structure or tissue next to or near another related structure
C. Pregnancy
D. Inner lining of the uterine cavity, which appears echogenic to hypoechoic on ultrasound, depending on the menstrual cycle
E. Across, or through, the labia
F. Refers to a horizontal plane through the longitudinal axis of the body to image structures from anterior to posterior
G. Bending backward
H. Any hornlike projection; refers to the fundus of the uterus, where the fallopian tube arises
I. Across, or through, the perineum
J. Middle layer of the uterine cavity that appears very homogeneous on ultrasound
K. Refers to a vertical plane through the longitudinal axis of the body that divides it into two portions
L. An opening or entrance into a canal or cavity, as the vagina
M. Time before the onset of menses
N. When menses have ceased permanently
O. Tipping forward

### Exercise 2

*Match the following sonographic evaluation terms with their definitions.*

G ___ 1. arcuate vessels
J ___ 2. internal os
A ___ 3. menstruation
H ___ 4. Pourcelot resistive index
C ___ 5. proliferative phase (early)
F ___ 6. proliferative phase (late)
I ___ 7. pulsatility index
D ___ 8. secretory phase
B ___ 9. sonohysterography
E ___ 10. S/D ratio

A. Days 1 to 4 of the menstrual cycle; endometrial canal appears as a hypoechoic central line representing blood and tissue
B. Technique that uses a catheter inserted into the endometrial cavity, with instillation of saline solution or contrast medium to fill the endometrial cavity for the purpose of demonstrating abnormalities within the cavity or uterine tubes
C. Days 5 to 9 of the menstrual cycle; endometrium appears as a single thin stripe with a hypoechoic halo encompassing it; creates the "three-line sign"
D. Days 15 to 28 of the menstrual cycle; the endometrium is at its greatest thickness and echogenicity with posterior enhancement
E. Difference between peak systole and end diastole
F. Days 10 to 14 of the menstrual cycle; ovulation occurs; the endometrium increases in thickness and echogenicity
G. Small vessels found along the periphery of the uterus
H. Doppler measurement that takes the highest systolic peak minus the highest diastolic peak divided by the highest systolic peak
I. Doppler measurement that uses peak systole minus peak diastole divided by the mean
J. Inner surface of the cervical os

## SAGITTAL AND CORONAL LANDMARKS

### Exercise 3

*Label the following illustration.*

1. Transvaginal sagittal plane.

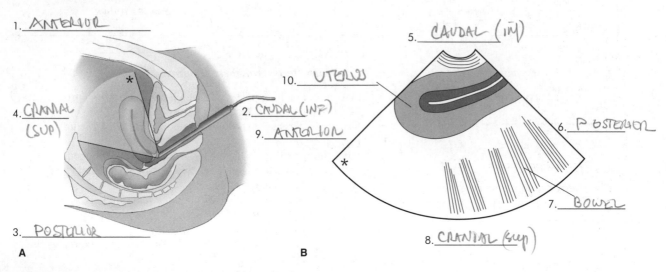

1. ANTERIOR
4. CRANIAL (SUP)
3. POSTERIOR

A

5. CAUDAL (INF)
10. UTERUS
2. CAUDAL (INF)
9. ANTERIOR
6. POSTERIOR
7. BOWEL
8. CRANIAL (sup)

B

## SONOGRAPHIC EVALUATION

### Exercise 4

*Fill in the blank(s) with the word(s) that best completes the statements about the sonographic and Doppler evaluation of the female pelvis.*

1. The full bladder ___DISPLACES___ the bowel and its contained gas from the field of view and ___FLATTENS___ the anteflexed uterus slightly so that it is more perpendicular to the transducer angle.

2. The bladder shape may be helpful because a well-distended bladder typically has a(n) ___TRIANGULAR___ or elongated shape on midline scans.

3. The ___ILIAC___ vessels can be used as a landmark to identify the lateral adnexal borders.

4. If pathology is present, documentation of the ___RUQ___ (Morison's pouch and subphrenic area) and bilateral ___RENAL___ areas must be obtained.

5. In transvaginal scanning, it is necessary to advance the transducer slightly, angling ___ANTERIOR___ to visualize the fundus, and to withdraw slightly, away from the external os, while angling ___POSTERIOR___ to see the cervix and the rectouterine recess.

6. These measurements of the uterus and ovaries should be documented: ___LENGTH___, ___WIDTH___, and ___TRANS (AXIAL)___.

7. The thickness of the endometrium should be measured in the ___SAGITTAL___ plane.

8. Pelvic muscles may be mistaken for ovaries, fluid collections, or masses. A(n) ___PAIRED (symmetric)___ bilateral arrangement indicates that they are muscles.

9. Sonographically, sections of the _____ muscle are seen at the posterior lateral corners of the bladder at the level of the vagina and cervix.

10. The muscle that is best visualized sonographically in a transverse plane with caudal angulation at the most inferior aspect of the bladder is the _____ muscle.

**334**

11. The muscles that are located on either side of the midline posterior to the upper half of the uterine body and fundus are the _____ muscles.

12. To assess the uterine vessels, the sonographer interrogates just _____ to the cervix and lower uterine segment at the level of the internal os.

13. A(n) _____, highly resistive flow pattern in the ovary is shown during the follicular phase of the menstrual cycle.

14. At ovulation, the maximum velocity increases, and the resistive index (RI) _____.

15. The middle uterine layer is the _____ of the uterus; this layer should have a homogeneous echotexture with smooth-walled borders.

16. The _____ of the uterus is hypoechoic and surrounds the relatively echogenic endometrial stripe, creating a subendometrial halo.

17. Calcifications may be seen in the _____ arteries in postmenopausal women and appear as peripheral linear echoes with shadowing.

18. The body of the uterus is separated from the cervix by the isthmus at the level of the _____ and is identified by narrowing of the canal.

19. The axis of the uterine body relative to the cervix is referred to as the _FLEXION_____, whereas _VERSION_____ refers to the axis of the cervix relative to the vagina.

20. The best way to measure the cervical-fundal dimension of the uterus in the longitudinal plane is the _____ technique.

21. During menstruation (days 1 to 4), the _ENDOMETRIAL___ canal appears as a hypoechoic central line representing blood and tissue reaching 4 to 8 mm, including the basal layer in this measurement.

22. As menses progress (days 3 to 7), the hypoechoic echo that represented blood disappears, and the endometrial stripe is a discrete thin _HYPERECHOIC____ line that is usually only 2 to 3 mm long.

23. In the early proliferative phase (days 5 to 9), the endometrial canal appears as a(n) _SINGLE THIN____ stripe.

24. The layer that is seen as a hyperechoic halo encompassing the stripe is the _FUNCTIONALIS___ layer.

25. The layer of the endometrium that represents the thin surrounding hyperechoic outermost echo is the _BASALIS_____ layer.

26. During the _SECRETORY____ (luteal) phase (days 15 to 28), the endometrium is at its greatest thickness and echogenicity with posterior enhancement.

27. Sonographically, the postmenopausal endometrial complex is seen as a thin _____ line measuring less than 8 mm, unless a hormone regimen is being followed.

28. If the tubes are distended with or surrounded by a sufficient amount of _____, they can be easily outlined by the contrasting fluid.

29. Typically, the ovary is located just _____ to the uterus and _____ to the internal iliac vessels, which can be used as a landmark to localize the ovary.

30. The best sonographic marker for the ovary is identification of a(n) _____, which has the classic appearance of being thin-walled and anechoic with through-transmission posteriorly.

31. The posterior cul-de-sac, or _____, is the most posterior and inferior reflection of the peritoneal cavity. It is located between the rectum and the vagina and is also known as the pouch of Douglas.

32. _____ involves the instillation of sterile saline solution into the endometrial cavity.

*Provide a short answer for each question after evaluating the images.*

1. Identify the locations of the fundus of the uterus and the cervix in this image.

_____

_____

_____

2. Identify the structure in the center of the uterine cavity.

_____

_____

3. Describe the structures seen within the ovary.

_____

_____

_____

4. Identify the stage of the menstrual cycle that this image demonstrates.

_____

_____

# 43 Pathology of the Uterus

## KEY TERMS

### Exercise 1

*Match the following cervical and vaginal pathology terms with their definitions.*

_____1. cervical polyp

_____2. cervical stenosis

_____3. dysmenorrhea

_____4. ectocervix

_____5. ectopic pregnancy

_____6. Gartner's duct cyst

_____7. leiomyoma

_____8. nabothian cyst

_____9. squamous cell carcinoma

A. Pain associated with menstruation
B. Small cyst within the vagina
C. Hyperplastic protrusion of the epithelium of the cervix; may be broad-based or pedunculated
D. Portion of the canal of the uterine cervix that is lined with squamous epithelium
E. Benign tiny cyst within the cervix
F. Acquired condition with obstruction of the cervical canal
G. Most common type of cervical cancer
H. Most common benign gynecologic tumor in women during their reproductive years
I. Pregnancy occurring outside the uterine cavity

### Exercise 2

*Match the following uterine pathology terms with their definitions.*

_____1. adenomyosis

_____2. curettage

_____3. intramural leiomyoma

_____4. metrorrhea

_____5. submucosal leiomyoma

_____6. subserosal leiomyoma

A. Type of leiomyoma found to deform the endometrial cavity and cause heavy or irregular menses
B. Benign invasive growth of the endometrium that may cause heavy, painful menstrual bleeding
C. Irregular, acyclic bleeding
D. Scraping with a curette to remove the contents of the uterus, as is done following inevitable or incomplete abortion; to obtain specimens for use in diagnosis; and to remove growths, such as polyps
E. Most common type of leiomyoma; deforms the myometrium
F. Type of leiomyoma that may become pedunculated and appear as an extrauterine mass

## Exercise 3

*Match the following endometrial pathology terms with their definitions.*

_____1. endometrial carcinoma

_____2. endometrial hyperplasia

_____3. endometrial polyp

_____4. endometritis

_____5. hematometra

_____6. hydrometra

_____7. pyometra

_____8. sonohysterography

_____9. tamoxifen

A. An antiestrogen drug used in treating some breast carcinomas; reported to cause growth in leiomyomas

B. Pedunculated or sessile well-defined mass attached to the endometrial cavity

C. Obstruction of the uterus and/or the vagina characterized by an accumulation of fluid

D. Malignancy characterized by abnormal thickening of the endometrial cavity; usually associated with irregular bleeding in perimenopausal and in postmenopausal women

E. Obstruction of the uterus and/or the vagina characterized by an accumulation of pus

F. Infection within the endometrium of the uterus

G. Injection of sterile saline into the endometrial cavity under ultrasound guidance

H. Obstruction of the uterus and/or vagina characterized by an accumulation of blood

I. Benign condition that results from estrogen stimulation to the endometrium without the influence of progestin; frequent cause of bleeding

## PATHOLOGY

## Exercise 4

*Fill in the blank(s) with the word(s) that best completes the statements about the pathology of the uterus.*

1. The most common finding, seen frequently in middle-aged women, is the presence of _____.

2. Clinical findings of irregular bleeding may be the result of _____, a condition that arises from the hyperplastic protrusion of the epithelium of the endocervix or ectocervix.

3. An acquired condition with obstruction of the cervical canal at the internal or external os resulting from radiation therapy, previous cone biopsy, postmenopausal cervical atrophy, chronic infection, laser surgery or cryosurgery, or cervical carcinoma is _____.

4. A vaginal _____ is seen in hysterectomy patients after surgery.

5. The most common cystic lesion of the vagina is the _____ cyst; it usually is found incidentally during sonographic examination.

6. The most common congenital abnormality of the female genital tract is a(n) _____, resulting in obstruction.

7. The benign tumor called a(n) _____ is the most common gynecologic tumor, occurring in approximately 20% to 30% of women over the age of 30 with a higher incidence in African American women.

8. Myomas are _____ dependent and may increase in size during pregnancy, although about one half of all myomas show little change during pregnancy.

9. Leiomyomas are characterized as _____ (displacing or distorting the endometrial cavity with subsequent irregular or heavy menstrual bleeding), _____ (confined to the myometrium, the most common type), or _____ (projecting from the peritoneal surface of the uterus, sometimes becoming pedunculated and appearing as extrauterine masses).

10. _____ myomas may erode into the endometrial cavity and cause irregular or heavy bleeding, which may lead to anemia.

11. The earliest sonographic finding of _____ shows uterine enlargement with a heterogeneous texture and contour distortion along the interface between the uterus and the bladder.

12. The most common cause of uterine calcification is _____; a less common cause is _____ artery calcification in the periphery of the uterus.

13. The ectopic occurrence of nests of endometrial tissue within the myometrium is _____ and is more extensive in the posterior wall.

14. Uterine _____ malformations (AVMs) consist of a vascular plexus of arteries and veins without an intervening capillary network.

15. The most common cause of abnormal uterine bleeding in both premenopausal and postmenopausal women that develops from unopposed estrogen stimulation is _____.

16. Ideally a woman using _____ hormones should be studied at the beginning or end of her hormone cycle, when the endometrium is theoretically at its thinnest.

17. Sonographically, _____ appear toward the end of the luteal phase and are represented by a hypoechoic region within the hyperechoic endometrium.

18. _____ most often occurs in association with pelvic inflammatory disease (PID), in the postpartum state, or following instrumentation invasion.

19. Intrauterine _____ (endometrial adhesions, Asherman's syndrome) are found in women with posttraumatic or postsurgical histories, including uterine curettage.

20. The earliest change associated with _____ is a thickened endometrium; it is also associated with endometrial hypertrophy and polyps.

21. Sonographically, a thickened endometrium (greater than 4 to 5 mm) must be considered _____ until proved otherwise.

22. The _____ device appears as highly echogenic linear structures in the endometrial cavity within the uterine body that are separate from normal, central endometrial echoes.

**Exercise 5**

*Provide a short answer for each question after evaluating the images.*

1. Identify the abnormality demonstrated in this transvaginal sagittal image of the cervical canal.

_____

_____

2. A 63-year-old asymptomatic woman on cyclic hormone replacement therapy demonstrates this abnormality of the lower uterine segment:

_____

_____

_____

3. What are the sonographic findings on this 3D coronal image of the uterus?

_____

_____

_____

4. Sagittal transvaginal images of the uterus demonstrate this finding:

_____

_____

_____

5. 3D coronal image of the uterine cavity demonstrates this finding:

_____

_____

_____

6. A patient presented with a recent spontaneous abortion. Identify the sonographic findings.

_____

_____

_____

# 44 Pathology of the Ovaries

## KEY TERMS

### Exercise 1

*Match the following ovarian function and ovarian pathology terms with their definitions.*

_____ 1. androgen

_____ 2. cystadenocarcinoma

_____ 3. cystadenoma

_____ 4. estrogen

_____ 5. corpus luteum cyst

_____ 6. dermoid tumor

_____ 7. endometriosis

_____ 8. follicular cyst

_____ 9. functional cyst

_____10. Meigs' syndrome

_____11. mucinous cystadenocarcinoma

_____12. mucinous cystadenoma

_____13. ovarian carcinoma

_____14. ovarian torsion

_____15. paraovarian cyst

_____16. polycystic ovarian syndrome

_____17. serous cystadenocarcinoma

_____18. serous cystadenoma

_____19. simple ovarian cyst

_____20. surface epithelial-stromal tumors

_____21. theca-lutein cysts

A. Second most common benign tumor of the ovary; unilocular or multilocular

B. Cyst that results from the normal function of the ovary

C. Partial or complete rotation of the ovarian pedicle on its axis

D. Multilocular cysts that occur in patients with hyperstimulation

E. Malignant tumor of the ovary with multilocular cysts

F. Smooth, well-defined cystic structure that is filled completely with fluid

G. Condition that occurs when functioning endometrial tissue invades sites outside the uterus

H. Endocrine disorder associated with chronic anovulation

I. Benign tumor of the ovary associated with ascites and pleural effusion

J. Gynecologic tumors that arise from the surface epithelium and cover the ovary and the underlying stroma

K. Malignant tumor of the ovary that may spread beyond the ovary and metastasize to other organs via the peritoneal channels

L. Benign tumor composed of hair, muscle, teeth, and fat

M. Cystic structure that lies adjacent to the ovary

N. Benign tumor of the ovary that contains thin-walled multilocular cysts

O. Most common type of ovarian carcinoma; may be bilateral with multilocular cysts

P. Benign cyst within the ovary that may occur and disappear on a cyclic basis

Q. Benign adenoma containing cysts

R. Small endocrine structure that develops within a ruptured ovarian follicle and secretes progesterone and estrogen

S. Substance that stimulates the development of male characteristics; the ovaries will synthesize some of these substances and convert them to estrogens

T. Female hormone produced by the ovary

U. Malignant tumor that forms cysts

**Exercise 2**

*Label the following illustration.*

1. Normal anatomy of the female pelvis.

cavity of the uterus

1. _____

2. _____

3. _____

4. _____

5. _____

6. _____

7. _____

8. _____

9. _____

10. _____

11. _____

12. _____

PATHOLOGY

**Exercise 3**

*Fill in the blank(s) with the word(s) that best completes the statements about the pathology and sonographic evaluation of the ovaries.*

1. In the anteflexed midline uterus, the ovaries are usually identified _____ or _____.

2. Following hysterectomy, the ovaries tend to be located more _____ and directly superior to the vaginal cuff.

3. The normal ovary has a(n) _____ echotexture, which may exhibit a central, more echogenic medulla with small anechoic or cystic follicles seen in the cortex.

4. Small anechoic or cystic follicles may be seen _____ in the cortex.

5. During the early _____ phase, many follicles develop and increase in size until about day 8 or 9 of the menstrual cycle.

6. The _____ may occasionally be detected as an eccentrically located, cystlike 1-mm internal mural protrusion.

7. If the fluid in the nondominant follicles is not reabsorbed, a(n) _____ cyst develops.

8. The occurrence of fluid in the cul-de-sac is commonly seen after ovulation and peaks in the early

   _____ phase.

9. Following ovulation in the luteal phase, a mature _____ develops and may be identified sonographically as a small hypoechoic or isoechoic structure peripherally within the ovary.

10. Any simple _____ that hemorrhages may appear as a complex mass.

11. The more sonographically complex the tumor, the more likely it is to be _____, especially if associated with ascites.

12. Patients with normal menstrual cycles are best scanned in the first _____ days of the cycle; this prevents confusion with normal changes in intraovarian blood flow because high diastolic flow occurs in the luteal phase.

13. A mass showing complete absence of or very little diastolic flow (very elevated resistive index and pulsatility index values) is usually _____.

14. Duplex Doppler reveals prominent _____ flow in corpus luteum cysts. This low-velocity waveform is present throughout the luteal phase of the cycle.

15. Echogenic, free intraperitoneal fluid in the cul-de-sac can help confirm the diagnosis of a(n) _____ or leaking hemorrhagic cyst.

16. The largest of the functional cysts are _____ and appear as very large, bilateral, multiloculated cystic masses. This mass is associated with high levels of human chorionic gonadotropin (hCG) and is seen most frequently in association with gestational trophoblastic disease.

17. A frequent iatrogenic complication of ovulation induction is _____. The ovaries are enlarged but measure less than 5 cm in diameter.

18. An endocrinologic disorder associated with chronic anovulation with an imbalance of luteinizing hormone and follicle-stimulating hormone resulting in abnormal estrogen and androgen production is _____.

19. Paraovarian cysts account for approximately 10% of adnexal masses; they arise from the _____ ligament and usually are of mesothelial or paramesonephric origin.

20. Endometriosis is a common condition in which functioning _____ tissue is present outside the uterus.

21. The localized form consists of a discrete mass called an endometrioma, or _____.

22. Endometriosis may appear as bilateral or unilateral ovarian cysts with patterns ranging from anechoic to solid, depending on the amount of _____ and its organization.

23. Torsion of the ovary is caused by partial or _____ rotation of the ovarian pedicle on its axis.

24. Ovarian torsion produces an enlarged _____ ovary, usually greater than 4 cm in diameter.

25. Unilocular or thinly septated cysts are more likely _____.

26. Multilocular thickly septated masses and masses with solid nodules are more likely _____.

27. Ovarian cancer can present as a complex, cystic, or solid mass, but it is more likely preponderantly _____.

28. The incidence of ovarian cancer is greatly _____ in women who have had breast and colon cancer.

29. Malignant tumor growth is dependent on _____ with the development of abnormal tumor vessels. This leads to decreased vascular resistance and higher diastolic flow velocity.

30. Sonography may demonstrate one of several patterns: (1) a completely cystic mass; (2) a cystic mass with a very echogenic nodule along the mural wall representing a(n) _____; (3) a(n) _____ level; (4) high-amplitude echoes with _____ (e.g., teeth or bone); or (5) a complex mass with _____ septations.

31. The _____ are more involved with metastatic disease than any other pelvic organ.

*Provide a short answer for each question after evaluating the images.*

1. Identify the abnormality that is most likely represented in these images.

   _____

   _____

   _____

2. A transvaginal ultrasound was performed on a 49-year-old woman whose presenting symptom was a palpable mass. What is your sonographic finding?

   _____

   _____

   _____

A

B

3. Describe your sonographic findings in this transvaginal image of the ovaries.

_____

_____

_____

_____

(From Rumack C, Wilson S, Charboneau W: Diagnostic ultrasound, ed 4, St. Louis, 2011, Mosby.)

4. A patient with severe pelvic pain. Describe the sonographic findings.

_____

_____

_____

_____

5. A 37-year-old female presented with mild abdominal distention and bloating for 1 month. Describe the sonographic findings.

_____

_____

_____

_____

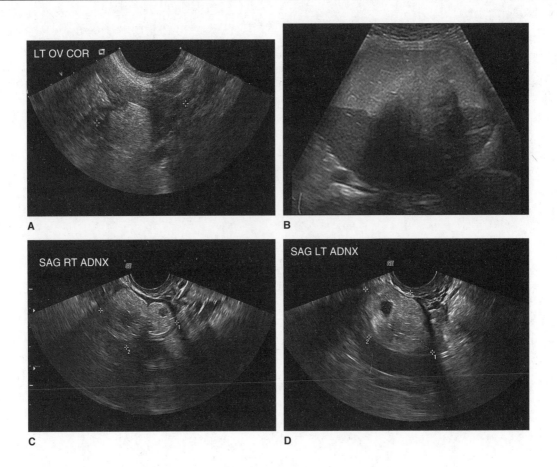

6. Which abnormality is most likely represented by these images?

_____

_____

# 45 Pathology of the Adnexa

## KEY TERMS

### Exercise 1

*Match the following adnexa pathology terms with their definitions.*

_____ 1. adenomyosis

_____ 2. *Chlamydia trachomatis*

_____ 3. endometrioma

_____ 4. endometriosis

_____ 5. endometritis

_____ 6. hydrosalpinx

_____ 7. myometritis

_____ 8. oophoritis

_____ 9. parametritis

_____10. pelvic inflammatory disease (PID)

_____11. periovarian inflammation

_____12. pyosalpinx

_____13. salpingitis

_____14. tubo-ovarian abscess

_____15. tubo-ovarian complex

A. Fluid within the fallopian tube
B. Infection that involves the fallopian tube and the ovary
C. Localized tumor of endometriosis most frequently found in the ovary, cul-de-sac, rectovaginal septum, and peritoneal surface of the posterior wall of the uterus
D. All-inclusive term that refers to all pelvic infections
E. Infection within the endometrium of the uterus
F. Infection within the fallopian tubes
G. Condition that occurs when functioning endometrial tissue invades sites outside the uterus
H. Infection within the ovary
I. Fusion of the inflamed dilated tube and ovary
J. Infection within the uterine serosa and broad ligaments
K. Enlarged ovaries with multiple cysts and indistinct margins
L. Organism that causes a great variety of diseases, including genital infections in men and women
M. Infection within the myometrium of the uterus
N. Benign invasive growth of the endometrium into the muscular layer of the uterus
O. Retained pus within the inflamed fallopian tube

## PATHOLOGY

### Exercise 2

*Fill in the blank(s) with the word(s) that best completes the statements about the pathology of the adnexa.*

1. Infrequently, a pelvic infection may ascend the right flank, causing perihepatic inflammation that may mimic liver, gallbladder, or right renal pain. This perihepatic inflammation is called the _____ syndrome.

2. Sexually transmitted PID is spread via the _____ of the pelvic organs through the cervix into the pelvic cavity.

3. Infection in the uterine endometrium is known as _____; inflammation in the fallopian tubes is called acute _____.

4. As the dilated tube becomes obstructed, it becomes filled with pus, a condition known as _____.

5. Clinically, patients with pelvic inflammatory disease may present with intense pelvic _____ and tenderness described as dull and aching, with constant _____ discharge.

6. An obstructed tube filled with serous secretions is a(n) _____; this can occur as a result of PID, endometriosis, or postoperative adhesions.

7. Severe and chronic pyosalpinx often contains _____, _____ mucoid pus, which does not transmit sound as well as serous fluid or blood.

8. When periovarian adhesions that distort anatomy form, the ovary cannot be separated from the inflamed, dilated tube and is called the _____ complex.

9. Inflammation of the peritoneum—the serous membrane lining the abdominal cavity and covering the viscera—is called _____.

10. Internal endometriosis is called _____ and occurs within the uterus. External endometriosis is called _____ and occurs outside the uterus; for example, it can be found in the pouch of Douglas, on the surface of the ovary and fallopian tube and uterus, on the broad ligaments, and on the rectovaginal septum.

11. Endometriomas may appear as bilateral or unilateral ovarian cysts with patterns ranging from _____ to _____, depending on the amount of blood and its organization.

12. Pain and the development of a pelvic mass after pelvic surgery can indicate complications such as postoperative _____, _____, or _____ formation.

## Exercise 3
*Provide a short answer for each question after evaluating the images.*

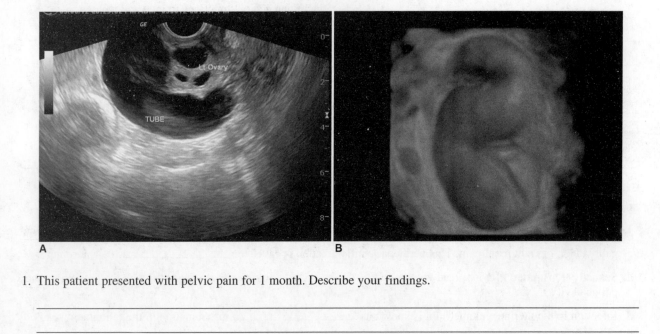

A                                        B

1. This patient presented with pelvic pain for 1 month. Describe your findings.

_____

_____

_____

A          B

2. A young woman presents with pain, adnexal tenderness, and fever for 2 weeks. What are your sonographic findings?

_____

_____

_____

3. Is this fluid intrauterine or extrauterine?

_____

_____

_____

SAG ML

A

TRV

B

TRV PELVIS

C

4. A 23-year-old female presented with fever, vaginal discharge, and acute pelvic pain for the past several days. Describe the sonographic findings.

_____

_____

_____

# 46 Role of Ultrasound in Evaluating Female Infertility

## KEY TERMS

### Exercise 1

*Match the following female infertility terms with their definitions.*

___D___ 1. assisted reproductive technology

___B___ 2. embryo transfer

___E___ 3. gonadotropin

___H___ 4. human chorionic gonadotropin (hCG)

___F___ 5. intrauterine insemination

___A___ 6. in vitro fertilization (IVF)

___C___ 7. ovarian hyperstimulation syndrome (OHSS)

___G___ 8. ovulation induction therapy

A. Method of fertilizing the human ova outside the body by collecting the mature ova and placing them in a dish with a sample of spermatozoa

B. Technique that follows IVF in which the fertilized ova are injected into the uterus through the cervix

C. Syndrome that presents sonographically as enlarged ovaries with multiple cysts, abdominal ascites, and pleural effusions. Often seen in patients who have undergone ovulation induction, post administration of follicle-stimulating hormone (FSH), or with a GnRH analog followed by hCG.

D. Technologies employed using male and female gametes to assist the infertility patient to become pregnant.

E. Hormonal substance that stimulates the function of the testes and ovaries

F. Introduction of semen into the uterus by mechanical or instrumental means rather than by sexual intercourse

G. Controlled ovarian stimulation with clomiphene citrate or parenterally administered gonadotropins

H. Glycoprotein secreted from placental trophoblastic cells; this chemical component is found in maternal urine during pregnancy

## FEMALE INFERTILITY

### Exercise 2

*Fill in the blank(s) with the word(s) that best completes the statements about female infertility.*

1. Infertility is the inability to conceive within ___12___ months with regular coitus.

2. The role of the cervix in fertility is to provide a(n) _____ environment to harbor sperm.

3. When assessing the endometrium, the sonographer wants to evaluate the _____ and _____ characteristics and to include evaluation for any _____ lesions.

4. The congenital anomalies most easily assessed with ultrasound require evaluation for _____ uterus and _____ uterus.

5. _____ uterus is associated with a low incidence of fertility complications.

6. The fallopian tubes can be examined by ultrasound to evaluate for a hydrosalpinx and assess _____ by injecting saline into the tube and looking for spillage of fluid into the cul-de-sac or by using contrast to evaluate for spillage.

7. A follicle is selected to develop into a(n) _____ follicle in response to FSH and an increase in estradiol.

8. The dominant follicle will grow at a rate of approximately 2 to 3 mm per day until it reaches an average diameter of _____ mm.

9. If serum estradiol is _____ and a large ovarian cyst is present, then oral contraceptives may be indicated to suppress follicular activity before ovarian stimulation therapy is started.

10. A normal endometrial response associated with ovarian stimulation is increasing thickness from 2 to 3 mm to _____ mm.

11. Complications associated with assisted reproductive technologies include ovarian _____ syndrome, multiple _____, and _____ pregnancy.

12. _____ is a syndrome that presents sonographically as enlarged ovaries with multiple cysts, abdominal ascites, and pleural effusions.

13. An ectopic pregnancy coexisting with an intrauterine pregnancy is a(n) _____ pregnancy.

## Exercise 3

*Provide a short answer for each question after evaluating the images.*

1. Identify the abnormality demonstrated in this infusion sonography image.

_____

_____

2. Which abnormality, demonstrated in this infusion sonography image, may interfere with implantation?

_____

_____

3. Identify the phase of the ovary shown in this image.

_____

4. This transvaginal image of the ovary is found in what condition?

_____

_____

_____

# 47 Role of Sonography in Obstetrics

## KEY TERMS

### Exercise 1

*Match the following terms related to indications for obstetric sonography with their definitions.*

_____ 1. abruptio placentae

_____ 2. amniocentesis

_____ 3. anencephaly

_____ 4. cerclage

_____ 5. embryonic age (or conception age)

_____ 6. gestational age

_____ 7. hydatidiform mole

_____ 8. incompetent cervix

_____ 9. intrauterine growth restriction (IUGR)

_____ 10. macrosomia

_____ 11. maternal serum alpha-fetoprotein (MSAFP)

_____ 12. oligohydramnios

_____ 13. placenta

_____ 14. placenta previa

_____ 15. polyhydramnios

_____ 16. aneuploidy

_____ 17. quad screen

A. Age of embryo stated as time from day of conception

B. Length of pregnancy defined in the United States as number of weeks from first day of last normal menstrual period (LNMP)

C. Neural tube defect characterized by absence of the brain, including the cerebrum, the cerebellum, and basal ganglia

D. One of several biochemical tests used to assess fetal risk for aneuploidy or fetal defect; a component of the "triple screen," the normal value of MSAFP, varies with gestational age, and assessment of gestational age is essential for accurate interpretation of results

E. Bleeding from a normally situated placenta as a result of its complete or partial detachment after the 20th week of gestation

F. Condition in which the cervix dilates silently during the second trimester; without intervention, the membranes bulge through the cervix and rupture, and the fetus drops out, resulting in a premature preterm delivery

G. Ligatures around the cervix uteri to treat cervical incompetence during pregnancy

H. Reduced growth rate or abnormal growth pattern of the fetus, resulting in a small-for-gestational-age fetus

I. Aspiration of a sample of amniotic fluid through the mother's abdomen for diagnostic analysis of fetal genetics, maturity, and/or disease

J. Exceptionally large infant with excessive fat deposition in the subcutaneous tissue; most frequently seen in fetuses of diabetic mothers

K. Abnormal conception in which there is partial or complete conversion of the chorionic villi into grapelike vesicles

L. Placental implantation encroaches upon the lower uterine segment; if the placenta presents first in late pregnancy, bleeding is inevitable

M. Organ of communication whereby nutrition and products of metabolism are interchanged between the fetal and maternal blood systems; is formed from the chorion frondosum with a maternal decidual contribution

N. Excessive amount of amniotic fluid

O. Reduced amount of amniotic fluid

P. Maternal serum biochemical levels in the second trimester of human chorionic gonadotropin, alpha-fetoprotein, estriol, and inhibin A

Q. Fetal syndrome associated with abnormal number of chromosomes

## Exercise 2

*Match the following terms related to obstetric sonography during the first, second, and third trimesters with their definitions.*

_____ 1. amnion

_____ 2. cervix

_____ 3. chorion

_____ 4. corpus luteum

_____ 5. ductus venosum

_____ 6. embryo

_____ 7. gestational sac

_____ 8. lower uterine segment

_____ 9. trimester

_____ 10. umbilical cord

_____ 11. yolk sac

_____ 12. zygote

A. Cellular, outermost extraembryonic membrane, composed of trophoblast lined with mesoderm

B. Products of conception from fertilization through implantation; the zygotic stage of pregnancy lasts for approximately 12 days after conception

C. Vascular structure within the fetal liver that connects the umbilical vein to the inferior vena cava and allows oxygenated blood to bypass the liver and return directly to the heart

D. Functional structure within the normal ovary that is formed from cells lining the graafian follicle after ovulation; it produces estrogen and progesterone and may become enlarged and appear cystic during early pregnancy

E. Inferior segment of the uterus, which normally is more than 3.5 cm long during pregnancy and decreases in length during labor

F. Connecting lifeline between the fetus and the placenta; it contains two umbilical arteries, which carry deoxygenated fetal blood, and one umbilical vein, which carries oxygenated fetal blood encased in Wharton's jelly

G. Developing individual from implantation to the end of the ninth week of gestation

H. Smooth membrane enclosing the fetus and amniotic fluid; it is loosely fused with the outer chorionic membrane except at the placental insertion of the umbilical cord, where it is contiguous with the membranes surrounding the umbilical cord

I. Thin expanded lower portion of the uterus that forms in the last trimester of pregnancy

J. Circular structure within the gestational sac seen sonographically between 4 and 10 weeks' gestational age; supplies nutrition, facilitates waste removal, and is the site of origin of early hematopoietic stem cells in the embryo

K. A 40-week pregnancy is divided into three 13-week periods from the first day of the last normal menstrual period

L. Structure lined by the chorion that normally implants within the uterine decidua and contains the developing embryo

## SONOGRAPHIC EVALUATION

## Exercise 3

List the recommended indications for obstetric sonographic examinations.

1. _____

2. _____

3. _____

4. _____

5. _____

6. _____

7. _____

8. _____

9. _____

10. _____

11. _____

12. _____

13. _____

14. _____

15. _____

16. _____

17. _____

18. _____

19. _____

20. _____

21. _____

22. _____

23. _____

24. _____

25. _____

26. _____

27. _____

## MATERNAL RISK FACTORS AND PATIENT HISTORY

### Exercise 4

*Fill in the blank(s) with the word(s) that best completes the statements, or provide a short answer about the maternal risk factors and patient information.*

1. List the maternal risk factors that increase the chances of producing a fetus with congenital anomalies.

_____

_____

_____

_____

2. Other risk factors include a previous child born with a(n) _____ disorder or exposure to a known _____ drug or infectious agent known to cause birth defects.

3. _____ is the total number of pregnancies, and _____ is the number of live births.

4. The sonographer should ask the patient several important questions before beginning the obstetric sonography evaluation. List these questions.

a. _____

b. _____

c. _____

d. _____

e. _____

## QUALITY STANDARDS

### Exercise 5

*Fill in the blank(s) with the word(s) that best completes the statements, or provide a short answer about the quality standards for the obstetric examination.*

1. Quality standards include not only the components of the examination protocol but also the following:

a. _____

b. _____

c. _____

d. _____

e. _____

f. _____

g. _____

2. The purpose of a national _____ or registry is to assure the public that the person performing sonography has the necessary knowledge, skills, and experience to provide this service.

3. Documentation standards require that a(n) _____ record of measurements and anatomic findings is maintained.

4. Images need to be labeled with the _____, _____, and _____ if appropriate.

5. Describe the ultrasound protocol for the first-trimester pregnancy.

a. _____

b. _____

c. _____

d. _____

6. Describe the ultrasound protocol for second- and third-trimester pregnancies.

a. _____

b. _____

c. _____

d. _____

e. _____

f. _____

7. List the normal anatomic structures that should be recorded in a standard obstetric examination in each region during the second or third trimester:

a. Head and neck

_____

b. Chest

_____

c. Abdomen

_____

d. Spine

_____

e. Extremities

_____

f. Gender

_____

# 48 Clinical Ethics for Obstetric Sonography

## KEY TERMS

### Exercise 1

*Match the following clinical ethics terms with their definitions.*

_____ 1. autonomy

_____ 2. beneficence

_____ 3. confidentiality

_____ 4. ethics

_____ 5. informed consent

_____ 6. integrity

_____ 7. justice

_____ 8. morality

_____ 9. nonmaleficence

_____10. respect for persons

_____11. veracity

A. The study of what is good and bad and of moral duty and obligation; systematic reflection on and analysis of morality

B. Bringing about good by maximizing benefits and minimizing possible harm

C. Truthfulness, honesty

D. Refraining from harming oneself or others

E. Incorporates both respect for the autonomy of individuals and the requirement to protect those with diminished autonomy

F. Self-governing or self-directing freedom and especially moral independence; the right of persons to choose and to have their choices respected

G. Adherence to moral and ethical principles

H. The protection of cherished values that relate to how persons interact and live in peace

I. Holding information in confidence; respect for privacy

J. The ethical principle that requires fair distribution of benefits and burdens

K. Providing complete information and ensuring comprehension and voluntary consent by a patient or subject to a required or experimental medical procedure

## PRINCIPLES OF MEDICAL ETHICS

### Exercise 2

*Fill in the blank(s) with the word(s) that best completes the statements about medical ethics.*

1. Ethics is defined as systematic reflection on and analysis of _____.

2. Morality concerns _____ conduct (what we ought or ought not do) and _____ character (the kinds of persons we should become and the virtues we should cultivate in doing so).

3. Morality reflects duties and _____.

4. To demonstrate values, a person has to have rights of expression, so _____ and

   _____ are also integral parts of morality.

5. Discussion, reflection, and discourse on morality are known as _____.

6. Hippocrates cautioned his students to *primum non nocere*, which means, "_____."

7. The principle of _____ directs the sonographer not to cause harm.

8. Application of the principle of nonmaleficence requires the sonographer to obtain appropriate _____ and clinical skills to ensure competence in performing each examination required.

9. Use of obstetric ultrasound must be justified by the goal of seeking the greater balance of clinical "goods" over "harms," not simply preventing harm to the patient at all cost. This ethical principle is called

_____ and provides a more comprehensive basis for ethics in sonography than is provided by nonmaleficence.

10. Beneficence encourages sonographers to go beyond the _____ standard protocol and to seek additional images and information if achievable and in the best interests of patients.

11. Beneficence requires sonographers to focus on small comforts for the patient, respecting their _____ and the inclusion of family.

12. Beneficence, similar to nonmaleficence, requires _____, _____, and

excellent _____ skills to ensure that the patient and the fetus receive the greatest benefit of the examination.

13. A person's capacity to formulate, express, and carry out value-based preferences is referred to as

_____.

14. Informed _____ is an autonomy-based right. Each health professional has autonomy-based obligations regarding this process.

15. If a practitioner asks a sonographer to perform an examination that he or she is not competent to do, it is essential for the sonographer to be truthful about his or her limitations to protect the patient. This is an example of

_____.

16. _____ means simply that sonographers must strive to treat all patients equally.

17. Justice and autonomy are the ethical principles that determine the _____ of routine obstetric sonography examinations.

18. The obligation of confidentiality derives from the principles of _____ (the patient will be more forthcoming) and respect for autonomy (the patient's privacy rights are protected).

# 49 The Normal First Trimester

## KEY TERMS

### Exercise 1

*Match the following terms related to a normal first trimester with their definitions.*

__E__ 1. diamniotic

__A__ 2. dichorionic

__D__ 3. embryologic age

__I__ 4. menstrual age

__G__ 5. monoamniotic

__B__ 6. monochorionic

__F__ 7. primary yolk sac

__C__ 8. secondary yolk sac

__H__ 9. zygote

A. Multiple pregnancy with two chorionic sacs
B. Multiple pregnancy with one chorionic sac
C. Formed at 23 days when the primary yolk sac is pinched off by the extraembryonic coelom
D. Age calculated from when conception occurs
E. Multiple pregnancy with two amniotic sacs
F. First site of formation of red blood cells that will nourish the embryo
G. Multiple pregnancy with one amniotic sac
H. Conceptus resulting from union of male and female gametes
I. Length of time calculated from the first day of the last normal menstrual period to the point at which the pregnancy is being assessed

### Exercise 2

*Match the following laboratory values and sonographic evaluation terms with their definitions.*

__K__ 1. amniotic cavity

__C__ 2. chorionic cavity

__N__ 3. chorionic villi sampling

__G__ 4. crown-rump length

__M__ 5. decidua basalis

__B__ 6. decidua capsularis

__J__ 7. double decidual sac sign

__E__ 8. embryonic period

__H__ 9. hematopoiesis

__D__ 10. human chorionic gonadotropin (hCG)

__L__ 11. IUP

__I__ 12. MSD

__A__ 13. transvaginal transducer

__F__ 14. yolk stalk

A. High-frequency transducer that is inserted into the vaginal canal to obtain better definition of first-trimester pregnancy
B. Uterine decidua on the surface of the implantation site
C. Surrounds the amniotic cavity and contains the yolk sac
D. Hormone secreted by the trophoblastic cells of the blastocyst; laboratory test indicates pregnancy when values are elevated
E. Time between 4 and 10 weeks' gestation
F. The umbilical duct connecting the yolk sac with the embryo
G. Most accurate measurement of the embryo in the first trimester
H. Production and development of blood cells
I. Mean sac diameter
J. Interface between the decidua capsularis and the echogenic, highly vascular endometrium
K. Cavity in which the fetus exists; forms early in gestation; fills with amniotic fluid to protect the fetus
L. Intrauterine pregnancy
M. Uterine decidual surface on the maternal side of the placenta
N. Invasive diagnostic genetic testing that involves sampling zygotic cells from developing placental tissue

## Exercise 3

*Label the following illustrations.*

1. Diagram illustrating normal conception.

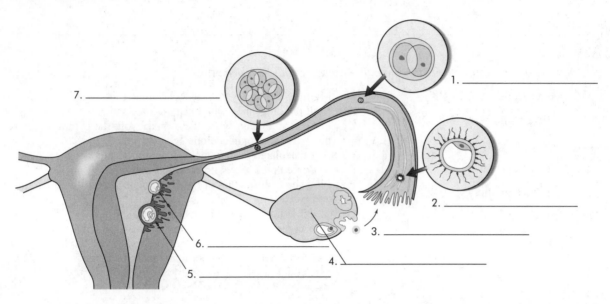

7. _____

1. _____

2. _____

3. _____

4. _____

5. _____

6. _____

2. Schema showing the relation of the fetal membranes and the wall of the uterus.

1. DECIDUA BASALIS

9. DECIDUA PARIETALIS

8. CHORIONIC CAVITY

7. AMNIOTIC CAVITY

6. DECIDUA CAPSULARIS

5. CHORION LAEVE

2. AMNIOTIC CAVITY

3. YOLK SAC

4. PLACENTA

A                                    B

3. Schematics demonstrating the development of amnion, yolk sac, and embryo.

1. AMNION
2. CONNECTING STALK
3. EMBRYONIC DISC
4. YOLK SAC
5. CHORION

6. CHORIONIC CAVITY
7. AMNIOTIC CAVITY
8. UMBILICAL CORD
9. YOLK SAC

10. AMNION
11. CONNECTING STALK
12. YOLK SAC
13. CHORIONIC CAVITY

14. SMOOTH CHORION
15. AMNION
16. AMNIOTIC SAC
17. UMBILICAL CORD
18. YOLK SAC REMNANT

## FIRST TRIMESTER

### Exercise 4

*Fill in the blank(s) with the word(s) that best completes the statements about early development in the first trimester.*

1. Clinicians and sonographers use _____ to date the pregnancy, with the first day of the last menstrual period as the beginning of gestation.

2. In the first 9 menstrual weeks, the conceptus is called a(n) _____.

3. For the time after the first 9 weeks, the embryo is called a(n) FETUS.

4. The *gestational age* (age known as postmenstrual age) is calculated by adding 2 weeks to conceptional age.

5. The fertilized ovum, which now should be referred to as a(n) _____, undergoes rapid cellular division to form the 16-cell morula.

6. The blastocyst typically enters the uterus 4 to 5 days after fertilization, with implantation occurring _____ days after ovulation.

7. Although the organ function remains as minimal, the _____ system is the first organ to develop rapidly, with the first heartbeats noted between 5.5 and 6 weeks.

8. Gestational sac size and hCG levels increase _____ until 8 menstrual weeks.

9. After 8 weeks, hCG levels _____ and subsequently decline while the gestational sac continues to grow.

10. A normal gestational sac can be consistently demonstrated when the hCG level ranges between 1000~2000 mIU/mL.

11. The sonographer must be aware that when the hCG level is elevated and the gestational sac is not seen within the uterus, a(n) _____ pregnancy should be considered.

Chapter **49** **The Normal First Trimester**

12. The interface between the decidua capsularis and the echogenic, highly vascularized endometrium forms the DOUBLE DECIDUAL SAC sign, which has been reported to be a reliable sign of a viable gestation.

13. The gestational sac size grows at a predictable rate of __1__ mm per day in early pregnancy.

14. The first intragestational sac anatomy seen is the sonographic __YOLK__ sac, which is routinely visualized between 5 and 5.5 weeks' gestation.

15. The limb buds are embryologically recognizable during the __6th__ week of gestation.

16. The spine is also developing during the embryonic period, particularly in the _____ week(s) of gestation.

17. The embryonic face undergoes significant evolution starting in the 5th week of gestation, with palate fusion beginning around the __10-12__ week of gestation.

18. At approximately 10 weeks' gestation, the midgut loop continues to grow and rotate before it descends into the fetal abdomen at about the _____ week.

19. The cystic rhomboid fossa can sonographically be imaged routinely from the _____ week of gestation.

20. It is important to note that the _____ ventricles completely fill the cerebral vault at this time in gestation.

## Exercise 5

*Fill in the blank(s) with the word(s) that best completes the statements about the first trimester of pregnancy.*

1. Sonographically, the gestational sac size or mean sac diameter is determined by calculating the average sum of the __L__, __W__, and __H__ of the gestational sac.

2. Failure to visualize the yolk sac, with a minimum of __12__ mm MSD using transvaginal sonography, should provoke suspicion of abnormal pregnancy.

3. Transabdominal studies have shown that the yolk sac should be seen within mean sac diameters of _____ mm and should always be visualized with a mean sac diameter of 20 mm.

4. The growth rate of the yolk sac has been reported to be approximately _____ mm per millimeter of growth of the MSD when the MSD is less than 15 mm.

5. The early embryo is not identified with transvaginal sonography until heart motion is detected and the crown-rump length measures approximately __3__ mm.

6. The embryonic period is the time between __4__ and 10 weeks' gestation.

7. The primitive neural tube closes by __6__ weeks' gestation.

8. At __8__ weeks, three primary vesicles are seen within the fetal brain: the prosencephalon, the mesencephalon, and the rhombencephalon.

9. During development, the midgut loop of the bowel continues to grow and rotate before it descends into the fetal abdomen at about the __11-12__ week.

**Exercise 6**

*Fill in the blank(s) with the word(s) that best completes the statements about multiple gestations.*

1. Using transvaginal sonography, multiple gestations can readily be diagnosed at very early stages, between

   _____ weeks.

2. Sonographically, dichorionic and diamniotic twins appear as _____2_____ separate gestational sacs with individual trophoblastic tissue, which allows the appearance of a thick dividing membrane.

3. Monochorionic-diamniotic twins appear to be contained within _____1_____ chorionic sac;

   _____2_____ amnion(s), yolk sac(s), and _____2_____ embryos are identified.

4. The monozygotic, monoamniotic-monochorionic twin gestation shows _____1_____ gestational sac with

   _____1_____ amniotic membrane, which may contain one or two yolk sacs and two embryos within the single amniotic membrane.

**Exercise 7**

*Provide a short answer for each question after evaluating the images.*

1. Identify the sonographic findings in this early pregnancy.

   _____

   _____

   _____

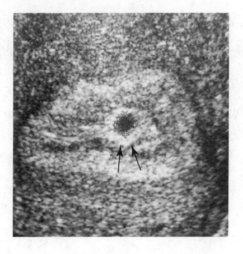

2. Identify the structure that the arrows are pointing to in this 6-week gestation.

_DECIDUA CAPSULARIS_

A

B

3. Identify the disclike structure adjacent to the yolk sac in image A. Identify what the letter "C" represents in image B.

_EMBRYO_               _C_   _CRL_

4. In this 8-week gestation, name the structure that the curved arrow is pointing to. Name the structure that the straight arrows are pointing to.

____AMNIOTIC MEMBRANE_____ ✓ UMBILICAL CORD____

5. What important fetal measurement does this image demonstrate?

____CRL_____

6. Name the type of multiple gestations you would predict from this image.

DICHORIONIC - DIAMNIOTIC

7. Name the type of multiple gestations demonstrated by this sonogram.

MONO CHORIONIC - DIAMNIOTIC    (2 YOLK SACS = 2 AMNIONS)

# 50 First-Trimester Complications

## KEY TERMS

### Exercise 1

*Match the following embryonic abnormality terms with their definitions.*

_____ 1. acrania

_____ 2. anencephaly

_____ 3. bowel herniation

_____ 4. cephalocele

_____ 5. cystic hygroma

_____ 6. gastroschisis

_____ 7. holoprosencephaly

_____ 8. iniencephaly

_____ 9. omphalocele

_____10. Turner's syndrome

_____11. ventriculomegaly

A. Congenital defect of the abdominal wall with protrusion of abdominal contents into the base of the umbilical cord; the cord appears to enter the mass

B. Protrusion of the brain from the cranial cavity

C. Congenital absence of the brain and cranial vault with the cerebral hemispheres missing or reduced to small masses

D. A nonlethal genetic abnormality in which chromosomal makeup is 45 XO instead of the normal 46 XX or XY

E. Congenital defective opening in the wall of the abdomen just to the right of the umbilical cord; bowel and other organs may protrude outside the abdomen from this opening

F. During the first trimester, the bowel normally herniates outside the abdominal cavity between 8 and 12 weeks

G. A rare neural tube defect in which brain tissue protrudes through a fissure in the occiput so that the brain and spinal cord occupy a single cavity characterized by extreme retroflexion of the head

H. Dilation of the cerebral ventricles without enlargement of the cranium

I. Partial or complete absence of the cranium

J. Fluid-filled structure, initially surrounding the neck; may extend upward to the head or laterally to the body

K. Failure of forebrain to divide into cerebral hemispheres, which results in a single large ventricle with varying amounts of cerebral cortex that has been known to occur with trisomies 13 to 15 and trisomy 18

### Exercise 2

*Match the following first-trimester terms with their definitions.*

_____1. anembryonic pregnancy

_____2. spontaneous pregnancy loss

_____3. corpus luteum cyst

_____4. ectopic pregnancy

_____5. gestational trophoblastic disease

_____6. heterotopic pregnancy

_____7. incomplete spontaneous abortion

_____8. interstitial pregnancy

_____9. pseudogestational sac

A. Pregnancy occurring in the fallopian tube near the cornu of the uterus

B. A physiologic cyst that develops within the ovary after ovulation and that secretes progesterone and prevents menses if fertilization occurs; may persist until the 16th to 18th week of pregnancy

C. Simultaneous intrauterine and extrauterine pregnancy

D. Gestational sac without an embryo

E. Pregnancy that implants somewhere other than the center of the uterus

F. Pregnancy loss with products of conception remaining in the uterus

G. Decidual reaction with fluid present within the uterus in a patient with an ectopic pregnancy

H. Additional term for missed abortion or miscarriage

I. Condition in which trophoblastic tissue overtakes the pregnancy and propagates throughout the uterine cavity

**377**

## Exercise 3

*Fill in the blank(s) with the word(s) that best completes the statements, or provide a short answer about the abnormal first trimester.*

1. The dominant structure seen within the embryonic cranium within the first trimester is that of the

   _____, which fills the lateral ventricles that in turn fill the cranial vault.

2. _____ of the cranial vault is not complete in the first trimester; the resulting false cranial border definition may give rise to a false-negative diagnosis for cranial anomaly.

3. An abnormality that may be seen near the end of the first trimester when there is absence of the cranium superior to the orbits with preservation of the base of the skull and facial features with the brain projected from the open

   cranial vault is _____.

4. In _____, the choroid plexus is shown to be "dangling" in the dilated dependent lateral ventricle.

5. On ultrasound, a large posterior fossa cyst that is continuous with the fourth ventricle, an elevated tentorium, and

   dilatation of the third and lateral ventricles may be seen in a fetus with _____.

6. The fetal urinary bladder becomes sonographically apparent at _____ weeks' gestation.

7. One of the most common abnormalities seen sonographically in the first trimester is _____.

8. Sonographically, placental hematomas may be difficult to distinguish from _____ hemorrhages.

9. By far the most common ovarian mass seen in the first trimester of pregnancy is a(n) _____ cyst.

10. List the associated risk factors for ectopic pregnancy.

    _____

    _____

    _____

11. The most important finding in scanning for ectopic pregnancy is to determine if there is a normal intrauterine gestation (thus ruling out the possibility of an ectopic pregnancy), or if the uterine cavity is

    _____ and an adnexal _____ is present.

12. As many as 20% of patients with ectopic pregnancy demonstrate an intrauterine saclike structure known as the

    _____.

13. Cornual pregnancy, or _____, is potentially the most life-threatening of all ectopic gestations.

14. Embryonic cardiac rates lower than _____ beats per minute at any gestational age within the first trimester have been shown to be a poor prognostic finding.

15. The most common occurrence of bleeding in the first trimester results from _____ hemorrhage.

16. Several sonographic findings may be shown with _____ abortion, ranging from an intact gestational sac with a nonliving embryo to a collapsed gestational sac that is grossly misshapen.

17. A proliferative disease of the trophoblast after a pregnancy is _____ disease.

18. In the above condition, serum levels of beta–human chorionic gonadotropin are dramatically _____, often to greater than 100,000 IU/mL.

19. The characteristic "_____" appearance of hydatidiform mole, which includes a moderately echogenic soft tissue mass filling the uterine cavity and studded with small cystic spaces representing hydropic chorionic villi, may be seen on ultrasound.

20. Bilateral _____ cysts have been reported in as many as half of molar pregnancies.

## Exercise 4

*Provide a short answer for each question after evaluating the images.*

A        B

1. The mother presented with an elevated maternal serum alpha-fetoprotein level, larger than appropriate for dates and bleeding. Describe the sonographic findings in this fetus.

_____

_____

_____

A        B

2. A young female in her first trimester presented in the emergency room with elevated human chorionic gonadotropin levels, bleeding, and pelvic pain. What are the sonographic findings?

_____

_____

_____

     Chapter **50** **First-Trimester Complications**

3. Sonogram of a first-trimester pregnancy demonstrates this condition:

_____

_____

_____

4. Name the structure that the arrows are pointing to in this 13-week embryo.

_____

_____

_____

5. This was an ultrasound on a 13.5-week fetus. Describe the sonographic findings.

_____

_____

_____

# 51 Sonography of the Second and Third Trimesters

## KEY TERMS

### Exercise 1

*Match the following terms related to fetal presentation and fetal anatomy with their definitions.*

____F____ 1. apex

____J____ 2. breech

____N____ 3. choroid plexus

____D____ 4. ductus arteriosus

____B____ 5. ductus venosus

____O____ 6. echogenic intracardiac focus

____H____ 7. frontal bossing

____L____ 8. hyperechoic bowel

____G____ 9. micrognathia

____A____ 10. midline echo

____K____ 11. nomogram

____E____ 12. normal situs

____M____ 13. nuchal skin fold

____C____ 14. transverse fetal lie

____I____ 15. vertex

A. Linear echoes located centrally in the fetal head that are produced by the borders of opposing cerebral hemispheres
B. Structure that carries oxygenated blood from the umbilical vein to the inferior vena cava
C. Indicates that fetus is lying transversely in the uterus, horizontal or perpendicular to the maternal sagittal axis
D. Structure that carries oxygenated blood from the pulmonary artery to the descending aorta
E. Typical position of the abdominal organs with the liver and inferior vena cava on the right, the stomach on the left, and the apex of the heart directed toward the left
F. Where the ventricles of the heart come to a point; normally directed toward the left hip
G. Abnormally small chin
H. Protrusion or bulging of the forehead
I. Indicates that the fetus is positioned head-down in the uterus
J. Indicates that the fetal head is toward the fundus of the uterus
K. Written representation by graphs, diagrams, or charts of the relationship between numeric variables
L. Increased echogenicity of the bowel associated with aneuploidy risk and fetal pathology
M. Thickness of the fetal skin at the back of the neck; may be visualized to assess aneuploidy risk
N. Echogenic tissue within the lateral ventricles that produces central nervous system fluid
O. Echo within a fetal heart chamber that is as bright as bone and persists despite changes in the sonographic plane

## SUGGESTED PROTOCOL

### Exercise 2

*Provide a short answer that best completes the statements about the protocol and guidelines for the second and third trimesters.*

1. The second- and third-trimester sonography examination should include the following:

   a. _____

   b. _____

   c. _____

   d. _____

   e. _____

f. _____

g. _____

h. _____

i. _____

j. _____

k. _____

## OBSTETRIC PARAMETERS

### Exercise 3

*Fill in the blank(s) with the word(s) that best completes the statements about obstetric parameters, gravidity, and parity of the first, second, and third trimesters.*

1. Pregnancy can be clinically verified approximately 6 to 8 days after ovulation by the presence of

   ___βhCG___ within the maternal urine or serum.

2. The number of pregnancies, including the present one, is ___GRAVIDITY___.

3. A numeric system that describes all possible pregnancies is used to report ___PARITY___.

4. A G4P2103 describes a patient undergoing her fourth pregnancy. She has had ___2___

   full-term deliveries, ___1___ premature births, ___0___ early pregnancy losses,

   and ___3___ living children.

## NORMAL FETOPLACENTAL ANATOMY

### Exercise 4

*Fill in the blank(s) with the word(s) that best completes the statements about the normal fetoplacental anatomy of the second and third trimesters.*

1. The sonographer should initially determine the position of the fetus in relationship to the position of the

   _____.

2. It is important to remember to view _____ activity at the beginning of each study to ensure that the fetus is alive.

3. After fetal position is conceptualized, the sonographer determines the _____ of the fetus.

4. The fetal position changes less frequently after _____ weeks.

5. If the fetus is lying perpendicular to the long axis of the mother, it is described as a(n) _____ fetal lie.

6. If the fetus is lying longitudinal or parallel to the maternal long axis, it is described as a(n) _____

   (head-down) presentation or a(n) _____ (head-up) presentation.

7. A(n) _____ breech occurs when the hips are extended and one or both feet are the presenting parts closest to the cervix.

8. If the fetus is in a vertex presentation with the fetal spine toward the maternal right side, the right side of the fetus

   is _____, and the left side is _____.

**Exercise 5**

*Fill in the blank(s) with the word(s) that best completes the statements about the normal fetoplacental anatomy of the cranium of the fetus.*

1. Fetal brain tissue, a solid structure, may appear _____ or cystic because of the low density of the tissue.

2. As the brain develops, structures change their sonographic appearances (e.g., the choroid plexuses seem _____ early in pregnancy), but as the brain grows, these structures appear _____ in relationship to the entire brain.

3. By the 12th week of gestation, the cranial bones _____.

4. Two types of brain tissues are highly echogenic, the _____ and the _____, which cover the inner and outer brain surfaces.

5. In a transverse plane, at the most cephalad level within the skull, the contour of the skull should be _____ (depending on exact level) and should have a(n) _____ surface.

6. At the most superior level in the skull, the interhemispheric fissure, or _____, is observed as a membrane separating the brain into two equal hemispheres.

7. The fetal ventricles are important to assess because ventriculomegaly, or hydrocephalus (dilated ventricular system), is a sign of _____ system abnormalities.

8. If the _____ appears to float or dangle within the cavity, measurements of ventricular size are recommended to exclude abnormally enlarged or dilated ventricles (ventriculomegaly).

9. Any ventricle measuring greater than _____ mm is considered outside of normal error ranges and therefore is abnormal, warranting further consultation and prenatal testing.

10. The widest transverse diameter of the skull is the _____ and is therefore the proper level at which to measure the biparietal diameter and to assess the development of midline brain structures.

11. Between the thalamic structures lies the cavity of the _____ ventricle.

12. The circle of _____ may be seen anterior to the midbrain and appears as a triangular region that is highly pulsatile as a result of the midline-positioned anterior cerebral artery and lateral convergence of the middle cerebral arteries.

13. The _____ is located in back of the cerebral peduncles within the posterior fossa.

14. The _____ (a posterior fossa cistern filled with cerebrospinal fluid) lies directly behind the cerebellum.

15. The normal cisterna magna measures _____ mm, with an average size of 5 to 6 mm.

16. In second-trimester sonographic examinations, the thickness of the nuchal skin fold is measured in a plane containing the cavum septi pellucidi, the _____, and the cisterna magna.

**Exercise 6**

*Fill in the blank(s) with the word(s) that best completes the statements, or provide a short answer about the face, spine, and thorax of the fetus.*

1. Facial morphology becomes more apparent in the second trimester, but visualization is heavily dependent on fetal _____, adequate amounts of _____, and excellent _____ window.

2. In a normally proportioned face, each of the segments containing the forehead, the eyes and nose, and the mouth and chin forms approximately _____ of the profile.

3. The oral cavity and the tongue are frequently outlined during fetal _____.

4. Fetal hair is often observed along the _____ of the skull and must not be included in the biparietal diameter measurement.

5. Standard antepartum obstetric examination guidelines require the sonographer to image and record the

_____, _____, and _____ spine.

6. There are _____ ossification points in each vertebra.

7. The double-line appearance of the spine is referred to as the "_____ sign" and is generated by echoes from the posterior and anterior laminae and the spinal cord.

8. In a transverse plane, all three ossification points are visible; the points are spaced _____, and the spinal column appears as a closed circle, indicating closure of the neural tube.

9. Three echoes form a circle that represents the _____ of the vertebral body and the posterior elements (laminae or pedicles).

10. Optimal viewing of the spine occurs when the fetus is lying on its side in a(n) _____ direction with its back a slight distance from the uterine wall.

11. The fluid-filled fetal lungs are observed as solid masses of _____ tissue bordered medially by the heart, inferiorly by the diaphragm, and laterally by the rib cage.

12. List the criteria that are used to assess the fetal heart.

_____

_____

_____

_____

_____

_____

**Exercise 7**

*Fill in the blank(s) with the word(s) that best completes the statements about the diaphragm, fetal circulation, and the abdomen.*

1. The diaphragm is the muscle that separates the thorax and abdomen and is commonly viewed in the

_____ plane.

2. The esophagus and oropharynx help determine the location of the carotid arteries and are outlined when amniotic

fluid is _____ by the fetus.

3. The sonographer should recognize the characteristic arterial _____ from the aorta and its branches.

4. The inferior vena cava is identified coursing to the _____ and parallel with the aorta.

5. Fetal _____ occurs in the placenta, where small fetal vessels on the surface of the villi are bathed by maternal blood within the intervillous spaces.

6. Concentrations of waste products, such as urea and creatinine, are _____ in fetal blood, and these products diffuse into the maternal circulation.

7. Fetal circulation _____ the lungs because fetal lungs do not oxygenate blood.

8. The ductus arteriosus shunts blood _____ from the lungs.

9. Fetal circulation shunts oxygenated blood arriving from the placenta away from the abdomen _____ to the heart and then to the brain.

10. The hepatobiliary system serves the important function of shunting oxygen-rich blood arriving from the placenta directly to the heart through the _____.

11. Oxygenated blood from the placenta flows through the _____ vein, within the umbilical cord, to the fetal cord insertion, where it enters the abdomen.

12. From the umbilicus, the umbilical vein courses cephalad along the _____ ligament to the liver, where it connects with the left portal vein.

13. This blood then filters into the liver sinusoids, returning to the inferior vena cava by drainage into the _____ veins.

14. Inferior vena cava blood flows from the right atrium through the left atrium by way of the _____ ovale.

15. After birth, the _____, the _____, and the _____ close, and fetal circulation converts to the pattern seen throughout the rest of life.

16. The _____ lobe of the liver is larger than the right lobe because of the large quantity of oxygenated blood flowing through it.

17. The fetal _____ appears as a cone-shaped or teardrop-shaped cystic structure located in the right upper abdomen just below the left portal vein.

18. The spleen may be observed by scanning transversely and posteriorly to the left of the _____.

19. The stomach becomes apparent as early as the _____ week of gestation as swallowed amniotic fluid fills the stomach cavity. The full stomach should be seen in all fetuses beyond the _____ week of gestation.

20. The large bowel typically contains _____ particles and may measure up to 20 mm in the preterm fetus and even larger near the time of birth or in the postdate fetus.

21. The kidneys are located on either side of the spine in the posterior abdomen and are apparent as early as the _____ week of pregnancy.

22. The _____ center may be difficult to define in early pregnancy, whereas with continued maturation of the kidneys, the borders become more defined and the renal pelvis becomes more distinct.

23. A renal pelvis that measures greater than _____ mm beyond 20 weeks' gestation is considered abnormal.

24. The center of the adrenal gland appears as a central _____ line surrounded by tissue that is less echogenic.

25. A fetus generally voids at least _____ an hour, so failure to see the bladder should prompt the investigator to recheck for bladder filling.

26. The bladder should be visualized in all _____ fetuses and is an important indicator of renal function.

27. Identification of the male and female genitalia is possible provided the fetal legs are _____ and a sufficient quantity of amniotic fluid is present.

28. The gender of the fetus may be appreciated as early as _____ weeks' gestation, although clear delineation may not be possible until the _____ week.

29. The male genitalia may be differentiated as early as the _____ week of pregnancy.

30. The scrotal sac is seen as a mass of _____ between the hips with the scrotal septum.

**Exercise 8**

*Fill in the blank(s) with the word(s) that best completes the statements about the musculoskeletal system of the fetus.*

1. The sonographer must attempt not only to measure fetal limb bones but also to survey the anatomic configurations

    of the individual bones whenever possible for evidence of _____, _____, or demineralization, as seen in several common forms of skeletal dysplasias.

2. The _____ is found in a sagittal plane by moving the probe laterally away from the ribs and scapula.

3. Epiphyseal ossification centers may be apparent around the _____ week of pregnancy.

4. The laterally positioned _____ projects deeper into the elbow, which is helpful in differentiating this bone from the medially located radius.

5. Coronally, the hands and fingers may be viewed when they are _____.

6. The distal femoral epiphysis is seen within the cartilage at the knee, and this signifies a gestational age beyond

    _____ weeks' gestation.


**Exercise 9**

*Provide a short answer for each question after evaluating the images.*

A                                                                         B

1. What position is the fetus lying in?

_____

2. What is the echogenic structure within the ventricle in image *A*? What is the hypoechoic structure in the center of the fetal head in image *B?* Name the structure that is being measured in image *C*. Identify the level at which the biparietal diameter should be measured.

_____

_____

_____

_____

3. Identify the anatomic parts denoted by *f*, *t*, and *c*.

_____

_____

_____

4. Which fetal side is lying closest to the transducer?

_____

_____

5. Identify what the letter *L* is pointing to in this fetus.

_____

_____

A                                    B

6. Which two anatomic structures are demonstrated here?

_____

_____

7. Name the two echogenic structures demonstrated in this fetus.

_____

_____

# 52 Obstetric Measurements and Gestational Age

## Exercise 1

*Match the following terms related to gestational age assessment with their definitions.*

- G  1. abdominal circumference
- J  2. age range analysis
- L  3. average age
- A  4. binocular distance
- D  5. biparietal diameter
- E  6. crown-rump length
- H  7. embryonic heart rate
- M  8. femoral length
- B  9. gestational sac diameter
- C 10. growth-adjusted sonar age
- I 11. humeral length
- F 12. last menstrual period
- K 13. small for gestational age

A. Measurement that includes both fetal orbits at the same time to predict gestational age
B. Used in the first trimester to estimate appropriate gestational age with menstrual dates
C. Method whereby the fetus is categorized into small, average, or large growth percentile
D. Fetal transverse cranial diameter at the level of the thalamus and cavum septum pellucidum
E. Most accurate measurement for determining gestational age; made in the first trimester
F. Used to determine the start date for human pregnancies
G. Measurement at the level of the stomach, left portal vein, and left umbilical sign
H. Heart rate before the 9th week of gestation
I. Measurement from the humeral head to the distal end of the humerus
J. Size and proportionality of the fetal parameter expressed as age
K. Normal fetus that measures smaller than dates
L. Average age of multiple fetal parameters
M. Measurement of the femoral diaphysis

## Exercise 2

*Match the following abnormal finding terms with their definitions.*

- E  1. anophthalmus
- C  2. banana sign
- I  3. brachycephaly
- F  4. dolichocephaly
- B  5. hypertelorism
- K  6. intrauterine growth restriction
- J  7. lemon sign
- H  8. microphthalmos
- G  9. oxycephaly
- A 10. platycephaly
- D 11. spina bifida

A. Flattening of the vertex of the skull
B. Condition in which the orbits are spaced far apart
C. Refers to the shape of the cerebellum when a spinal defect is present
D. Failure of the vertebrae to close
E. Absence of one or both eyes
F. Fetal head is relatively narrow in the transverse plane and is elongated in the anteroposterior plane
G. Condition of having a relatively high cranial vault with a high or peaked appearance
H. Abnormally small eyes
I. Fetal head is relatively wide in the transverse diameter and shortened in the anteroposterior plane
J. Occurs with spina bifida; frontal lobes collapse inward
K. Condition in which fetus is not growing as fast as normal; usually considered malnourished or abnormal

### Exercise 3

*Fill in the blank(s) with the word(s) that best completes the statements about gestational age assessment in the first trimester.*

1. Sonographically, the earliest sign of intrauterine pregnancy is the ___DECIDUA___, which appears as an echogenic, thickening filling of the fundal region of the endometrial cavity occurring at approximately 3 to 4 weeks' gestation.

2. At 5 weeks, the average of the three perpendicular internal diameters of the gestational sac, calculated as the mean of the ___A-P___ diameter, the ___TRANSVERSE___ diameter, and the ___LONGITUDINAL___ diameter, can provide an adequate estimation of menstrual age.

3. The sac grows rapidly in the first ___10___ weeks, with an average increase of 1 mm per day.

4. When the gestational sac exceeds ___8___ mm in mean internal diameter, a yolk sac should be seen.

5. Normal yolk sac size should be less than ___6___ mm; greater than ___8___ mm has been associated with poor pregnancy outcome.

6. When the mean gestational sac diameter exceeds ___16___ mm, an embryo with definite cardiac activity should be well visualized with transvaginal scanning.

7. The embryonic echoes can be identified as early as 38 to 39 days' menstrual age, and the crown-rump length is usually ___1-2___ mm at this stage.

8. The most accurate sonographic technique for establishing gestational age in the first trimester is ___CRL___.

9. In general, the crown rump length (CRL) should increase at a rate of _____ mm per day.

10. Absence of an embryo by 7 to 8 weeks' gestation is consistent with an embryonic demise or a(n) _____ pregnancy.

11. If a nomogram is not readily available to identify gestational age, a convenient formula is gestational age in weeks equals _____.

## GESTATIONAL AGE ASSESSMENT: SECOND AND THIRD TRIMESTERS

### Exercise 4

*Fill in the blank(s) with the word(s) that best completes the statements about gestational age assessment in the second and third trimesters.*

1. In the second trimester, the gestational age parameters extend to ___BIPARIETAL___ diameter, ___HEAD___ circumference, and ___FEMUR___ length.

2. The reproducibility of the biparietal diameter (BPD) is ± _____ mm (±2 standard deviations).

3. Growth of the fetal skull slows from _____ mm per week in the second trimester to _____ mm per week in the third trimester.

4. The fetal head should be imaged in a transverse _____ section, ideally with the fetus in a direct occiput transverse position.

5. The BPD should be measured perpendicular to the fetal skull at the level of the ___THALAMUS___ and ___CSP___.

6. Intracranial landmarks should include the _____ anteriorly and posteriorly, the

   _____ anteriorly in the midline, and the _____ in the atrium of each lateral
   ventricle.

7. The head shape should be _____, not round, because this can lead to overestimation of
   gestational age, just as a flattened or compressed head can lead to underestimation of gestational age.

8. The calipers should be placed from the _____ edge of the parietal bone to the

   _____ edge of the opposite parietal bone, or "outer edge to inner edge."

9. The _____ head circumference is less affected than BPD by head compression; therefore the
   head circumference (HC) is a valuable tool in assessing gestational age.

10. The proper coronal view should be _____ to the standard transverse HC view passing through
    the thalamus.

11. One can _____ gestational age from a dolichocephalic head or _____ with
    brachycephaly.

12. The AC is very useful in monitoring normal fetal growth and in detecting fetal growth disturbances, such as

    intrauterine growth restriction (IUGR) and macrosomia; however, it is more useful as a(n) _____
    than in predicting gestational age.

13. The fetal abdomen should be measured in a transverse plane at the level of the _____ where the

    _____ vein branches into the left portal sinus.

14. The abdomen should be more _____ than oval because an oval shape indicates an oblique cut
    resulting in a false estimation of size.

15. The ___FEMUR___ length is an especially useful parameter that can be used to date a pregnancy when a
    fetal head cannot be measured because of position, or when there is a fetal head anomaly.

16. Often an echo from the near side of the cartilaginous distal femoral condyles will be seen, called the

    "_____"; this should not be included in the measure of the diaphysis.

17. The tibia and fibula can be measured by first identifying the _____, then following it down until
    the two parallel bones can be identified.

18. Humerus length is sometimes more difficult to measure than femur length because the humerus usually is found

    very close to the fetal _____ but can exhibit a wide range of motion.

19. The ulna can be distinguished from the radius because it penetrates much more deeply into the _____.

## Exercise 5

*Provide a short answer for each question after evaluating the images.*

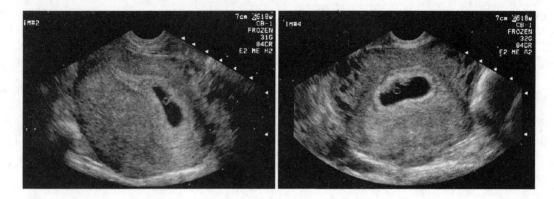

1. Identify the small sonolucent structure within the gestational sac and estimate the gestational age.

_____

_____

2. Identify *f*, *t*, and *c* in this image of the fetal biparietal diameter.

_____

_____

3. Identify *sp* and *st*. Which measurement should be made at this level?

_____

_____

# 53 Fetal Growth Assessment by Sonography

## KEY TERMS

### Exercise 1

*Match the following fetal growth terms with their definitions.*

_____ 1. amniotic fluid index

_____ 2. biophysical profile

_____ 3. estimated fetal weight

_____ 4. intrauterine growth restriction (IUGR)

_____ 5. large for gestational age

_____ 6. macrosomia

_____ 7. nonstress test

_____ 8. placental grade

_____ 9. postterm

_____ 10. preterm

_____ 11. pulsed wave Doppler

_____ 12. small for gestational age

A. Type of Doppler used in most fetal examinations; the transducer can both send and receive signals
B. Technique of grading the placenta for maturity
C. Decreased rate of fetal growth; may be symmetrical or asymmetrical
D. Fetus born earlier than the normal 38- to 42-week gestational period
E. Assessment of fetus to determine fetal well-being; includes evaluation of cardiac nonstress test, fetal breathing movement, gross fetal body movements, fetal tone, and amniotic fluid volume
F. Birth weight greater than 4000 g or above the 90th percentile for the estimated gestational age
G. Fetus born later than the 42-week gestational period
H. Incorporation of all fetal growth parameters
I. Normal fetus measures smaller than dates
J. Uses Doptone to record the fetal heart rate and its reactivity to the stress of uterine contraction
K. Sum of the four quadrants of amniotic fluid
L. Fetus measures larger than dates (diabetic fetus)

## FETAL GROWTH ASSESSMENT

### Exercise 2

*Fill in the blank(s) with the word(s) that best completes the statements, or provide a short answer about intrauterine growth restriction.*

1. Intrauterine growth restriction is most commonly defined as a fetal weight at or below _____% for a given gestational age.

2. Identify the most significant maternal factors for IUGR.

   _____

   _____

   _____

3. Identify the structures that should be measured to determine gestational age during the second or third trimester.

   _____

   _____

   _____

4. _____ IUGR is usually the result of a first-trimester insult, such as a chromosomal abnormality or infection.

5. _____ IUGR begins late in the second or third trimester and usually results from placental insufficiency.

6. Symmetrical growth restriction is characterized by a fetus that is _____ in all physical parameters (e.g., biparietal diameter [BPD], head circumference [HC], abdominal circumference [AC], femur length [FL]).

7. Asymmetrical IUGR is characterized by an appropriate BPD and HC and a disproportionately small

_____.

## Exercise 3
*Fill in the blank(s) with the word(s) that best completes the statements, or provide a short answer about ultrasound diagnostic criteria for fetal growth parameters.*

1. Fetal blood is shunted away from other vital organs to nourish the fetal brain, giving the fetus an appropriate BPD

   (±1 standard deviation) for the true gestational age in the _____ theory.

2. A problem with using the BPD as a predictor of IUGR is the potential alteration in fetal _____ shape secondary to oligohydramnios.

3. In IUGR, the fetal _____ is one of the most severely affected body organs, which alters the circumference of the fetal abdomen.

4. The association between IUGR and _____ is well recognized and has been associated with fetal renal anomalies, rupture of the intrauterine membranes, and postdate pregnancy.

## Exercise 4
*Fill in the blank(s) with the word(s) that best completes the statements, or provide a short answer about the biophysical profile and intrauterine growth restriction.*

1. List the five requirements in the biophysical profile.

   _____

   _____

   _____

   _____

   _____

2. Doppler ultrasound has shown that in fetuses with asymmetrical IUGR, the vascular resistance _____

   in the aorta and umbilical artery and _____ in the fetal middle cerebral artery.

3. In the umbilical circulation, extreme cases of elevated _____ causing absent or reverse end-diastolic flow velocity waveforms are associated with high rates of morbidity and mortality.

4. Macrosomia has classically been defined as a birth weight of _____ g or greater or above the 90th percentile for estimated gestational age.

5. Macrosomia is also a common result of poorly controlled maternal _____.

## Exercise 5

*Provide a short answer for each question after evaluating the images.*

A    B

C    D

1. Name the fetal assessment that these images are demonstrating.

_____

_____

_____

_____

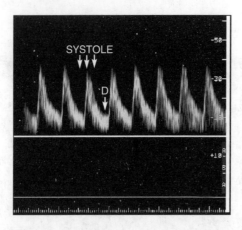

2. Does this flow velocity pattern of the fetal umbilical artery represent normal or abnormal flow?

_____

_____

3. Determine whether this flow velocity pattern represents a high-resistance or low-resistance profile. Describe the follow-up and possible complications for this fetus.

_____

_____

_____

# 54 Sonography and High-Risk Pregnancy

## Exercise 1

*Match the following terms related to high-risk pregnancy with their definitions.*

_____ 1. anasarca

_____ 2. caudal regression syndrome

_____ 3. conjoined twins

_____ 4. dizygotic

_____ 5. eclampsia

_____ 6. fetus papyraceus

_____ 7. hydrops fetalis

_____ 8. hyperemesis gravidarum

_____ 9. maternal serum alpha-fetoprotein

_____ 10. maternal serum quad screen

_____ 11. monozygotic

_____ 12. nonimmune hydrops

_____ 13. oligohydramnios

_____ 14. polyhydramnios

_____ 15. preeclampsia

_____ 16. pregnancy-induced hypertension

_____ 17. premature rupture of the membranes

_____ 18. Rh blood group

_____ 19. Spalding's sign

_____ 20. systemic lupus erythematosus

_____ 21. twin–twin transfusion syndrome

A. Too little amniotic fluid; fluid measures less than 5 on the amniotic fluid index

B. Coma and seizures in the second- or third-trimester patient secondary to pregnancy-induced hypertension

C. System of antigens that may be found on the surface of red blood cells

D. Occurs when division of the egg takes place after 13 days

E. Blood test conducted during the second trimester to identify pregnancies at higher risk for chromosomal anomalies and neural tube defects

F. Elevation of maternal blood pressure that may put fetus at risk

G. Inflammatory disease involving multiple organ systems

H. Fluid occurring in at least two areas: pleural effusion, pericardial effusion, ascites, or skin edema

I. Group of conditions in which hydrops is present in the fetus but not as a result of fetomaternal blood group incompatibility

J. Twins that arise from two separately fertilized ova

K. Too much amniotic fluid; fluid measures greater than 22 on the amniotic fluid index

L. Lack of development of the caudal spine and cord that may occur in the fetus of a diabetic mother

M. Overlapping of the skull bones; indicates fetal death

N. Twins that arise from a single fertilized egg, which divides to produce two identical fetuses

O. Excessive vomiting that leads to dehydration and electrolyte imbalance

P. Fetal death that occurs after the fetus has reached a certain growth that is too large to resorb into the uterus

Q. Complication of pregnancy characterized by increasing hypertension, proteinuria, and edema

R. Antigen present in the fetus

S. Leaking or breaking of the amniotic membranes causing loss of amniotic fluid that may lead to premature delivery or infection

T. Severe generalized massive edema often seen with fetal hydrops

U. Monozygotic twin pregnancy with single placenta and arteriovenous shunt within the placenta

**Exercise 2**

*Fill in the blank(s) with the word(s) that best completes the statements, or provide a short answer about infertility.*

1. A patient who will be 35 or older at the time of delivery is described as _____.

2. In the first trimester, testing is performed by looking for the pattern of biochemical markers associated with plasma protein A (PAPP-A) and free **BhCG3. These laboratory values are used in conjunction with an ultrasound (performed between 11 and 14 weeks) to measure the _____ translucency.

3. Second-trimester screening can be performed with the maternal serum _____ screen laboratory value and a targeted ultrasound examination.

4. A detailed evaluation of all fetal anatomy that can be seen at the time between 18 and 20 weeks' gestation is the _____ sonogram.

5. A condition in which excessive fluid accumulates within the fetal body cavities is _____.

6. Excessive fluid accumulation may result in _____, _____, _____, _____, _____, or _____.

7. Any substance that elicits an immunologic response, such as production of an antibody to that substance, is a(n) _____.

8. Sonographic findings of hydrops are _____ edema, _____ effusion, _____ effusion, _____, _____, and _____ placenta.

9. A procedure in which a needle is placed into the fetal umbilical vein and a blood sample is obtained is _____.

10. Infants with _____ are at increased risk for intracerebral hemorrhage in utero and spontaneous bleeding.

11. A group of conditions in which hydrops is present in the fetus but is not a result of fetomaternal blood group incompatibility is _____.

12. Cardiovascular lesions are often the most frequent causes of non-immune hydrops. Congestive heart failure may result from _____ cardiac problems, such as dysrhythmias, tachycardias, and myocarditis, and from _____ anomalies, such as hypoplastic left heart and other types of congenital heart disease.

13. If glucose levels are very high and uncontrolled, the fetus may also become _____.

14. If delivery of a macrosomic infant is attempted vaginally, the physician may have difficulty delivering the shoulders of the baby after the head has delivered. This is termed _____.

15. Anomalies associated with diabetes include congenital heart and neural tube defects. The most common cardiac problems in the diabetic fetus include _____ and _____.

16. Caudal regression syndrome (lack of development of the caudal spine and cord) is seen almost exclusively in _____ individuals.

17. Hypertensive pregnancies may be associated with _____ placentas because of the effects of hypertension on the blood vessels.

18. The occurrence of seizures or coma in a preeclamptic patient is representative of _____.

19. A chronic autoimmune disorder that can affect almost all organ systems in the body is _____.

20. _____ exists when a pregnant woman vomits so much that she develops dehydration and electrolyte imbalance.

21. Describe the combination of effects that may cause hydronephrosis.

_____

_____

_____

## PREGNANCY COMPLICATIONS

### Exercise 3

*Fill in the blank(s) with the word(s) that best completes the statements, or provide a short answer about complications of pregnancy.*

1. Intrauterine fetal death accounts for roughly _____ of all perinatal mortality.

2. Fetal heart tones should be heard with Doppler at approximately _____ weeks' gestation.

3. At 20 weeks' gestation, the uterine fundal height should have risen to the umbilicus, and the uterus should measure approximately _____ cm above the symphysis pubis.

4. The mother should also perceive fetal movements on a daily basis beginning between _____ weeks' gestation

5. List five sonographic findings that are associated with fetal death.

_____

_____

_____

_____

_____

## MULTIPLE GESTATION PREGNANCY

### Exercise 4

*Fill in the blank(s) with the word(s) that best completes the statements about multiple gestation pregnancy.*

1. The mother with a multiple gestation is at increased risk for obstetric complications, such as _____, _____ bleeding, and _____ cord.

2. A twin has a(n) _____ times greater chance of perinatal death than a singleton fetus.

3. During the first trimester, multiple pregnancy can be identified by visualizing more than one _____ sac within the uterus.

4. _____ twins arise from two separately fertilized ova. Each ovum implants separately in the uterus and develops its own placenta, chorion, and amniotic sac (_____, _____).

5. Identical or _____ twins arise from a single fertilized egg, which divides, resulting in two genetically identical fetuses.

6. Depending on whether the fertilized egg divides _____ or _____, there may be one or two placentas, chorions, and amniotic sacs.

7. If division occurs _____ 0 to 4 days post conception, two amnions and two chorions (dichorionic, diamniotic) will be present.

8. If division occurs at _____ days, one chorion and two amniotic sacs (monochorionic, diamniotic) will be present.

9. If division occurs after 8 days, two fetuses will be present but only one chorion and one amnion. This is called a _____ chorionic, _____ amniotic twin pregnancy.

10. If division occurs after 13 days, the division may be incomplete and _____ twins may result.

11. Stuck twin syndrome, or _____ sequence, is characterized by a diamniotic pregnancy with polyhydramnios in one sac and severe oligohydramnios and a smaller twin in the other sac.

12. Twin–twin transfusion syndrome exists when a(n) _____ shunt is placed within the placenta.

13. By definition, a rare anomaly occurring in monochorionic twins in which one twin develops without a heart and often with absence of the upper half of the body is _____ anomaly.

14. When scanning multiple gestations, the sonographer should always attempt to determine whether one or two _____ sacs are present by locating the membrane that separates the sacs.

15. It is important to keep in mind that a fetus from a multiple gestation is usually _____ than a singleton fetus.

16. No flow and _____ flow during diastole are signs of fetal jeopardy that may prompt the obstetrician to do further fetal well-being testing or even to deliver the fetuses.

### Exercise 5

*Provide a short answer for each question after evaluating the images.*

A

B

C

1. Erythroblastosis fetalis is a condition marked by several sonographic findings. Identify which abnormality is shown in each image (**A, B, C**).

   _____

   _____

   _____

   _____

2. Name the abnormality demonstrated in this image.

_____

_____

3. Identify the abnormality demonstrated in this fetus with nonimmune hydrops. Identify *v* in image **B**.

_____

_____

_____

A=2.36cm
B=2.72cm
DIST=1.63cm

4. Describe the abnormality seen in this patient, who is pregnant with triplets.

_____

_____

_____

5. This sonogram represents what type of twin gestation?

_____

_____

**409**

6. This sonogram depicts what type of twinning?

_____

_____

7. This patient presented with a gestation larger than dates. Describe the sonographic findings.

_____

_____

_____

_____

# 55 Prenatal Diagnosis of Congenital Anomalies

## KEY TERMS

### Exercise 1

*Match the following prenatal diagnosis terms with their definitions.*

_____ 1. alpha-fetoprotein (AFP)

_____ 2. amniocentesis

_____ 3. cystic hygroma

_____ 4. hypertelorism

_____ 5. hypoplasia

_____ 6. hypotelorism

_____ 7. intrauterine growth restriction

_____ 8. micrognathia

_____ 9. omphalocele

_____10. polydactyly

_____11. TORCH

A. Abnormally small chin; commonly associated with other fetal anomalies

B. Transabdominal removal of amniotic fluid from the amniotic cavity using ultrasound

C. Underdevelopment of a tissue, organ, or body

D. An acronym originally coined from the first letters of toxoplasmosis, rubella, cytomegalovirus, and herpesvirus type 2

E. Dilatation of jugular lymph sacs caused by improper drainage of the lymphatic system into the venous system

F. Anterior abdominal wall defect in which abdominal organs are atypically located within the umbilical cord; highly associated with cardiac, central nervous system, renal, and chromosomal anomalies

G. Abnormally wide-spaced orbits usually found in conjunction with congenital anomalies and mental retardation

H. Abnormally closely spaced orbits; associated with holoprosencephaly, chromosomal and central nervous system disorders, and cleft palate

I. Anomalies of the hands or feet in which there is an addition of a digit; may be found in association with certain skeletal dysplasias

J. Decreased rate of fetal growth, usually fetal weight below the 10th percentile for a given gestational age

K. Protein manufactured by the fetus, which can be studied in amniotic fluid and maternal serum

## GENETIC TESTING

### Exercise 2

*Fill in the blank(s) with the word(s) that best completes the statements about genetic testing.*

1. A major congenital anomaly is found in _____ of every 100 births, and an additional 10% to 15% of births are complicated by minor birth defects.

2. An ultrasound-directed biopsy of the placenta or chorionic villi (chorion frondosum) is _____.

3. A specialized prenatal test that permits direct viewing of the developing embryo using a transcervical endoscope

   inserted into the extracoelomic cavity during the first trimester of pregnancy is _____.

4. The technique first used to relieve polyhydramnios, to predict Rh isoimmunization, and to document fetal lung maturity is _____.

5. The amniocentesis technique for multiple gestations is similar to the singleton method, except that _____ fetal sac is entered.

6. Another method in which chromosomes are analyzed is _____.

7. The major protein in fetal serum that is also produced by the yolk sac in early gestation and later by the fetal liver is _____.

8. AFP is transported into the _____ by fetal urination and reaches maternal circulation or blood through the fetal membranes.

9. Common reasons for high AFP levels are _____, such as anencephaly and open spina bifida.

10. Two common abdominal wall defects, _____ and _____, produce elevations of AFP.

11. It is expected that the AFP level in a twin pregnancy will be _____ that of a singleton pregnancy.

12. The quadruple screen was formerly known as the triple test or triple screen; this biochemical screening test combined three serum markers: _____, _____, and _____, plus another maternal serum marker, dimeric inhibin.

## MEDICAL GENETICS

### Exercise 3
*Fill in the blank(s) with the word(s) that best completes the statements about medical genetics.*

1. A normal karyotype consists of _____ chromosomes, _____ pairs of autosomes, and a pair of sex chromosomes.

2. An abnormality of the number of chromosomes is _____.

3. One of the most common aneuploid conditions is _____ syndrome, in which an individual has an extra chromosome number 21.

4. An inherited dominant disorder carries a(n) _____% chance that each time pregnancy occurs, the fetus will have the condition.

5. A recessive disorder is caused by a pair of defective genes, one inherited from each parent. With each pregnancy, the parents have a(n) _____% chance of having a fetus with the disorder.

6. X-linked disorders are inherited by _____ from their mothers.

7. Each of the _____ of female carriers of X-linked disorders has a 50% chance of being affected, and each of the _____ has a 50% chance of being a carrier.

8. An abnormal event that arises because of the interaction of one or more genes and environmental factors is a(n) _____ condition.

9. The occurrence of a gene mutation or chromosomal abnormality in a portion of an individual's cells is _____.

**Exercise 4**

*Fill in the blank(s) with the word(s) that best completes the statements, or provide a short answer about chromosomal abnormalities.*

1. An abnormal fluid collection behind the fetal neck has been strongly associated with _____.

2. A nuchal translucency of _____ mm or greater has been used to define an abnormal thickness.

3. The translucency should be oriented perpendicular to the ultrasound beam, and the measurement should be taken from inside the fetal _____ to inside the _____ membrane.

4. A measurement of _____ mm increases the risk of aneuploidy four times, and nuchal translucencies of _____ mm and greater carry an even greater risk.

5. List the anomalies associated with Down's syndrome.

   _____

   _____

   _____

   _____

6. List the anomalies associated with trisomy 18.

   _____

   _____

   _____

   _____

7. List the anomalies associated with trisomy 13.

   _____

   _____

   _____

   _____

8. List the anomalies associated with triploidy.

   _____

   _____

   _____

   _____

9. A genetic abnormality marked by absence of the X or Y chromosome is _____ syndrome (45,X).

10. The most pathognomonic finding for the above disorder is _____. Other physical features include cardiac anomalies, which are commonly present, with _____ being the most common.

**413**

## Exercise 5

*Provide a short answer for each question after evaluating the images.*

A

B

C

SINGLE AV VALVE

D

(Image **A** from Henningsen C: *Clinical guide to ultrasonography,* St Louis, 2004, Mosby.) (Image **C** courtesy G. Goreczky, RDMS, Maternal Fetal Center at Florida Hospital, Orlando, Fla.)

1. Describe the sonographic findings in each of these images of different fetuses with trisomy 21.

A. _____

B. _____

C. _____

D. _____

2. A fetus with trisomy 13 presented with alobar holoprosencephaly. Describe the other sonographic findings.

_____

_____

_____

_____

_____

Chapter **55** **Prenatal Diagnosis of Congenital Anomalies**

(From Henningsen C: *Clinical guide to ultrasonography,* St Louis, 2004, Mosby.)

3. A fetus with trisomy 13 is presented for ultrasound examination. Describe the sonographic findings.

_____

_____

_____

_____

_____

4. A fetus with Turner's syndrome is presented. Describe the sonographic findings.

_____

_____

# 56 Placenta

## KEY TERMS

### Exercise 1

*Match the following terms related to embryogenesis with their definitions.*

_____ 1. basal plate

_____ 2. battledore placenta

_____ 3. chorion frondosum

_____ 4. chorionic plate

_____ 5. chorionic villi

_____ 6. decidua basalis

_____ 7. decidua capsularis

_____ 8. placenta previa

A. Portion of the chorion that develops into the fetal portion of the placenta

B. Placenta grows in the lower uterine segment and covers all or part of the cervix

C. Microscopic vascular projections from the chorion that combine with maternal uterine tissue to form the placenta

D. Maternal surface of the placenta that lies contiguous with the decidua basalis

E. Part of the decidua that surrounds the chorionic sac

F. Part of the decidua that unites with the chorion to form the placenta

G. Cord insertion into the margin of the placenta

H. Part of the chorionic membrane that covers the placenta

### Exercise 2

*Match the following terms associated with sonographic evaluation of the umbilical cord and placenta with their definitions.*

_____ 1. abruptio placentae

_____ 2. Braxton Hicks contractions

_____ 3. circum-marginate placenta

_____ 4. circumvallate placenta

_____ 5. ductus venosus

_____ 6. ligamentum venosum

_____ 7. lower uterine segment (LUS)

_____ 8. molar pregnancy

_____ 9. placenta accreta

_____10. placenta increta

_____11. placenta percreta

_____12. placental migration

_____13. succenturiate placenta

_____14. vasa previa

_____15. Wharton's jelly

A. Also known as gestational trophoblastic disease; abnormal proliferation of trophoblastic cells in the first trimester

B. Fibrous remains of the ductus venosus from fetal circulation

C. Growth of the chorionic villi superficially to the myometrium; does not penetrate through the myometrium

D. Spontaneous painless uterine contractions that occur throughout a pregnancy

E. Occurs when the intramembranous vessels course across the internal cervical os

F. The placenta is attached to the uterine wall; as the uterus enlarges, the placenta "moves" with it. Therefore a low-lying placenta may move out of the uterine segment in the second trimester.

G. Lower part of the uterine cavity, which expands during pregnancy and joins with the cervical canal

H. Mucoid connective tissue that surrounds the vessels within the umbilical cord

I. Growth of the chorionic villi deep into the myometrium

J. Placental condition in which the chorionic plate is smaller than the basal plate; the margin is raised with a rolled edge

K. One or more accessory lobes connected to the body of the placenta by blood vessels

L. Connection that is patent during fetal life from the left portal vein to the systemic veins (inferior vena cava)

M. Premature detachment of the placenta from the maternal wall

N. Growth of the chorionic villi through the myometrium to the uterine serosa

O. Placental condition in which the chorionic plate is smaller than the basal plate, with a flat interface between the fetal membranes and the placenta

## Exercise 3

*Label the following illustrations.*

1. The placenta.

9. _____

8. _____

7. _____

6. _____

1. _____

2. _____

3. _____

4. _____

5. _____

2. The chorionic villi.

1. _____

8. _____

7. _____

6. _____

5. _____

2. _____

3. _____

4. _____

3. The major functioning unit of the placenta.

1. _____  2. _____  3. _____

4. _____

5. _____

6. _____

12. _____

11. _____

10. _____

7. _____

8. _____

9. _____

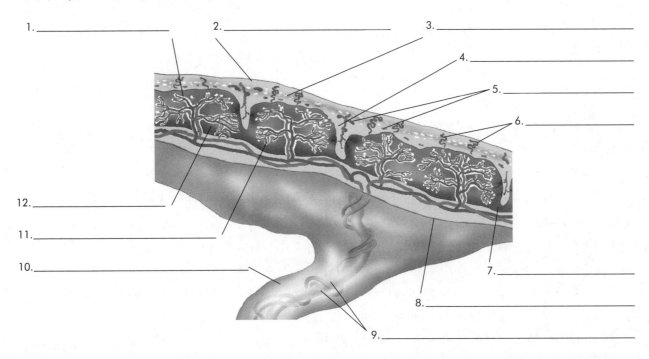

## Exercise 4

*Fill in the blank(s) with the word(s) that best completes the statements, or provide a short answer about the anatomy and physiology of the placenta.*

1. The major role of the placenta is to permit the exchange of _____ maternal blood (rich in oxygen and nutrients) with _____ fetal blood.

2. Maternal vessels course _____ to the placenta and circulate blood into the placenta, whereas blood from the fetus reaches this point through the _____.

3. The fetal surface of the placenta, which is contiguous with the surrounding chorion, is termed the _____.

4. The maternal portion of the placenta that lies contiguous with the decidua basalis is termed the _____.

5. The major functioning unit of the placenta is the _____.

6. Before birth, the fetal membranes and the placenta perform the following functions and activities: _____, _____, _____, and _____.

7. Oxygenated maternal blood is brought to the placenta through 80 to 100 end branches of the uterine arteries—the _____ arteries.

8. The maternal placental circulation may be reduced by a variety of conditions that decrease uterine blood flow, such as severe _____, _____ disease, or _____ infarction.

9. List the three main functions of the placenta.

_____

_____

_____

10. The attachment of the cord is usually near the _____ of the placenta.

11. Most of the amniotic fluid comes from the maternal _____ by diffusion across the amnion from the decidua parietalis and intervillous spaces of the placenta.

12. In the first trimester, the fetus begins to _____ urine into the sac to fill the amniotic cavity; the fetus _____ this fluid, and the cycle continues throughout pregnancy.

## PATHOLOGY

### Exercise 5

*Fill in the blank(s) with the word(s) that best completes the statements, or provide a short answer about the pathology of the placenta.*

1. The placenta is separated from the myometrium by a(n) _____ venous complex.

2. Although the placenta increases in size and volume with gestational age, the maximum thickness does not exceed _____.

3. The sonographer should always describe the _____ of the placenta.

4. For the sonographer to visualize the internal os of the cervix, the patient should have a _____.

5. When the sonographer sees two separate parts of the placenta that do not appear to communicate, a(n) _____ placenta should be considered.

6. Before 20 weeks, uterine artery Doppler typically shows a(n) _____ flow, _____ resistance pattern, particularly for the uterine artery on the same side as the placenta.

7. Maternal diabetes and Rh incompatibility are primary causes for _____.

8. Placenta _____ is the implantation of the placenta in the lower uterine segment in advance of the fetus.

9. With _____ previa, the cervical internal os is completely covered by placental tissue.

10. Other approaches that are useful in evaluating the lower uterine segment with ultrasound when the definition of the placenta needs to be clarified include _____ and _____.

11. A potentially life-threatening fetal complication of the placenta that occurs when large fetal vessels run in the fetal membranes across the cervical os is _____ previa, which places them at risk of rupture and hemorrhage.

12. Abnormal adherence of part or all of the placenta with partial or complete absence of the decidua basalis is _____ accreta.

13. The risk of placenta accreta increases in patients with placenta previa and uterine scar from previous _____.

14. Placenta _____ results from underdeveloped decidualization of the endometrium.

15. The attachment of the placental membranes to the fetal surface of the placenta rather than to the placental margin is a(n) _____ placenta.

16. The separation of a normally implanted placenta before term delivery is referred to as placental _____.

17. _____ abruption results from the rupture of spiral arteries and is a "high-pressure" bleed.

18. _____ abruption results from tears of the marginal veins and represents a "low-pressure" bleed.

19. A focal discrete lesion caused by ischemic necrosis is placental _____.

20. In _____ disease, the sonogram shows a uterine size larger than dates, no identifiable parts, and an inhomogeneous texture with variously sized cystic structures of the placenta that represent multiple vesicular changes throughout the placenta.

21. The second most common tumor of the placenta is known as _____.

## Exercise 6

*Provide a short answer for each question after evaluating the images.*

1. Where is the cord insertion in this sonographic image?

_____

_____

A                                                              B

2. Describe the findings in these two images of the placenta.

_____

_____

3. What structure is the arrow pointing to?

_____

_____

A                                                                                    B

4. This is an image of the lower uterine segment in a patient who has been bleeding for 3 days with bright red blood. Describe the sonographic finding.

_____

_____

5. What structure is the arrow pointing to in this image of the placenta?

_____

_____

6. This patient presented with a posterior placenta. What are the arrows pointing to?

_____

_____

# 57 | Umbilical Cord

## Exercise 1

*Match the following terms related to the umbilical cord with their definitions.*

_____ 1. allantoic duct

_____ 2. battledore placenta

_____ 3. ductus venosus

_____ 4. false knots of the umbilical cord

_____ 5. gastroschisis

_____ 6. hemangioma of the cord

_____ 7. membranous (velamentous) insertion of the cord

_____ 8. nuchal cord

_____ 9. omphalocele

_____ 10. omphalomesenteric cyst

_____ 11. single umbilical artery

_____ 12. superior vesical arteries

_____ 13. true knots of the umbilical cord

_____ 14. umbilical herniation

_____ 15. vasa previa

_____ 16. Wharton's jelly

_____ 17. yolk stalk

A. Cord inserts into the membranes before it enters the placenta

B. Failure of the bowel, stomach, and liver to return to the abdominal cavity; completely covered by a peritoneal-amniotic membrane

C. The smaller, shorter, and posterior of the two branches into which the umbilical vein divides after entering the abdomen. It empties into the inferior vena cava

D. Marginal or eccentric insertion of the umbilical cord into the placenta

E. Umbilical duct connecting the yolk sac with the embryo

F. Failure of the anterior abdominal wall to close completely at the level of the umbilicus

G. Myxomatous connective tissue that surrounds the umbilical vessels and varies in size

H. Elongated duct that contributes to development of the umbilical cord and placenta during the first trimester

I. High association of congenital anomalies with this

J. Occurs when blood vessels are longer than the cord; they fold on themselves and produce nodulations on the surface of the cord

K. Cystic lesion of the umbilical cord

L. Occurs when the cord is wrapped around the fetal neck

M. Vascular tumor within the umbilical cord

N. Arise from fetal movements and are more likely to develop during early pregnancy, when relatively more amniotic fluid is present; associated with advanced maternal age, multiparity, and long umbilical cords

O. Occurs when the umbilical cord vessels cross the internal os of the cervix

P. Anomaly in which part of the bowel remains outside the abdominal wall without a membrane

Q. After birth, the umbilical arteries are known as these

## Exercise 2

*Fill in the blank(s) with the word(s) that best completes the statements about the development and normal anatomy of the umbilical cord.*

1. The umbilical cord is the essential link for _____ and important nutrients among the fetus, the placenta, and the mother.

2. The intestines grow at a faster rate than the abdomen and _____ into the proximal umbilical cord at approximately 7 weeks, where they remain until approximately 10 weeks.

3. The umbilical cord includes _____ umbilical arteries and _____ umbilical vein and is surrounded by a homogeneous substance called _____ jelly.

4. The intraabdominal portions of the umbilical vessels degenerate after birth; the umbilical arteries become the lateral ligaments of the _____, and the umbilical vein becomes the round ligament of the

    _____.

5. From the left portal vein, the umbilical blood flows through the _____ to the systemic veins, bypassing the liver, or through the right portal sinus to the right portal vein.

6. The ductus venosus forms the conduit between the _____ system and the _____ veins.

7. The ductus venosus is patent during fetal life until shortly after birth, when transformation of the ductus into the ligamentum _____ occurs (beginning in the second week after birth).

8. The umbilical arteries run along the _____ margin of the fetal bladder and are well imaged with color flow Doppler. In the postpartum stage, the umbilical arteries become the superior vesical arteries.

9. The diameter of the umbilical cord has been measured to be between _____ and _____ cm; variations in cord diameter are usually attributed to diffuse accumulation of Wharton's jelly.

## PATHOLOGY

## Exercise 3

*Fill in the blank(s) with the word(s) that best completes the statements about the pathology of the umbilical cord.*

1. _____ knots of the umbilical cord have been associated with long cords, polyhydramnios, intrauterine growth restriction, and monoamniotic twins.

2. _____ knots of the umbilical cord are seen when the blood vessels are longer than the cord.

3. The most common cord entanglement in the fetus is _____ cord.

4. When the cord implants into the edge of the placenta instead of into the middle, the condition is called _____ placenta.

5. Membranous, or _____, insertion of the cord occurs when the cord inserts into the membranes before it enters the placenta, rather than inserting directly into the placenta.

6. When the cord lies below the presenting part, _____ of the umbilical cord occurs.

7. _____ of the cord reduces or cuts off the blood supply to the fetus and may result in fetal demise.

8. The sonographic detection of a _____ umbilical artery should prompt the investigation of further fetal anomalies.

**Exercise 4**

*Provide a short answer for each question after evaluating the images.*

1. Describe the findings in these images in a third-trimester fetus.

   A. _____

   B. _____

   C. _____

2. Identify which image has a right/left twist to the umbilical cord.

   _____

   _____

3. This mass was seen to project outside the fetal abdomen. The abnormality you suspect is:

_____

_____

4. Which abnormality is visible on this image of a fetal abdomen?

_____

_____

5. How would you describe this cord insertion?

_____

_____

A

B

6. Identify the normal and abnormal Doppler flow pattern of the umbilical cord in these two images.

A. _____

B. _____

# 58 Amniotic Fluid and Fetal Membranes

## KEY TERMS

### Exercise 1

*Match the following terms related to amniotic fluid assessment and abnormal volumes with their definitions.*

_____1. amniotic cavity

_____2. amniotic fluid

_____3. amniotic fluid index (AFI)

_____4. maximum vertical pocket

_____5. placental insufficiency

_____6. polyhydramnios

_____7. oligohydramnios

_____8. subjective assessment of fluid

_____9. vernix caseosa

A. Sonographer surveys uterine cavity for visual determination of amniotic fluid present
B. Produced by the umbilical cord and membranes, the fetal lung, skin, and kidney
C. Each of the four uterine quadrants is evaluated with the transducer perpendicular to the table in the deepest vertical pocket without fetal parts; the four quadrants are added together to determine this
D. Too little amniotic fluid; associated with intrauterine growth restriction, renal anomalies, premature rupture of membranes, postdate pregnancy, and other factors
E. Fatty material found on fetal skin and in amniotic fluid late in pregnancy
F. Method used to determine the amount of amniotic fluid
G. Structure that forms early in gestation and surrounds the embryo
H. Too much amniotic fluid; associated with central nervous system disorders, gastrointestinal anomalies, fetal hydrops, skeletal anomalies, renal disorders, and other factors
I. Inability of the placenta to provide adequate blood/nutrient supply to the fetus because of underlying maternal disease

### Exercise 2

*Match the following terms related to fetal membranes with their definitions.*

_____ 1. amniotic band syndrome

_____ 2. anasarca

_____ 3. ascites

_____ 4. Asherman's syndrome

_____ 5. chorioamnionitis

_____ 6. corticosteroid therapy

_____ 7. hydrops fetalis

_____ 8. immune hydrops fetalis

_____ 9. nonimmune hydrops fetalis

_____10. pericardial effusion

A. Condition in which the amniotic bag breaks, labor has not begun, and the pregnancy is less than 37 weeks' gestation
B. Condition in which the amniotic bag breaks with labor or just after labor begins
C. Scars within the uterus secondary to previous gynecologic surgery
D. Abnormal serous fluid collection found in the abdomen or pelvis
E. Accumulation of abnormal fluid collections caused by Rhesus factor incompatibility
F. Generalized swelling and edema of skin throughout the body
G. Abnormal collection of fluid surrounding the heart measuring greater than 2 mm

**431**

_____11. pleural effusion

_____12. premature rupture of membranes

_____13. spontaneous premature rupture of membranes

_____14. uterine synechiae

H. Multiple fibrous strands of amnion that develop in utero that may entangle fetal parts to cause amputations or malformations of the fetus

I. Bacterial infection of the fetal membranes usually due to upward ascent of a vaginal infection

J. Accumulation of abnormal fluid collections not caused by Rhesus factor incompatibility

K. Abnormal fluid collection in the thoracic cavity

L. Administered to pregnant women to help accelerate fetal lung maturity

M. Abnormal accumulation of fluid or edema found in at least two fetal areas

N. Acquired uterine condition characterized by the presence of intrauterine scars

## AMNIOTIC FLUID

### Exercise 3

_Fill in the blank(s) with the word(s) that best completes the statements about amniotic fluid._

1. _____ allows the fetus to move freely within the amniotic cavity while also maintaining intrauterine temperature and protecting the developing fetus from injury.

2. The amnion can be visualized with transvaginal sonography in the early first trimester between 4 and 5 weeks' gestation as a thin membrane separating the _____ cavity (which contains the fetus) from the extraembryonic coelom and the secondary _____ sac.

3. Amniotic fluid is produced by the umbilical cord, the _____, _____, skin, and _____.

4. As the fetus and placenta mature, amniotic fluid production and consumption change to include movement of fluid across the _____ and fetal skin, fetal urine output and fetal swallowing, and gastrointestinal absorption.

5. Fetal production of urine and the ability to swallow begin between _____ and _____ weeks of gestation and become the major pathway for amniotic fluid production and consumption after this time period.

6. The fetus _____ amniotic fluid, which is absorbed by the digestive tract. The fetus also _____ urine, which is passed into the surrounding amniotic fluid.

7. Fetal urination into the amniotic sac accounts for nearly the total volume of amniotic fluid by the second half of pregnancy, so that the quantity of fluid is directly related to _____ function.

8. Normal lung development depends critically on the _____ of amniotic fluid within the lungs.

9. Inadequate lung development may occur when severe _____ is present, placing the fetus at high risk for developing small or hypoplastic lungs.

10. The volume of amniotic fluid increases progressively until about 33 weeks' gestation, with average increment per week of _____ mL from the 11th to the 15th week and _____ mL from the 15th to the 28th week of gestation.

11. At 20 to 30 weeks' gestation, amniotic fluid may appear somewhat _____, although this typically represents a normal amniotic fluid variant.

12. At the end of pregnancy, the amniotic fluid is scanty, and _____ fluid pockets may be the only visible areas of fluid.

13. The small-for-age fetus has _____ amniotic fluid; the large-for-age fetus has _____ volume of fluid.

14. Amniotic fluid generally appears _____ sonographically, although fluid particles (particulate matter) may be seen occasionally.

## Exercise 4

*Fill in the blank(s) with the word(s) that best completes the statements about the sonographic assessment of amniotic fluid.*

1. When the sonographer initially scans the entire uterus to get an overall visual assessment of the fluid present, the lie of the fetus, and the position of the placenta, this is called a(n) _____.

2. With the _____ method, the uterine cavity is divided into four equal parts by two imaginary lines perpendicular to each other.

3. The largest vertical pocket of amniotic fluid, excluding fetal limbs or umbilical cord loops, is measured in the four quadrants and added together for the _____.

4. Subjective assessment of normal amniotic fluid correlates with AFI of 10 to 20 cm; borderline values of _____ cm indicate low fluid, and values of _____ cm indicate increased fluid.

5. The sonographer must be careful to hold the transducer _____ to the table (not the curved skin surface) when assessing these pockets of fluid.

6. The _____ (i.e., fluid should measure greater than 1 cm "rule") assessment of amniotic fluid is done by identifying the largest pocket of amniotic fluid.

7. In twin pregnancies, the two-dimensional pocket measurement appears to be a better predictor of _____ than the AFI or the largest vertical pocket.

## Exercise 5

*Fill in the blank(s) with the word(s) that best completes the statements, or provide a short answer about the abnormalities of amniotic fluid.*

1. Hydramnios, or _____, is defined as an amniotic fluid volume greater than 2000 mL.

2. Polyhydramnios is often associated with _____ disorders and/or _____ problems.

3. This central nervous system disorder causes _____ swallowing.

4. With gastrointestinal abnormalities, often a(n) (atresia) of the esophagus, stomach, duodenum, and small bowel results in ineffective swallowing.

5. An overall reduction in the amount of amniotic fluid resulting in fetal crowding and decreased fetal movement is _____.

6. Oligohydramnios may be defined as a single pocket of fluid with a depth less than _____ cm or an AFI less than _____ cm.

7. Identify one of the five causes that may be attributed to the development of oligohydramnios.

8. The association between _____ and decreased amniotic fluid (oligohydramnios) is well recognized.

9. Evaluation of _____ in the umbilical cord, the placenta, and the cerebral vascular system with color and Doppler techniques is critical to determine the presence or absence of intrauterine growth restriction.

10. Cord _____ by the fetus is another potential cause for fetal asphyxia leading to oligohydramnios.


**Exercise 6**

*Fill in the blank(s) with the word(s) that best completes the statements about amniotic band syndrome.*

1. A common, nonrecurrent cause of various fetal malformations involving the limbs, craniofacial region, and trunk is

   the _____.

2. The site where the amniotic band cuts across the fetus is usually evident after _____.

3. Amniotic sheets are believed to be caused by uterine scars, or _____, from previous instrumentation of the uterus (usually curettage), cesarean section, or episodes of endometritis.


**Exercise 7**

*Provide a short answer for each question after evaluating the images.*

1. Identify the sonographic finding in this 30-week fetus.

   _____

   _____

2. Describe the amniotic fluid assessment in this twin pregnancy.

_____

_____

_____

3. Describe the abnormality (arrow) seen in this 3D image.

_____

_____

4. Describe the abnormality demonstrated in this fetus.

_____

_____

5. Identify the abnormality in this 30-week fetus.

_____

_____

# 59 Fetal Face and Neck

## KEY TERMS

### Exercise 1

*Match the following fetal face and neck abnormality terms with their definitions.*

_____ 1. anophthalmia

_____ 2. arrhinia

_____ 3. cephalocele

_____ 4. craniosynostoses

_____ 5. dacryocystocele

_____ 6. exophthalmia

_____ 7. fetal cystic hygroma

_____ 8. fetal goiter (thyromegaly)

_____ 9. holoprosencephaly

_____10. hypertelorism

_____11. microcephaly

_____12. micrognathia

_____13. nuchal lucency

_____14. phenylketonuria (PKU)

_____15. Treacher Collins syndrome

A. Malformation of the lymphatic system that leads to single or multiloculated lymph-filled cavities around the neck
B. Premature closure of cranial sutures
C. Underdevelopment of the jaw and cheekbone and abnormal ears
D. Head smaller than the body
E. Cystic dilatation of the lacrimal sac at the nasocanthal angle
F. Absent eyes
G. Small chin
H. Congenital defect caused by an extra chromosome, which causes a deficiency in the forebrain
I. Absence of the nose
J. Increased thickness in the nuchal fold area in the back of the neck associated with trisomy 21
K. Abnormal protrusion of the eyeball
L. Protrusion of the brain from the cranial cavity
M. Enlargement of the thyroid gland
N. Hereditary disease caused by failure to oxidize an amino acid (phenylalanine) to tyrosine because of a defective enzyme; can lead to mental retardation
O. Eyes too far apart

### Exercise 2

*Match the following fetal face and neck abnormality terms with their definitions.*

_____ 1. Beckwith-Wiedemann syndrome

_____ 2. branchial cleft cyst

_____ 3. epignathus

_____ 4. hemifacial microsomia

_____ 5. hypotelorism

_____ 6. macroglossia

_____ 7. microphthalmia

A. Underdevelopment of the eyes, fingers, and mouth
B. A cylindrical protuberance of the face that in cyclopia or ethmocephaly represents the nose
C. Underdevelopment of the jaw that causes the ears to be located close together toward the front of the neck
D. Cystic defect that arises from the primitive branchial apparatus
E. Solid tumor
F. Eyes too close together
G. Small eyes

_____ 8. oculodentodigital dysplasia

_____ 9. otocephaly

_____10. Pierre Robin sequence

_____11. proboscis

_____12. strabismus

_____13. teratoma

_____14. trigonocephaly

H. Premature closure of the metopic suture
I. Abnormal smallness of one side of the face
J. Group of disorders having in common the coexistence of an omphalocele, macroglossia, and visceromegaly
K. Micrognathia and abnormal smallness of the tongue, usually with a cleft palate
L. Eye disorder in which optic axes cannot be directed to the same object
M. Teratoma located in the oropharynx
N. Hypertrophied tongue

## ANATOMY

### Exercise 3

_Label the following illustrations._

1. Lateral view of the embryo at 28 days.

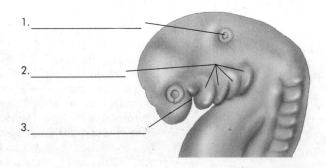

1._____

2._____

3._____

2. Frontal view of the embryo at 24 days.

1._____

2._____

3._____

4._____

5._____

3. Frontal view of the embryo at 33 days.

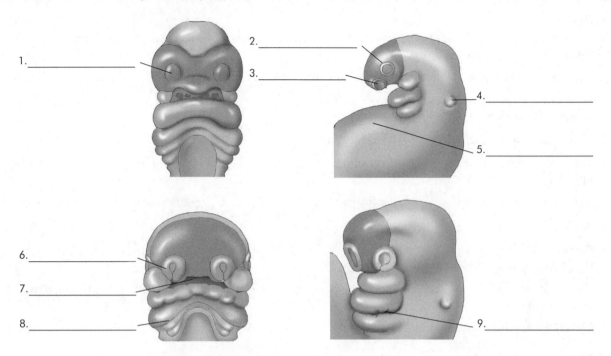

1._____

2._____

3._____

4._____

5._____

6._____

7._____

8._____

9._____

**Exercise 4**

*Fill in the blank(s) with the word(s) that best completes the statements about the embryology of the fetal face and neck.*

1. The embryo in the 4th week has characteristic external features of the head and neck area in the form of a series of

   branchial arches, pouches, grooves, and membranes that are referred to as the _____ and bear a resemblance to gills.

2. There are _____ branchial arches.

3. The first branchial arch is also known as the _____ arch; it forms the jaw, zygomatic bone, ear, and temporal bone.

4. The _____ crest cells develop the skeletal parts of the face, and the _____ of each arch develops the musculature of the face and neck.

5. The primitive mouth is an indentation on the surface of the _____ (referred to as the *stomodeum*).

6. The maxillary prominences grow _____ between the 5th and 8th weeks. This growth compresses the medial nasal prominences together toward the midline. The two medial nasal prominences and the two

   maxillary prominences lateral to them fuse together to form the _____ lip.

## Exercise 5

*Fill in the blank(s) with the word(s) that best completes the statements about sonographic evaluation and abnormalities of the fetal face.*

1. Fetal facial evaluation is not routinely included in a basic fetal scan, but when there is a(n) _____ history of craniofacial malformation or when another _____ anomaly is found, the face should be screened for a coexisting facial malformation.

2. Many fetuses with a facial defect also have _____ abnormalities.

3. The fetal forehead (frontal bone) appears as a(n) _____ surface with differentiation of the nose, lips, and chin seen inferiorly.

4. Anterior cephaloceles may arise from the frontal bone or midface, causing widely spaced orbits, a condition called _____.

5. Premature closure of any or all six of the cranial sutures, a condition known as _____, causes the fetal cranium to become abnormally shaped.

6. Cloverleaf skull or _____ appears as an unusually misshapen skull with a cloverleaf appearance in the anterior view.

7. Cloverleaf skull has been associated with numerous skeletal dysplasias, most notably _____ and _____.

8. _____ (premature closure of the metopic suture) may cause the forehead to have an elongated (tall) appearance in the sagittal plane and to appear triangular in the axial plane.

9. _____ may be observed in a fetus with a lemon-shaped skull (from spina bifida) or with skeletal dysplasias.

10. Underdevelopment of the middle structures of the face is _____ or _____ hypoplasia with depressed or absent nasal bridge.

11. Midface hypoplasia may be seen in fetuses with chromosome anomalies such as trisomy _____, in craniosynostosis syndromes such as Apert's syndrome, or in limb and skeletal abnormalities such as achondroplasia, chondrodysplasia punctata, asphyxiating thoracic dysplasia, and others.

12. A median-cleft face syndrome consisting of a range of midline facial defects involving the eyes, forehead, and nose is _____.

13. The optimum gestational age for the measurement of fetal nuchal translucency is _____ weeks' gestation to _____ weeks _____ days' gestation.

14. Fetal crown-rump length should be within the range of _____ mm to _____ mm.

15. Tongue protrusion may suggest macroglossia (enlarged tongue), a condition found in _____ syndrome (congenital overgrowth of tissues).

16. Mandibular width is measured in an axial plane laterally from _____ to _____.

17. Mandibular length, or AP diameter, is assessed by measuring from the _____ of the mandible to the _____ of the lateral width line.

18. Micrognathia is associated with many conditions that can be subdivided into three groups of anomalies: _____ anomalies, dysplasias, and primary _____ disorders.

19. The sonographer must document the presence of both eyes and must assess the overall size of the eyes to exclude

_____ (small eyes) and _____ (absent eyes).

20. A condition characterized by decreased distance between the orbits is _____.

21. _____ is characterized by abnormally widely spaced orbits.

22. The contour of the nose, upper and lower lips, and chin is observed in a(n) _____ plane.

23. Evaluation of the nasal triad should assess _____, _____, and _____.

24. _____ lip with or without cleft palate represents the most common congenital anomaly of the face.

25. Defects range from clefting of the lip alone to involvement of the _____ palate, which may extend into the nose and, in rare cases, to the inferior border of the orbit.

26. Isolated cleft lip may occur as a unilateral or bilateral defect; when unilateral, it commonly originates on the

_____ side of the face.

27. In fetuses with epignathus, _____ may be impaired, resulting in hydramnios.


## ABNORMALITIES

### Exercise 6

*Fill in the blank(s) with the word(s) that best completes the statements about abnormalities of the neck.*

1. Cleft _____ represents the most common congenital anomaly of the face.

2. When a large neck tumor exists, delivery of the infant is complicated because the tumor may cause delivery

_____, the inability to deliver the trunk once the head has been delivered.

3. A(n) _____ observed prenatally suggests that the mother may have thyroid disease.

4. When cystic hygroma is found, there is a high risk for _____ syndrome (45,X).

5. Malformation of the lymphatic system that leads to single or multiloculated lymph-filled cavities around the neck

results in _____.

6. An accumulation of lymph in the fetal tissues may lead to fetal _____.

7. A fetal _____ usually appears as a symmetrical (bilobed), solid, homogeneous mass arising from the anterior fetal neck in the region of the fetal thyroid gland.

## Exercise 7

*Provide a short answer for each question after evaluating the images.*

1. What does the letter *l* denote in image **A**? What are the arrows pointing to in image **B**?

_____

_____

2. What does the *t* stand for in image **A** (a sagittal view of the facial profile)? Identify the view that is demonstrated in image **B**.

_____

_____

3. Describe this abnormality of the fetal skull.

_____

_____

4. Identify what the arrow is pointing to and what it indicates.

_____

_____

A

B

C

5. Describe the abnormality in this fetal head.

_____

_____

6. Describe the abnormality in this fetal face.

_____

_____

A

B

C

7. Describe the abnormality in each of these fetal images.

_____

_____

# 60 Fetal Neural Axis

Fetal Neural Axis

## KEY TERMS

### Exercise 1

*Match the following fetal head and spine anomaly terms with their definitions.*

_____ 1. acrania

_____ 2. alobar holoprosencephaly

_____ 3. anencephaly

_____ 4. anomaly

_____ 5. cebocephaly

_____ 6. cyclopia

_____ 7. cystic hygroma

_____ 8. holoprosencephaly

_____ 9. hydranencephaly

_____ 10. hydrocephalus

_____ 11. macrocephaly

_____ 12. meningocele

_____ 13. meningomyelocele

_____ 14. spina bifida

_____ 15. spina bifida occulta

_____ 16. ventriculomegaly

A. Enlargement of the fetal cranium as a result of ventriculomegaly

B. Most severe form of holoprosencephaly characterized by a single common ventricle and a malformed brain

C. Increase in size of the jugular lymphatic sacs caused by abnormal development

D. Neural tube defect of the spine in which the dorsal vertebrae fail to fuse together, allowing the protrusion of meninges and/or spinal cord through the defect

E. Abnormal accumulation of cerebrospinal fluid within the cerebral ventricles leading to dilatation of the ventricles; compression of developing brain tissue and brain damage may result; commonly associated with additional fetal anomalies

F. An abnormality or congenital malformation

G. Congenital absence of the cerebral hemispheres caused by occlusion of the carotid arteries; midbrain structures are present, and fluid replaces cerebral tissue

H. Open spinal defect characterized by protrusion of meninges and spinal cord through the defect, usually within a meningeal sac

I. Ventriculomegaly in the neonate; abnormal accumulation of cerebrospinal fluid within the cerebral ventricles resulting in compression and, frequently, destruction of brain tissue

J. Form of holoprosencephaly characterized by a common ventricle, hypotelorism, and a nose with a single nostril

K. Closed defect of the spine without protrusion of meninges or spinal cord

L. Neural tube defect characterized by lack of development of the cerebral and cerebellar hemispheres and cranial vault; this abnormality is incompatible with life

M. Condition associated with anencephaly in which there is complete or partial absence of the cranial bones

N. Severe form of holoprosencephaly characterized by a common ventricle, fusion of the orbits with one or two eyes present, and a proboscis

O. Open spinal defect characterized by protrusion of the spinal meninges

P. Range of abnormalities resulting from abnormal cleavage of the forebrain

## Exercise 2

*Fill in the blank(s) with the word(s) that best completes the statements, or provide a short answer about the fetal neural axis.*

1. The cephalic neural plate develops into the _____, and the caudal end forms the _____ cord.

2. The forebrain will continue to develop into the _____, the midbrain will become the

   _____, and the hindbrain will form the _____.

3. Failure of closure of the neural tube at the cranial end is _____.

4. List the sonographic features of anencephaly.

   _____

   _____

   _____

5. List the sonographic features of acrania.

   _____

   _____

   _____

6. A neural tube defect in which the meninges alone or the meninges and brain herniate through a defect in the

   calvarium is a(n) _____.

7. The term used to describe herniation of the meninges and brain through the defect is _____.

8. Cranial _____ describes the herniation of only meninges.

9. Fetuses with myelomeningoceles often present with the cranial defects associated with the _____ malformation, which is identified in 90% of patients.

10. List the sonographic features of spina bifida.

    _____

    _____

    _____

11. List the sonographic features of Dandy Walker Malformation.

    _____

    _____

    _____

12. _____ holoprosencephaly is characterized by a monoventricle; brain tissue that is small and may have a cup, ball, or pancake configuration; fusion of the thalamus; and absence of the interhemispheric fissure, cavum septi pellucidi, corpus callosum, optic tracts, and olfactory bulbs.

13. _____ holoprosencephaly presents with a single ventricular cavity with partial formation of the occipital horns, partial or complete fusion of the thalamus, a rudimentary flex and interhemispheric fissure, and absent corpus callosum, cavum septi pellucidi, and olfactory bulbs.

14. Almost complete division of the ventricles is seen with a corpus callosum that may be normal, hypoplastic, or absent, although the cavum septi pellucidi will still be absent in _____ holoprosencephaly.

15. A fibrous tract that connects the cerebral hemispheres and aids in learning and memory is the

_____.

16. List the sonographic features of agenesis of the corpus callosum.

_____

_____

_____

17. _____ results from obstruction, atresia, or stenosis of the aqueduct of Sylvius, causing ventriculomegaly.

18. Porencephaly or _____ cysts are cysts filled with cerebrospinal fluid.

19. A rare disorder characterized by clefts in the cerebral cortex is _____.

20. Enlargement of the ventricles occurs with _____ of cerebrospinal fluid flow.

21. Fetal ventriculomegaly typically progresses from the _____ horns into the temporal and then to the _____ ventricular horns.

22. A ventricle is considered dilated when its diameter exceeds _____ mm.

**Exercise 3**
*Provide a short answer for each question after evaluating the images.*

1. Describe your findings in this second-trimester sonogram.

_____

_____

2. Describe the abnormality demonstrated in this sagittal view of the fetal head.

_____

_____

3. Identify the abnormality seen in this sagittal view of the fetus.

_____

_____

4. Identify this abnormality of the fetal head.

_____

_____

5. Describe this abnormality of the fetal head.

_____

_____

6. Describe this abnormality of the fetal head.

_____

_____

7. Describe the abnormality shown in this fetal head.

_____

_____

# 61 Fetal Thorax

## KEY TERMS

**Exercise 1**

*Match the following fetal thorax terms with their definitions.*

_____ 1. asphyxiating thoracic dystrophy

_____ 2. bronchogenic cyst

_____ 3. congenital bronchial atresia

_____ 4. congenital cystic adenomatoid malformation

_____ 5. congenital diaphragmatic hernia

_____ 6. foramen of Bochdalek

_____ 7. foramen of Morgagni

_____ 8. lymphangiectasia

_____ 9. pleural effusion

_____10. pulmonary hypoplasia

_____11. pulmonary sequestration

A. Dilatation of a lymph node
B. Abnormality in the formation of the bronchial tree with secondary overgrowth of mesenchymal tissue from arrested bronchial development
C. Small, underdeveloped lungs with resultant reduction in lung volume; secondary to prolonged oligohydramnios or as a consequence of a small thoracic cavity
D. Most common lung cyst detected prenatally
E. Type of diaphragmatic defect that occurs posterior and lateral in the diaphragm; usually found in the left side
F. Accumulation of fluid within the thoracic cavity
G. Pulmonary anomaly that results from focal obliteration of a segment of the bronchial lumen
H. Extrapulmonary tissue present within the pleural lung sac or connected to the inferior border of the lung within its own pleural sac
I. Significantly narrow diameter of the chest in the fetus
J. Opening in the pleuroperitoneal membrane that develops in the first trimester
K. Diaphragmatic hernia that occurs anterior and medial in the diaphragm that may communicate with the pericardial sac

## EMBRYOLOGY AND SONOGRAPHIC CHARACTERISTICS

### Exercise 2

*Fill in the blank(s) with the word(s) that best completes the statements about the embryology and sonographic characteristics of the thoracic cavity.*

1. The lungs at birth are about half filled with _____ derived from the amniotic cavity, tracheal glands, and lungs.

2. The normal thoracic cavity is symmetrically _____ shaped, with the _____ forming the lateral margins, the _____ forming the upper margins, and the _____ forming the lower margins.

3. The thorax is normally slightly _____ than the abdominal cavity.

4. In the presence of oligohydramnios, resultant pulmonary _____ may be seen with a reduction in overall thoracic size.

5. The location of the heart is important to document in a routine sonographic examination because detection of abnormal position may indicate the presence of a chest _____, pleural _____, or cardiac _____.

6. The fetal lungs appear homogeneous on ultrasound with moderate _____.

7. Early in gestation, the lungs are similar to or slightly less echogenic than the _____, and as gestation progresses, there is a trend toward increased pulmonary echogenicity relative to the liver.

8. Fetal breathing becomes most prominent in the _____ and _____ trimesters.

9. Fetal breathing movements are documented as present if characteristic seesaw movements of the fetal chest or abdomen are sustained for at least _____ seconds.

## ABNORMALITIES

### Exercise 3

*Fill in the blank(s) with the word(s) that best completes the statements, or provide a short answer about the abnormalities of the thoracic cavity.*

1. What three things should a sonographer document when evaluating the fetus for a lung mass?

   _____

   _____

   _____

2. A decrease in the numbers of lung cells, airways, and alveoli, with a resulting decrease in organ size and weight, causes pulmonary _____.

3. Pulmonary hypoplasia may occur when there is an extreme _____ in amniotic fluid volume.

4. The sonographer may be able to check for pulmonary hypoplasia by measuring the thoracic circumference at the level of the _____ heart view, excluding the skin and subcutaneous tissues.

5. _____ cysts occur as a result of abnormal budding of the foregut and lack of any communication with the trachea or bronchial tree.

6. Accumulation of fluid within the pleural cavity that may appear as isolated lesions or secondary to multiple fetal anomalies is called a(n) _____, or _____.

7. In pulmonary _____, extrapulmonary tissue is present within the pleural lung sac

   (_____) or is connected to the inferior border of the lung within its own pleural sac

   (_____).

8. The arterial supply referred to in question 7 is usually derived from the _____, with venous drainage into the vena cava.

9. In reference to question 7, a(n) _____ solid mass resembling lung tissue is observed sonographically, usually in the lower lobe of the lung.

10. A multicystic mass within the lung consisting of primitive lung tissue and abnormal bronchial and bronchiolar-like

    structures is _____ malformation.

11. Congenital diaphragmatic hernia (CDH) is a herniation of the _____ viscera into the chest, which results from a congenital defect in the fetal diaphragm.

12. The most common type of diaphragmatic defect by far occurs posteriorly and laterally in the diaphragm

    (herniation through foramen of _____).

13. Diaphragmatic hernias may occur anteriorly and medially in the diaphragm through the foramen of

    _____ and may communicate with the pericardial sac.

14. Hydrops usually is not present with left-sided congenital diaphragmatic hernias unless associated fetal

    _____ are present.

15. On sonographic examination, a(n) _____ congenital diaphragmatic hernia usually is found when the cardiac silhouette is displaced to the right, and an ectopic stomach is in the chest.

16. The sonographer will see the liver in the chest; collapsed bowel may be present, and the heart may be deviated far

    to the left in a _____ -sided diaphragmatic hernia.

17. At birth, a majority of infants with congenital diaphragmatic hernia have pulmonary _____ and secondary respiratory insufficiency.

18. Development of the _____ procedure has allowed babies with severe diaphragmatic hernia a chance for survival immediately post delivery.

*Provide a short answer for each question after evaluating the images.*

1. State whether the lungs are more or less echogenic than the liver.

   _____

   _____

2. Describe where the apex of the fetal heart is in this image. State whether the fetal heart axis is normal in this image.

   _____

   _____

**A**    **B**

3. Describe the abnormalities seen in these images.

_____

_____

4. Which type of cystic adenomatoid malformation is shown in this fetal lung?

_____

_____

A          B

5. Describe the complication in this fetus with a known omphalocele.

_____

_____

6. Describe the sonographic findings in this 25-week fetus.

_____

_____

# 62 Fetal Anterior Abdominal Wall

**Exercise 1**

*Match the following terms related to abnormalities of the anterior abdominal wall with their definitions.*

_____ 1. amniotic band syndrome

_____ 2. Beckwith-Wiedemann syndrome

_____ 3. cloacal exstrophy

_____ 4. encephalocele

_____ 5. exencephaly

_____ 6. gastroschisis

_____ 7. limb–body wall complex

_____ 8. omphalocele

_____ 9. pentalogy of Cantrell

_____ 10. scoliosis

A. Opening in the layers of the abdominal wall with evisceration of the bowel

B. Rupture of the amnion that leads to entrapment or entanglement of fetal parts by the "sticky" chorion

C. Develops when a midline defect of the abdominal muscles, fascia, and skin results in herniation of intraabdominal structures into the base of the umbilical cord

D. Defect in the lower abdominal wall and anterior wall of the urinary bladder

E. Anomaly with large cranial defects, facial cleft, large body wall defects, and limb abnormalities

F. Abnormal lateral curvature of the spine

G. Group of disorders having in common the coexistence of an omphalocele, macroglossia, and visceromegaly

H. Abnormal condition in which the brain is located outside the cranium

I. Rare anomaly with five defects: omphalocele, ectopic heart, lower sternum, anterior diaphragm, and diaphragmatic pericardium

J. Protrusion of the brain through a cranial fissure

## Exercise 2

*Fill in the blank(s) with the word(s) that best completes the statements about the fetal anterior abdominal wall.*

1. The embryo is a flat disc consisting of three layers—_____, _____, and _____—that form by the end of the 5th week of development.

2. Umbilical hernia of the _____ occurs during the 8th week of development as the midgut extends to the extraembryonic coelom in the proximal portion of the umbilical cord.

3. The intestines return to the abdominal cavity by the _____ week of gestation.

4. The most common types of abdominal wall defects are _____, _____, and _____.

5. Abdominal wall defects cause _____ of the normal contour of the ventral or anterior surface of the fetal abdomen.

6. When bowel loops fail to return to the abdomen, a bowel-containing _____ occurs.

7. Omphalocele herniation is covered by a(n) _____ that is composed of amnion and peritoneum.

8. Fetuses with an omphalocele that contains only bowel have a higher risk for _____ abnormalities and other anomalies.

9. _____ omphaloceles may contain bowel and may demonstrate a relatively large abdominal wall defect in comparison with the abdominal diameter.

10. Gastroschisis is a periumbilical defect that nearly always is located to the _____ of the umbilicus.

11. _____ bowel is always found in the herniation.

12. _____ levels are significantly higher in gastroschisis compared with omphalocele because of the exposed bowel.

13. In gastroschisis, the edges of the bowel are irregular and free floating _____ a covering membrane, as is seen with omphalocele.

14. Rupture of the amnion, which leads to entrapment or entanglement of fetal parts by the "sticky" chorion, is the _____.

15. A rare group of disorders having in common the coexistence of an omphalocele, macroglossia, and visceromegaly is the _____ syndrome.

16. A defect in the lower abdominal wall and the anterior wall of the urinary bladder is a characteristic of bladder _____.

17. The _____, which is rare, is the association of a cleft distal sternum, diaphragmatic defect, midline anterior ventral wall defect, defect of the apical pericardium with communication into the peritoneum, and an internal cardiac defect.

18. The exposed heart presents outside the chest wall through a cleft sternum in _____.

19. _____ anomaly is associated with large cranial defects; facial cleft; body wall complex defects involving the thorax, abdomen, or both; and limb defects.

*Provide a short answer for each question after evaluating the images.*

1. Name the structure that the arrows are pointing to in this 14-week fetus.

_____

**A**                                                    **B**

2. This is a fetus with trisomy 18. What abnormalities are seen in these images?

_____

_____

3. Describe the abnormalities seen in this fetus.

_____

_____

A

B

4. Describe the abnormality seen in this 34-week fetus.

_____

_____

# 63 Fetal Abdomen

## KEY TERMS

### Exercise 1

*Match the following embryology and sonographic evaluation terms with their definitions.*

_____1. duodenal stenosis

_____2. esophageal atresia

_____3. esophageal stenosis

_____4. gastroschisis

_____5. haustral folds

_____6. hematopoiesis

_____7. Meckel's diverticulum

_____8. omphalocele

_____9. peristalsis

A. Abnormality of the abdominal wall in which the bowel without a covering membrane protrudes outside of the wall
B. Abnormality of the abdominal wall in which bowel and liver, both covered by a membrane, protrude outside the wall
C. Congenital hypoplasia of the esophagus; usually associated with a tracheoesophageal fistula
D. Narrowing of the esophagus, usually in the distal third segment
E. Remnant of the proximal part of the yolk stalk
F. One of the sacculations of the colon caused by longitudinal bands that are shorter than the gut
G. Narrowing of the pyloric sphincter
H. Formation of blood
I. Movement of the bowel

### Exercise 2

*Match the following terms related to abnormalities of the hepatobiliary system with their definitions.*

_____ 1. anorectal atresia

_____ 2. asplenia

_____ 3. choledochal cyst

_____ 4. cholelithiasis

_____ 5. cystic fibrosis

_____ 6. duodenal atresia

_____ 7. Hirschsprung's disease

_____ 8. jejunoileal atresia

_____ 9. meconium ileus

_____10. partial situs inversus

_____11. polysplenia

_____12. pseudoascites

_____13. situs inversus

_____14. VACTERL

A. Cystic growth of the common bile duct
B. Sonolucent band near the fetal anterior abdominal wall from the abdominal wall muscles in the fetus over 18 weeks
C. A congenital disorder in which there is abnormal innervation of the large intestine
D. Small-bowel disorder marked by the presence of thick echogenic meconium in the distal ileum
E. No development of splenic tissue
F. Complete blockage at the pyloric sphincter
G. Heart and abdominal organs are completely reversed
H. Gallstones
I. More than one spleen; associated with cardiac malformations
J. Vertebral defects, heart defects, renal and limb abnormalities
K. Blockage of the jejunum and ileal bowel segments that appears as multiple cystic structures within the fetal abdomen
L. Congenital condition characterized by mucus buildup within the lungs and other areas of the body
M. Complex disorder of the bowel and genitourinary tract
N. Condition in which only the heart or the abdominal organs are reversed

## Exercise 3

*Fill in the blank(s) with the word(s) that best completes the statements about the fetal gastrointestinal tract.*

1. The derivatives of the _____ are the pharynx, lower respiratory system, esophagus, stomach, part of the duodenum, liver and biliary apparatus, and pancreas.

2. When _____ occurs, amniotic fluid cannot pass to the intestines for absorption, and hydramnios results.

3. The stomach appears as a fusiform dilatation of the caudal part of the _____.

4. The dorsal mesogastrium is carried to the left during rotation of the stomach and formation of a cavity known as the omental bursa or _____ of peritoneum.

5. The lesser sac communicates with the main peritoneal cavity or greater peritoneal sac through a small opening, called the _____.

6. The duodenum develops from the _____ part of the foregut and the cranial part of the _____.

7. The junction of the two embryonic parts of the duodenum in the adult is just _____ to the entrance of the common bile duct.

8. Normally the duodenum is recanalized by the end of the 8th week. Partial or complete failure of this process results in duodenal _____ (narrowing) or duodenal _____ (blockage).

9. The liver grows rapidly and intermingles with the vitelline and _____ veins, divides into _____ parts, and fills most of the abdominal cavity.

10. During the 6th week, _____ (blood formation) begins and accounts for the large size of the liver between the 7th and 9th weeks of development.

11. The derivatives of the _____ are the small intestines (including most of the duodenum), the cecum and vermiform appendix, the ascending colon, and most of the transverse colon. All of these structures are supplied by the superior mesenteric artery.

12. A remnant of the proximal part of the yolk stalk that fails to degenerate and disappear during the early fetal period is a _____.

## Exercise 4

*Fill in the blank(s) with the word(s) that best completes the statements about the stomach, small bowel, and colon.*

1. The stomach should be identified as a(n) _____ structure in the left upper quadrant inferior to the diaphragm.

2. If no fluid is apparent, the stomach should be reevaluated in _____ to _____ minutes to rule out the possibility of a central nervous system problem (swallowing disorders), obstruction, oligohydramnios, or atresia.

3. The abdominal circumference is measured at the level of the _____ sinus and the _____ portion of the left portal vein ("hockey stick" appearance on the sonogram).

4. The insertion of the umbilical cord must be imaged with _____ because it inserts both into the fetal abdomen and into the placenta.

5. The fetus is capable of _____ sufficient amounts of amniotic fluid to permit visualization of the stomach by 11 menstrual weeks.

6. After the 15th to 16th week, _____ begins to accumulate in the distal part of the small intestine as a combination of desquamated cells, bile pigments, and mucoproteins.

7. The region of the small bowel can be seen because it is slightly _____ compared with the liver and may appear "masslike" in the central abdomen and pelvis.

8. After 27 weeks, _____ of normal small bowel is increasingly observed.

9. The _____ of the colon help to differentiate it from the small bowel.

10. The _____ does not have peristalsis as the small bowel does.

11. The meconium within the lumen of the colon appears _____ relative to the fetal liver and in comparison with the bowel wall.

12. The _____ lobe of the liver is larger than the _____ in utero secondary to the greater supply of oxygenated blood.

13. The normal gallbladder may be seen sonographically after _____ weeks of gestation.

## Exercise 5

*Fill in the blank(s) with the word(s) that best completes the statements about abnormalities of the fetal abdomen.*

1. _____ may present as a total reversal of the thoracic and abdominal organs or as a partial reversal.

2. The stomach may or may not be reversed in _____.

3. True ascites is identified within the peritoneal recesses, whereas _____ is always confined to an anterior or anterolateral aspect of the fetal abdomen.

4. A bowel obstruction results in _____ bowel dilatation that is characteristically recognized as one or more tubular structures within the fetal abdomen.

5. The most reliable criterion for diagnosing dilated bowel is the bowel _____, not the sonographic appearance.

6. A congenital blockage of the esophagus resulting from faulty separation of the foregut into its respiratory and digestive components is _____.

7. In reference to the diagnosis in question 6, the sonographer may observe the _____ stomach and _____.

8. Blockage of the jejunum and ileal bowel segments (jejunoileal atresia or stenosis) appears as multiple cystic structures _____ to the site of atresia within the fetal abdomen.

9. A small-bowel disorder marked by the presence of thick meconium in the distal ileum is _____.

10. _____ may present as part of the VACTERL association or in caudal regression.

11. Hyperechoic bowel is a(n) _____ impression of unusually echogenic bowel, typically seen during the second trimester.

12. True ascites in the fetal abdomen is always _____; it usually outlines the falciform ligament and umbilical vein.

*Provide a short answer for each question after evaluating the images.*

1. This image is representative of the level at which the abdominal circumference should be taken. Identify the following structures: *p, lpv, s,* and *S.*

   _____

   _____

2. List the causes of a double bubble, as seen in this image.

   _____

   _____

A

B

C

3. This fetus was known to have gastroschisis. Describe the additional sonographic findings demonstrated in these images.

_____

_____

**A**  **B**

4. Describe the appearance of the fetal abdomen in these images.

_____

_____

**A**  **B**

5. Describe the sonographic findings in these images of the fetal abdomen.

_____

_____

# 64 Fetal Urogenital System

## KEY TERMS

### Exercise 1

*Match the following terms related to sonographic findings suggesting abnormalities and congenital malformations with their definitions.*

_____ 1. cloacal exstrophy

_____ 2. epispadias

_____ 3. horseshoe kidney

_____ 4. hydroureters

_____ 5. hypospadias

_____ 6. pelvic kidney

_____ 7. posterior urethral valve

_____ 8. Potter's syndrome

_____ 9. renal agenesis

_____ 10. urachal cyst

_____ 11. ureterocele

A. Characterized by a group of findings associated with oligohydramnios and renal failure or bilateral renal agenesis

B. Occurs when the kidney does not migrate upward into the retroperitoneal space

C. Small part of the lumen of the allantois that persists while the urachus forms

D. Anatomic structure that occurs only in male fetuses

E. Renal system fails to develop

F. Forms when the inferior poles of the kidney fuse while they are in the pelvis

G. Complex malformation involving lower limb anomalies, spinal defect, anal atresia, and lower abdominal wall defect (exstrophy of the bladder and protrusion of the intestines)

H. Dilated ureters

I. Congenital outpouching of the distal ureter into the bladder

J. Abnormal congenital opening of the male urethra on the undersurface of the penis

K. Abnormal congenital opening of the male urethra on the top side of the penis

### Exercise 2

*Match the following terms related to obstructive abnormalities, renal cystic disease, and other pelvic masses with their definitions.*

_____ 1. cryptorchidism

_____ 2. fetal hydronephrosis

_____ 3. fetal ovarian cyst

_____ 4. hermaphroditism

_____ 5. hydrometrocolpos

_____ 6. infantile polycystic kidney disease

_____ 7. megacystis

_____ 8. megaureter

_____ 9. multicystic dysplastic kidney disease

_____ 10. Potter's sequence

_____ 11. prune belly syndrome

_____ 12. pyelectasis

_____ 13. ureteropelvic junction

_____ 14. ureterovesical junction

_____ 15. urethral atresia

A. Dilated renal pelvis without involvement of the calyces

B. Autosomal recessive disease that affects the fetal kidneys and liver

C. Collection of fluid in the vagina and uterus

D. Junction where the ureter enters the bladder

E. Failure of the testes to descend into the scrotum

F. Dilatation of the fetal abdomen secondary to severe hydronephrosis and fetal ascites

G. Level of the urethra where the urinary tract may become obstructed

H. Junction of the ureter entering the renal pelvis; most common site of obstruction

I. Condition in which both ovarian and testicular tissues are present

J. Condition that causes a massively distended bladder

K. Multiple cysts replace normal renal tissue throughout the kidney

L. Dilated renal pelvis in the fetus

M. Term used to describe renal diseases other than renal agenesis that result in renal failure and facial or structural abnormalities caused by oligohydramnios

N. Dilation of the lower end of the ureter

O. Ovarian mass that results from maternal hormone stimulation

**469**

## Exercise 3

*Fill in the blank(s) with the word(s) that best completes the statements about the fetal urinary system.*

1. A complete ultrasound examination includes evaluation of both _____, documentation of the urinary _____, and assessment of _____.

2. The urinary system and the genital system develop from the intermediate _____, and the excretory ducts of both systems initially enter a common cavity called the cloaca.

3. The part of the urogenital ridge that gives rise to the urinary system is known as the nephrogenic cord or _____ ridge.

4. The part that gives rise to the genital system is known as the gonadal ridge or _____ ridge.

5. The permanent kidneys or _____ begins to develop early in the 5th week while the mesonephric ducts are still developing.

6. Urine formation begins toward the end of the first trimester, around the _____ or _____ week, and continues actively throughout fetal life.

7. Urine is excreted into the amniotic cavity and forms a major part of the _____.

8. The kidneys do not need to function in utero because the _____ eliminates waste from the fetal blood.

9. The kidneys initially lie very close together in the _____; gradually, they migrate into the abdomen and become separated from one another.

10. In adolescent and adult patients, persistence of the fetal lobulation and groove may be seen on ultrasound as a(n) _____ triangular notch along the anterior wall of the _____ kidney.

## Exercise 4

*Fill in the blank(s) with the word(s) that best completes the statements about the development of the fetal urinary system.*

1. Complete absence of the kidneys is known as renal _____.

2. Division of the ureteric bud at an early stage results in a double or _____ kidney.

3. When the inferior poles of the kidney fuse while they are in the pelvis, a(n) _____ kidney is formed.

4. The fetal urinary bladder is derived from the hindgut derivative known as the _____ sinus.

5. _____ of the bladder occurs primarily in males and is characterized by protrusion of the posterior wall of the urinary bladder, which contains the trigone of the bladder and the ureteric orifices.

6. Early in development, the urinary bladder is continuous with the _____.

7. The allantois regresses to become a fibrous cord known as the _____.

8. If the lumen of the allantois persists while the urachus forms, a urachal _____ develops, which causes urine to drain from the bladder to the umbilicus.

9. If only a small part of the lumen of the allantois persists, it is called a(n) _____.

**Exercise 5**

*Fill in the blank(s) with the word(s) that best completes the statements about sonographic evaluation of the urinary system.*

1. The fetal kidneys and bladder may be seen on ultrasound by _____ weeks' gestation.

2. At this time period, the kidneys appear as bilateral _____ structures in the paravertebral regions.

3. By _____ weeks, it is possible to distinguish the renal cortex from the medulla, to outline the renal capsule clearly, and to see a central echogenic area in the renal sinus region.

4. The upper limit of normal for the renal pelves is _____ mm up to 33 weeks' gestation and _____ mm from 33 weeks' gestation until term.

5. If the bladder appears too large, it should be evaluated again at the end of the study (assuming the examination takes at least _____ minutes) to see if normal emptying has occurred.

6. When obstruction occurs at the level of the urethra, the bladder wall becomes _____.

7. Dilatation of the posterior _____ is highly suggestive of an obstructive process, such as posterior urethral valve syndrome, known as the "keyhole" sign on sonography because the dilated bladder has the shape of a keyhole superior to the obstructed urethra.

8. It is possible to have unilateral renal agenesis, but the contralateral kidney is usually quite _____ to compensate for this abnormality.

9. The _____ kidney shows a large central cyst with multiple small peripheral cysts that appear as a pelviureteric junction obstruction; however, these cysts do not communicate with one another, as is seen with hydronephrosis.

10. When the kidneys appear enlarged and echogenic, the sonographer should think of infantile _____ disease (with oligohydramnios).

11. Dilatation of the renal collecting system suggests either _____ or _____.

12. Pelviureteric junction obstruction shows dilatation of the renal _____, whereas ureteric dilatation suggests either a(n) _____ junction obstruction or reflux.

13. When the hydronephrosis is _____, the possibility of bladder outlet obstruction should be considered.

**Exercise 6**

*Fill in the blank(s) with the word(s) that best completes the statements about the pathophysiology of the fetal urinary system.*

1. A critical marker in the assessment of renal function is _____.

2. The fetal kidneys begin to excrete urine after the _____th week but do not become the major contributor of fetal urine (hence, amniotic fluid volume) until _____ to _____ weeks of pregnancy.

3. It usually takes at least _____ minutes to fill and empty the fetal bladder.

4. Renal agenesis and infantile polycystic kidney disease are fetal conditions _____ with life.

5. In renal agenesis, the _____ glands may be large and may mimic the kidneys.

6. _____ kidneys should be considered when the kidneys are not in their normal retroperitoneal location.

7. _____ syndrome is characterized by renal agenesis, oligohydramnios, pulmonary hypoplasia, abnormal facies, and malformed hands and feet.

8. Infantile polycystic kidney disease (IPKD) is an autosomal recessive disorder that affects the fetal

_____ and _____.

9. In the most severe cases of IPKD, renal failure occurs with _____ and a(n) _____ urinary bladder.

10. Multicystic dysplastic kidney disease is the most common form of renal _____ disease in childhood and represents one of the most common abdominal masses in the neonate.

11. Multicystic dysplastic kidney disease is composed of multiple smooth-walled, nonfunctioning, _____ cysts of variable size and number.

12. In autosomal dominant (adult) polycystic kidney disease, the fetal kidneys appear _____ and

_____, and, rarely, cysts may be observed prenatally.

13. In obstructive cystic dysplasia, renal _____ occurs secondary to obstruction in the first or early second trimester of pregnancy.

14. The urinary tract may be obstructed at the junction of the ureter entering the renal pelvis (_____

junction), at the junction of the ureter where it enters the bladder (_____ junction), or at the level

of the urethra (_____).

15. If the obstruction is _____, a multicystic kidney may develop.

16. Late obstruction causes _____.

## Exercise 7

*Fill in the blank(s) with the word(s) that best completes the statements about the dilatation of the fetal urinary system.*

1. Measurements of the renal pelvis have a wide discrepancy, varying between _____

and _____ mm in the second trimester and between _____ and

_____ mm in the third trimester.

2. The dilated anechoic renal pelvis is centrally located and distended with urine. If only the pelvis is seen, the term

_____ is used. Hydronephrosis will be identified with dilatation of the renal pelvis and the

_____.

3. Unilateral renal hydronephrosis commonly results from an obstruction at the junction of the renal pelvis and the

ureter; this is called a(n) _____ obstruction.

4. _____ obstruction commonly presents with dilatation of the lower end of the ureter (megaureter).

5. A dilatation of the intravesical (bladder) segment of the distal ureter is a(n) _____.

6. _____ outlet obstruction is produced by a membrane within the posterior urethra; the bladder wall

is severely thickened with a dilated posterior urethra, the "_____ sign."

7. Sonographic findings in prune belly syndrome include _____, mild to severe bilateral

hydronephrosis, fetal _____, and hypoplastic lungs.

**Exercise 8**

*Fill in the blank(s) with the word(s) that best completes the statements about fetal genital development.*

1. The phallus elongates to form the penis; this sonographic finding is known as the "_____ sign."

2. Both the urethra and the vagina open into the urogenital sinus, the vestibule of the vagina. The urogenital folds become the labia minora, the labioscrotal swellings become the labia majora, and the phallus becomes the clitoris; this sonographic finding is known as the "_____ sign."

3. The female fetus with _____ has a 46,XX karyotype. The most common cause is congenital virilizing adrenal hyperplasia that causes masculinization of the external genitalia.

4. _____ represent the most common cystic mass in female fetuses.

5. _____ occurs in the male fetus and is seen as an accumulation of serous fluid surrounding the testicle resulting from a communication with the peritoneal cavity.

6. Failure of the testes to completely descend into the scrotal sac results in a condition called _____.

7. _____ is the sonographic finding that describes the inability to delineate fetal gender. There are several congenital malformations that attribute to this finding; the malformations typically result from chromosomal defects or abnormal hormone levels.

8. A collection of fluid in the vagina and uterus is _____.

*Provide a short answer for each question after evaluating the images.*

1. From these images of the fetal urinary system, describe the abnormalities.

_____

_____

A

B

1 D 4.81cm
2 D 4.49cm

RT  LT

C

2. Describe the sonographic findings on this image.

_____

_____

A                      B

3. Describe the sonographic findings in this 28-week gestation.

_____

_____

4. This fetus was known to have Beckwith-Wiedemann syndrome. Describe the sonographic findings in this image.

_____

_____

A

B

C

D

5. Describe the sonographic findings of these fetal kidneys.

_____

_____

6. Discuss the sonographic findings in this fetal abdomen.

_____

_____

# 65 Fetal Skeleton

## KEY TERMS

### Exercise 1

*Match the following fetal skeletal terms with their definitions.*

___E___ 1. achondrogenesis

___C___ 2. achondroplasia

___A___ 3. craniosynostosis

___H___ 4. heterozygous achondroplasia

___F___ 5. homozygous achondroplasia

___B___ 6. hypophosphatasia

___I___ 7. osteogenesis imperfecta

___D___ 8. polydactyly

___G___ 9. thanatophoric dysplasia

A. Early ossification of the calvarium with destruction of the sutures; hypertelorism frequently found in association; sonographically the fetal cranium may appear brachycephalic

B. Congenital condition characterized by decreased mineralization of the bones resulting in "ribbon-like" and bowed limbs, underossified cranium, and compression of the chest; early death often occurs

C. A defect in the development of the cartilage at the epiphyseal centers of the long bones producing short, square bones

D. Anomalies of the hands or feet in which there is an addition of a digit; may be found in association with certain skeletal dysplasias

E. Lethal autosomal recessive short-limb dwarfism marked by long-bone and trunk shortening, decreased echogenicity of the bones and spine, and "flipper-like" appendages

F. Short-limb dwarfism affecting fetuses of achondroplastic parents

G. Lethal short-limb dwarfism characterized by a notable reduction in the length of the long bones, pear-shaped chest, soft-tissue redundancy, and frequently cloverleaf skull deformity and ventriculomegaly

H. Short-limb dysplasia that manifests in the second trimester of pregnancy; conversion abnormality of cartilage to bone affecting the epiphyseal growth centers; extremities are notably shortened at birth, with a normal trunk and frequent enlargement of the head

I. Metabolic disorder affecting the fetal collagen system that leads to varying forms of bone disease: intrauterine bone fractures, shortened long bones, poorly mineralized calvaria, and compression of the chest found in type II forms

**479**

## Exercise 2

*Fill in the blank(s) with the word(s) that best completes the statements, or provide a short answer about the fetal musculoskeletal system.*

1. The majority of the musculoskeletal system is formed from the primitive ___MESODERM___ arising from mesenchymal cells that are the embryonic connective tissues.

2. The vertebral column and ribs arise from the _____, and the limbs arise from the lateral plate

   _____.

3. Initially the limbs have a paddle shape with a ridge of thickened _____, known as the apical ectodermal ridge, at the apex of each bud.

4. The fingers are distinctly evident by day 49, although they are still webbed, and by the _____ week of development, the fingers are longer.

5. Development of the feet and toes is essentially complete by the _____ week, although the soles of the feet are still turned inward at this time.

6. The term used to describe abnormal growth and density of cartilage and bone is skeletal ___DYSPLASIA___.

7. When skeletal dysplasia is suspected, the protocol of the obstetric ultrasound examination should be adjusted to include the following criteria:

   a. ___ASSESS LIMB SHORTENING___

   b. ___ASSESS BONE CONTOUR - thickness, bowing, Fx___

   c. ___ESTIMATE DEGREE OF OSSIFICATION (cranium, ribs, spine, long bones)___

   d. ___EVALUATE THORACIC CIRCUMFERENCE/SHAPE___

   e. ___LOOK FOR HAND/FOOT ANOMALIES___

   f. ___EVALUATE FACE/PROFILE - cleft, bossing, micrognathia, hypertelorism, etc.___

   g. ___SURVEY FOR OTHER ANOMALIES - hydrocephaly, heart defect, hydrops___

## Exercise 3

*Fill in the blank(s) with the word(s) that best completes the statements, or provide a short answer about the fetal skeleton.*

1. Type I ___THANATOPHORIC DYSP___ is characterized by short, curved femurs and flat vertebral bodies.

2. Type II is characterized by straight, ___SHORT___ femurs, flat vertebral bodies, and a(n) ___CLOVERLEAF___ skull.

3. The most common nonlethal skeletal dysplasia is ___HETEROZYGOUS ACHONDROPLASIA___

4. The sonographic features of achondroplasia may not be evident until after 22 weeks of gestation when biometry becomes abnormal. Sonographic findings include the following:

   ___RHIZOMELIA___

   ___MACROCEPHALY___

   ___TRIDENT HANDS (short proximal and middle phalanges)___

   ___DEPRESSED NASAL BRIDGE___

   ___FRONTAL BOSSING___

   ___MILD VENTRICULOMEGALY___

5. Achondrogenesis is caused by cartilage abnormalities that result in abnormal ___BONE___ formation and ___HYPOMINERALIZATION___

6. Osteogenesis imperfecta is a rare disorder of collagen production leading to ___BRITTLE___ bones; manifestations in the teeth, skin, and ligaments; and blue ___SCLERA___.

7. Type II osteogenesis is considered the most severe form of ___OI___, having a lethal outcome.

8. A condition that presents with diffuse hypomineralization of the bone caused by an alkaline phosphatase deficiency is congenital ___HYPOPHOSPHATASIA___

9. Camptomelic (bent bone) dysplasia is a group of lethal skeletal dysplasias that are characterized by ___BOWING___ of the long bones.

10. Short-rib polydactyly syndrome is a lethal skeletal dysplasia characterized by short ribs, short ___LIMBS___, and polydactyly.

11. Ellis–van Creveld syndrome may present with a(n) ___NARROW___ thorax, causing pulmonary hypoplasia, and heart defects, the most common of which is the ___ASD___.

12. An anomaly in which there is fusion of the lower extremities is ___SIRENOMELIA___.

13. For the VACTERL association to be considered, ___3+___ features must be identified; a(n) ___SINGLE___ umbilical artery may also be identified.

14. Amputation defects may be identified as total or partial absence and may be associated with ___AMNIOTIC BAND___ syndrome.

15. Clubfoot, also known as ___TALIPES___, describes deformities of the foot and ankle.

16. ___ROCKER-BOTTOM___ foot is characterized by a prominent heel and a convex sole.

*Provide a short answer for each question after evaluating the images.*

1. Discuss the sonographic findings in this fetus with a lethal skeletal dysplasia.

_____

_____

_____

(From Henningsen C: *Clinical guide to ultrasonography,* St Louis, 2004, Mosby.)

2. Discuss the sonographic findings in this fetus with achondrogenesis.

_____

_____

A    B

3. This fetus had osteogenesis imperfecta, type II. Describe the sonographic findings.

_____

_____

A    B

4. Images of both femurs in a 22-week fetus. Describe the sonographic findings.

_____

_____

A          B

5. Describe the sonographic findings of the lower extremities.

_____

_____

6. Describe the sonographic findings in these images of the fetal feet.

_____

_____

# Cardiovascular Anatomy Review

Select the answer that best completes the following questions or statements.

1. The tricuspid valve opens when
   a. the right ventricular pressure drops below the right atrial pressure
   b. the papillary muscle contracts
   c. the velocity of blood flow in the right ventricle exceeds the velocity of flow in the right atrium
   d. the pulmonic valve opens

2. Blood normally flows from the right ventricle to the
   a. pulmonary artery
   b. aorta
   c. right atrium
   d. pulmonary vein

3. Which of the following statements about cardiac anatomy is false?
   a. The heart tends to assume a more vertical position in tall, thin people and a more horizontal position in short, heavy people.
   b. The ligamentum arteriosum runs from the left pulmonary artery to the descending aorta.
   c. The coronary arteries arise from the sinuses within the cusps of the aortic valve.
   d. The left ventricle constitutes most of the ventral surface of the heart.

4. The most posterior chamber to the left of the sternum is the
   a. right atrium
   b. left atrium
   c. right ventricle
   d. left ventricle

5. The medial wall of the right atrium contains the
   a. interventricular septum
   b. interatrial septum
   c. right upper pulmonary vein
   d. right lower pulmonary vein

6. The inferior vena cava is guarded by a fold of tissue called the _____ valve, whereas the coronary sinus is guarded by the _____ valve.
   a. eustachian, coronary
   b. thebesian, eustachian
   c. eustachian, thebesian
   d. eustachian, atrial

7. The interventricular septum is divided primarily into two major sections: membranous and muscular. Which of the terms below would be identified with the muscular septum?
    a. inflow
    b. outflow
    c. infundibular
    d. trabecular

8. The wall of the aorta bulges slightly at each semilunar cusp to form
    a. coronary arteries
    b. the sinus of Valsalva
    c. chordae tendineae
    d. Arantius nodule

9. The _____ valve lies behind the right half of the sternum opposite the 4th intercosal space.
    a. mitral
    b. aortic
    c. tricuspid
    d. pulmonic

10. The pulmonary artery may be distinguished from the aorta by all of the following except that
    a. it runs upward and to the left, anterior to the aorta
    b. the cusps are thinner than the aorta
    c. it bifurcates into right and left branches
    d. it runs upward and to the right, posterior to the aorta

11. The point at which the ductus joins the aorta is near the
    a. left common carotid artery
    b. left subclavian artery
    c. brachiocephalic artery
    d. crux of the heart

12. Most coronary venous drainage is into the
    a. coronary veins
    b. coronary sinus
    c. thebesian veins
    d. atrial sinus

13. Atrial contraction follows the _____ on the ECG.
    a. T wave
    b. P wave
    c. QRS
    d. ST segment

14. The brightest returning echo signal on the echocardiogram is from the
    a. anterior wall of the heart
    b. anterior leaflet of the mitral valve
    c. aortic semilunar cusps
    d. pericardium

15. To image the aortic root with semilunar cusps in the parasternal long axis view, the sonographer should angle the transducer
    a. toward the right shoulder
    b. toward the left shoulder
    c. inferior toward the left hip
    d. toward the 4th left ICS

16. The coronary sinus is often identified as a(n)
    a. vertical tubular structure posterior to the heart
    b. oblique tubular structure posterior and lateral to the heart
    c. vertical tubular structure lateral to the heart
    d. horizontal tubular structure posterior to the left atria of the heart

17. The Doppler shift would best be explained in the following way:
    a. If the source is moving toward the listener, it is "catching up" with the wave it just generated; the wavelength becomes shorter, and the listener hears a higher frequency.
    b. If the source is moving away, the wavelength becomes longer, and the listener hears a higher frequency.
    c. If the source is moving toward the listener, the wavelength becomes longer, and the listener hears a higher frequency.
    d. The difference between the frequency generated by the source and that observed by the listener is the Doppler shift.

18. The inflammatory process of the cardiac muscle is known as
    a. endocarditis
    b. pericarditis
    c. epicarditis
    d. myocarditis

19. The term *dyspnea* refers to the condition of
    a. difficulty in digesting food
    b. difficulty in breathing
    c. rapid breathing
    d. deep breathing

20. The amplitude of aortic root motion has been used to assess
    a. the vigor of left ventricular contraction
    b. the degree of aortic stenosis
    c. the degree of aortic insufficiency
    d. the size of the left atrium

21. The best window to image the area of the fossa ovalis is the
    a. apical
    b. subcostal four chamber
    c. parasternal long axis
    d. subcostal short axis

22. Atrial septal defects are classified on the basis of their position in the septum and their embryologic origin. The most common defect is the
    a. ostium primum defect
    b. ostium secundum defect
    c. sinus venosus defect
    d. primum secundum defect

23. The structure that plays a significant role in the development of the septum primum, atrioventricular valves, and membranous septum is the
    a. endocardial cushion
    b. ventral septal endocardium
    c. atrial septal endocardium
    d. endocardial fibroelastocushion

24. The heart is lined by a serous visceral membrane called the
    a. pericardium
    b. endocardium
    c. myocardium
    d. epicardium

25. The middle muscular layer of the heart is the
    a. pericardium
    b. endocardium
    c. myocardium
    d. epicardium

26. The _____ is located inside the pericardium and the myocardium and is most prominent around the inflow and outflow arteries of the heart.
    a. epicardium
    b. visceral pericardium
    c. pericardial fat
    d. endocardium

27. Risk factors identified for stroke include all of the following except
    a. age
    b. sex
    c. hypertension
    d. pregnancy

28. The warning signs of stroke include all of the following except
    a. symptoms of weakness or numbness
    b. sudden confusion, trouble speaking or understanding
    c. hypotension
    d. difficulty seeing or walking

29. An ischemic neurologic deficit that lasts less than 24 hours is known as
    a. CVA
    b. TIA
    c. RIND
    d. BEND

30. Blood supply to the brain is provided by the _____ arteries.
    a. internal and external
    b. carotid and vertebral
    c. ophthalmic and posterior communicating
    d. middle cerebral and anterior cerebral

31. Symptoms of lower-extremity occlusive arterial disease include
    a. claudication and rest pain
    b. shoulder pain
    c. thoracic pain
    d. lower abdominal pain

32. Characteristics of a normal Doppler arterial waveform include all of the following except
    a. triphasic
    b. high-velocity forward flow during systole
    c. low-velocity forward flow during systole
    d. short flow reversal in early diastole

33. A potentially lethal complication of acute DVT is
    a. pulmonary embolism
    b. claudication
    c. abscess
    d. fistula

34. Dilated, elongated, tortuous superficial veins are
    a. perforating veins
    b. varicose veins
    c. abscessed veins
    d. tortellini veins

# General Sonography Review

*Select the answer that best completes the following questions or statements.*

1. Useful clinical history and clinical symptoms the sonographer should be aware of in a patient who presents with acute abdominal pain include all of the following except
   a. past history
   b. previous diagnostic examinations and pertinent laboratory findings
   c. age and present condition
   d. weight

2. Which of the following would be most useful to the sonographer trying to define the nature of a patient's pain?
   a. Has the pain shifted?
   b. Locate the pain with your hand.
   c. Is there any radiation of the pain?
   d. Is the pain related to food ingestion?

3. All of the following questions relate to vomiting except
   a. Is it related to pain?
   b. How often does it occur?
   c. Is it related to inspiration?
   d. Is it associated with nausea?

4. When a pelvic examination is performed, all of the following questions regarding menstruation should be asked except
   a. What was the date of the LMP?
   b. Was the LMP normal?
   c. How long have you been pregnant?
   d. Do you have pain associated with your period?

5. All of the following terms relate to the past history of a patient except
   a. apnea
   b. jaundice
   c. weight loss
   d. fatigue

6. Central upper abdominal pain most likely would be associated with which of the following diseases?
   a. Crohn's disease
   b. diverticulitis
   c. acute pancreatitis
   d. pelvic inflammatory disease

7. Central pain with shock may be seen in all of the following conditions except
   a. cholelithiasis
   b. ectopic pregnancy
   c. internal hemorrhage
   d. dissecting aneurysm

**493**

8. An acute abdomen in a pregnant patient may represent any of the following conditions except
    a. degeneration of a fibroid
    b. hydatid disease
    c. ovarian torsion
    d. pelvic peritonitis

9. Patients who present with RUQ pain may have any of the following conditions except
    a. gallbladder disease
    b. hepatitis
    c. Baker's cyst
    d. renal stones

10. An abdominal trauma case may present with any of the following conditions except
    a. rupture of the cerebellum
    b. rupture of the liver, spleen, or kidney
    c. rupture of the bladder
    d. rupture of the intestine

11. Common clinical findings in patients with renal disease include any of the following except
    a. urinary pain, frequency, retention
    b. hematuria
    c. flank pain
    d. pectoralis pain

12. The most specific laboratory value in detecting acute pancreatitis is
    a. serum amylase
    b. serum lipase
    c. BUN
    d. bilirubin

13. Clinical signs of urinary tract infection may include any or all of the following except
    a. fever
    b. tremors
    c. nausea
    d. flank pain

14. Alkaline phosphatase is markedly increased in patients with
    a. hepatocellular disease
    b. early obstruction
    c. hydatid disease
    d. polycystic disease

15. If there is an interruption of the IVC, which vascular structure will take over its "job"?
    a. SVC
    b. azygos
    c. lumbar
    d. iliac

16. Distribution of blood to the liver, spleen, and stomach occurs via the
    a. portal vein
    b. celiac trunk vessels
    c. gastroduodenal artery
    d. superior mesenteric vein

17. Distribution of the proximal half of the colon and small intestine occurs via the
    a. splenic artery
    b. IMA
    c. SMA
    d. hepatic vein

18. A patient who presents with a clot in the main portal vein and hepatopetal flow in the collaterals most likely has
    a. hepatic vein thrombosis
    b. transformation of the portal vein
    c. renal vein thrombosis
    d. Budd-Chiari syndrome

19. When venous obstruction occurs within the liver or in extrahepatic portal veins, which condition exists?
    a. pulmonary hypertension
    b. portal hypertension
    c. superior mesenteric artery obstruction
    d. renal vein thrombosis

20. The most common collaterals in portal hypertension are
    a. left gastric and paraumbilical veins
    b. retroperitoneal and short gastric veins
    c. splenorenal and omental veins
    d. splenoperitoneal and retroperitoneal veins

21. The shunt that is performed via a transjugular approach is called
    a. PITS
    b. SIPS
    c. JITS
    d. TIPS

22. As portal venous flow to the liver decreases, hepatic arterial flow
    a. decreases
    b. increases
    c. stabilizes
    d. remains the same

23. Clinical signs of hepatic vein obstruction are characterized by all of the following except
    a. hepatomegaly
    b. shrunken liver
    c. ascites
    d. pain

24. Ultrasound excels over CT in its ability to image
    a. fascial planes and fat-containing structures
    b. ascites and intraperitoneal abscesses
    c. mesenteric infiltration
    d. omental seeding

25. Intraperitoneal fluid first accumulates in
    a. cul-de-sac or retrovesical fossa
    b. mesentery
    c. omental bursa
    d. pericolic ligaments

26. The location and distribution of intraperitoneal fluid are influenced by all of the following except
    a. patient position
    b. viscosity of the fluid
    c. respiration
    d. peritoneal adhesions

27. When ascites is found unexpectedly, the abdomen must be surveyed to detect all of the following except
    a. malignancy
    b. renal hypertension
    c. portal hypertension
    d. hepatic or portal vein thrombosis

28. Serous fluid is
    a. echogenic
    b. inhomogeneous
    c. anechoic
    d. complex

29. Peritoneal fluid that contains septations, low-level echoes, or debris suggests all of the following except
    a. portal vein thrombosis
    b. infection
    c. hemorrhage
    d. carcinomatosis

30. Which statement is false?
    a. Long-standing ascites may contain internal septations and may be loculated.
    b. Uninfected ascites usually has no mass effect and passively conforms to intraperitoneal compartments.
    c. Abscesses never displace adjacent bowel or organs.
    d. Abscesses usually have significant mass effect.

31. Acute intraperitoneal hemorrhage most often is caused by all of the following except
    a. lymphadenopathy
    b. blunt trauma
    c. ruptured ectopic pregnancy
    d. interventional procedures

32. This layer is a constant anatomic feature of the GI tract and serves as a useful landmark to identify a loop of bowel:
    a. muscularis propria
    b. submucosal layer
    c. muscularis mucosa
    d. adventitial surface

33. Neoplastic invasion of the bowel may cause a target or _____ appearance.
    a. sandwich sign
    b. comet tail
    c. pseudokidney
    d. mirror image

34. Landmarks the sonographer should use to image the appendix include all of the following except
    a. right colon
    b. cecum
    c. left colon
    d. psoas muscle

35. Complications of appendicitis may include all of the following except
    a. gangrenous infection
    b. periappendiceal abscess
    c. appendicolith
    d. cholecystitis

36. A mucocele is the result of
    a. acute appendicitis
    b. phlegmon
    c. chronic obstruction of the appendix
    d. intramural hemorrhage

37. Optimal color flow and spectral Doppler sonography of the liver requires
    a. high-frequency scanning
    b. low-frequency scanning
    c. high PRF
    d. increased scan angle

38. Flash artifact is associated with
    a. wraparound
    b. diaphragm interface
    c. color related to tissue motion
    d. decreased respiration

39. Thicker septations seen within a cyst are usually
    a. complicated cyst or neoplasm
    b. adenoma
    c. polycystic disease
    d. focal nodular hyperplasia

40. The most common benign hepatic neoplasm is
    a. adenoma
    b. hepatoma
    c. cavernous hemangioma
    d. angiomyolipoma

41. The most common liver metastases originate from all of the following except
    a. lung
    b. colon
    c. pancreas
    d. brain

42. The most common primary liver cancer in the United States is
    a. hemangioma
    b. hepatoblastoma
    c. liposarcoma
    d. hepatocellular carcinoma

43. The type of tumor that arises from the bile ducts to account for 10% of all primary liver cancers is
    a. cholangioma
    b. cholangiocarcinoma
    c. cholangiosarcoma
    d. cholangiolipoma

44. This type of abscess should be suspected when a patient presents from a high-risk population (e.g., recent immigrant from an endemic area, patients living in poor sanitary conditions, HIV-positive patients):
    a. pyogenic
    b. echinococcal
    c. fungal microabscess
    d. amebic

45. The most common symptomatic liver tumor in children younger than 5 years is
    a. Wilms' tumor
    b. hepatoblastoma
    c. neuroblastoma
    d. nephroblastoma

46. In chronic viral hepatitis, hepatomegaly and inhomogeneous patchy or diffuse increased echogenicity are common and are related to the
    a. amount of fatty infiltration and fibrosis present
    b. amount of fibrosis present
    c. amount of portal hypertension present
    d. amount of vascular compression present

47. Fatty liver is a nonspecific response to liver injury and may occur in dysnutritional states including any of the following except
    a. obesity
    b. hyperlipidemia
    c. dehydration
    d. diabetes mellitus

48. Fatty infiltration is often patchy or focal. A less affected region of the liver is called
    a. spared
    b. infiltrated
    c. hyperfused
    d. revascularized

49. In sonographic evaluation of patients with cirrhosis of the liver, all of the following should be considered except
    a. ratio of LLL to RLL
    b. nodularity of the liver surface
    c. attenuation of the ultrasound transmission
    d. increased size of the caudate lobe

50. The thyroid gland can be located at the level of the
    a. thyroid cartilage
    b. manubrium
    c. hyoid bone
    d. cricoid cartilage

51. Which of the following is typically the largest vascular structure located in the neck?
    a. common carotid artery
    b. internal jugular vein
    c. internal carotid artery
    d. external jugular vein

52. Which muscle divides the neck into anterior and posterior triangles?
    a. trapezius
    b. platysma
    c. longissimus dorsi
    d. sternocleidomastoid

53. The superior vena cava is formed by the junction of the
    a. internal jugular veins
    b. external jugular veins
    c. subclavian veins
    d. brachiocephalic veins

54. Which of the following makes up the apex of the heart?
    a. right atrium
    b. left atrium
    c. right ventricle
    d. left ventricle

55. Collateral circulation between the IVC and the SVC is supplied by the
    a. thoracic veins
    b. subclavian veins
    c. azygos veins
    d. intercostal veins

56. Which of the following is not considered a mediastinal structure?
    a. heart
    b. lungs
    c. trachea
    d. thymus gland

57. What vein passes anterior to the third part of the duodenum and posterior to the neck of the pancreas?
    a. portal
    b. splenic
    c. superior mesenteric
    d. inferior mesenteric

58. The gastroepiploic artery is a branch of the
    a. left gastric artery
    b. hepatic artery
    c. splenic artery
    d. pancreatic artery

59. Distribution of blood to the liver, spleen, and stomach occurs via the
    a. portal vein
    b. celiac trunk vessels
    c. gastroduodenal artery
    d. superior mesenteric vein

60. Distribution of blood to the proximal half of the colon and small intestine occurs via the
    a. splenic artery
    b. IMA
    c. SMA
    d. hepatic vein

61. The most common cause for abdominal aneurysm is
    a. cystic medial necrosis
    b. syphilis
    c. atheroma
    d. arteriosclerosis

62. An aneurysm that is connected to the vascular lumen by a neck that varies in size is
    a. fusiform
    b. saccular
    c. berry
    d. cylindroid

63. The triphasic waveform seen in the hepatic veins reflects the contractility of the
    a. right atrium
    b. left atrium
    c. right ventricle
    d. left ventricle

64. Which structure is retroperitoneal?
    a. gallbladder
    b. spleen
    c. pancreas
    d. stomach

65. Which of the following arteries is NOT one of the branches of the celiac axis?
    a. hepatic artery
    b. splenic artery
    c. gastric artery
    d. cystic artery

66. Which part of the pancreas is located in the curve of the duodenum?
    a. head
    b. neck
    c. body
    d. tail

67. What is the smallest lobe of the liver?
    a. right
    b. left
    c. caudate
    d. Riedel's

68. Which thin, tendinous structure connects the two rectus abdominis muscles at the midline?
    a. linea alba
    b. transversus abdominis
    c. internal oblique
    d. ligamentum teres

69. Morison's pouch is located in the
    a. subhepatic space
    b. subphrenic space
    c. paracolic gutter
    d. retroperitoneal space

70. Which of the following does not unite to form the portal vein?
    a. superior mesenteric vein
    b. inferior mesenteric vein
    c. hepatic vein
    d. splenic vein

71. The peritoneum is divided into the _____ layer, which lines the abdominal walls, and the _____ layer, which covers the organs.
    a. parietal, visceral
    b. visceral, parietal
    c. serous, mucous
    d. outer, inner

72. The major renal calyces empty urine into the
    a. pyramids
    b. arteries
    c. papilla
    d. pelvis

73. What anatomic area would you examine to rule out a rectus sheath hematoma?
    a. posterior abdominal wall
    b. anterior chest wall
    c. lateral wall
    d. anterior abdominal wall

74. The interlobar arteries of the kidneys can be found
    a. at the base of the medullary pyramids
    b. branching at right angles from the arcuate arteries
    c. coursing toward the cortex along the lateral borders of the pyramids
    d. along the capsule of the kidney

75. The glomerulus is
    a. contained in the loop of Henle
    b. a network of capillaries encased in Bowman's capsule
    c. located in the renal papilla
    d. found in the renal pelvis

76. The apices of the renal pyramids project into the minor calyces as the
    a. convoluted tubules
    b. renal columns of Bertin
    c. renal papillae
    d. glomerulus

77. Which of the following statements is true regarding the sonographic appearance of the neonatal kidney?
    a. The medullary pyramids are larger in relation to the cortex than in adult life.
    b. The kidneys are generally much more echogenic than the liver in the newborn and become increasingly less echogenic with age.
    c. In the normal newborn, the kidneys are often echogenic compared with the liver and spleen.
    d. The kidneys are generally smaller in relation to the other organs than they will appear in adult life.

78. The right adrenal gland is located
    a. anterior to the IVC, superior and medial to the upper pole of the right kidney, and posterior to the crus of the diaphragm
    b. posterior to the IVC, superior and lateral to the upper pole of the right kidney, and anterior to the crus of the diaphragm
    c. medial to the IVC, superior and medial to the upper pole of the right kidney, and posterior to the crus of the diaphragm
    d. posterior to the IVC, superior and medial to the upper pole of the right kidney, and anterior to the crus of the diaphragm

79. Arcuate arteries in the kidney are branches of the
    a. segmental arteries
    b. interlobar arteries
    c. renal arteries
    d. papillary arteries

80. The left renal vein courses
    a. posterior to the IVC
    b. anterior to the IVC
    c. anterior to the AO
    d. anterior to the SMA

81. The common bile duct can be seen at the _____ aspect of the pancreatic head.
    a. anterolateral
    b. superior
    c. anteromedial
    d. posteromedial

82. A choledochal cyst is an abnormality of the
    a. sphincter of Oddi
    b. gallbladder
    c. common bile duct
    d. pancreatic duct

83. The major renal calyces empty urine into the
    a. minor calyces and/or pyramids
    b. arteries
    c. papilla
    d. pelvis

84. Which of the following statements is TRUE regarding the common bile duct?
    a. It crosses the duodenum anteriorly before reaching the pancreas.
    b. It extends from the neck of the gallbladder to the duodenum.
    c. It is formed by the confluence of the cystic and common hepatic ducts.
    d. It courses posterior to the portal vein.

85. A thickened gallbladder wall may be encountered in any of the following states except
    a. ascites
    b. acute cholecystitis
    c. hydrops
    d. cholangiocarcinoma

86. In a 50-year-old female, the intraluminal diameter of the normal distal common bile duct should not exceed
    a. 4 mm
    b. 5 mm
    c. 6 mm
    d. 7 mm

87. Which of the following statements is NOT true regarding the spleen?

    a. The stomach lies on the posterior border of the spleen.

    b. The spleen is positioned posteriorly in the left upper quadrant.

    c. The spleen is bordered posteriorly by the ribs and the left kidney.

    d. The splenic artery is a branch of the portal trunk.

88. Which of the following is NOT true regarding multicystic dysplastic kidney?

    a. The reniform contour of the kidney is maintained.

    b. The cysts are of variable size and have a random distribution.

    c. Contralateral disease occurs in approximately one third of patients.

    d. The normal central echo pattern of the renal pelvis is generally absent.

89. An 8-year-old boy presents with a recent sore throat, hematuria and proteinuria, urinary red cell casts, and a slightly elevated BUN. His history is very suggestive of acute poststreptococcal glomerulonephritis. Which of the following is false?

    a. The renal sonogram may demonstrate a diffuse increase in cortical echogenicity similar to that of the renal sinus.

    b. Acute glomerulonephritis is usually an incidental finding.

    c. The kidneys may be enlarged in acute glomerulonephritis.

    d. The disease may reverse or progress to end-stage renal disease.

90. Which of the following is NOT a true statement about renal allograft rejection?

    a. The allograft increases in size at a greater rate than that associated with compensatory hypertrophy.

    b. Shrinking and increased echogenicity of the renal medullary pyramids occur.

    c. The size and echogenicity of the central renal sinus fat are diminished.

    d. The allograft may lose its elliptical configuration and become more globular in shape.

91. Which of the following is NOT a sign of renal transplant rejection?

    a. enlargement and decreased echogenicity of the pyramids

    b. hyperechoic cortex

    c. localized area of renal parenchyma presenting with an anechoic appearance

    d. hydronephrosis

92. Sonographic findings of acute cholecystitis include all of the following except

    a. positive Murphy's sign

    b. thickened gallbladder wall

    c. hydrops

    d. contracted gallbladder filled with stones

93. A tumor of the adrenal medulla that produces intermittent hypertension is

    a. neuroblastoma

    b. adenoma

    c. pheochromocytoma

    d. hyperplasia

94. A fluid collection that tends to occur 2 to 6 weeks posttransplantation and is associated with a chronic diminution in renal function rather than an acute decrease in urine output is the
   a. seroma
   b. abscess
   c. urinoma
   d. lymphocele

95. Which of the following describes the Doppler criteria used to diagnose acute vascular rejection of a renal allograft?
   a. In acute vascular rejection, diastolic flow in the renal, arcuate, and interlobar arteries rises significantly in relation to the systolic value.
   b. In acute vascular rejection, the diastolic value in the renal artery decreases in relation to the systolic value in the interlobar and arcuate arteries.
   c. In acute vascular rejection, the systolic-to-diastolic ratio decreases in the arcuate, interlobar, and renal arteries.
   d. In acute vascular rejection, the diastolic flow decreases, reverses, or becomes absent in the renal, arcuate, and interlobar arteries, increasing the systolic-to-diastolic ratio.

96. Which of the following would most likely cause anterior displacement of the superior mesenteric artery and vein?
   a. pancreatic neoplasm
   b. para-aortic lymphadenopathy
   c. cholelithiasis
   d. small-bowel obstruction

97. Courvoisier's gallbladder is associated with
   a. cholesterolosis
   b. multiple cholesterol polyps
   c. pancreatic head mass
   d. chronic cholecystitis

98. A form of infection seen in patients with obstruction secondary to long-standing calculi and chronic renal infection is
   a. acute lobar nephronia
   b. acute bacterial nephritis
   c. xanthogranulomatous pyelonephritis
   d. chronic atrophic pyelonephritis

99. A localized process in the kidney that forms a wedge-shaped phlegmonous lesion in which no true abscess exists is a(n)
   a. renal carbuncle
   b. acute lobar nephronia
   c. xanthogranulomatous pyelonephritis
   d. chronic atrophic pyelonephritis

100. Empyema of the gallbladder refers to
   a. gas in the gallbladder wall
   b. pus-filled gallbladder
   c. distention of the gallbladder with mucus and stones
   d. calcified gallbladder

101. Which of the following is NOT a true statement regarding adult polycystic disease?

    a. It is a form of primary renal disease transmitted as an autosomal dominant trait.

    b. Patients typically present with a large kidney, which contains multiple cysts of varying sizes, loss of the reniform contour, and no definable central echo complex.

    c. Associated cysts may be found in the liver and pancreas.

    d. Clinically, patients present with deteriorating renal function.

102. The blood supply to the gallbladder is accomplished by the

    a. gastroduodenal artery

    b. right gastric artery

    c. portal vein

    d. cystic artery

103. Cholangitis refers to

    a. inflammation of a bile duct

    b. inflammation of the gallbladder

    c. inflammation of a choledochal cyst

    d. inflammation of the bladder

104. A high level of serum amylase may be a result of

    a. liver disease

    b. dilated intrahepatic ducts

    c. pancreatitis

    d. insulinoma

105. Which of the following is NOT a retroperitoneal structure?

    a. pancreas

    b. kidney

    c. adrenal

    d. liver

106. The *primary* hormones produced in the pancreas are

    a. glucagon and insulin

    b. collagen and fibrin

    c. lipase and cholase

    d. pancreatin and secretin

107. The membrane that lines the abdominal cavity is the

    a. retroperitoneum

    b. omentum

    c. mesentery

    d. peritoneum

108. Chronic pancreatitis is usually associated with all of the following sonographic patterns except

    a. hyperechoic, more echogenic than liver

    b. generalized decrease in size

    c. bright, discrete echoes from calcification, dilated pancreatic duct

    d. hypoechoic with diffuse swelling

109. The target-like structure anterior to the aorta and posterior to the left lobe of the liver represents the normal
    a. appendix
    b. pylorus
    c. antrum
    d. esophagogastric junction

110. Which of the following statements about the right crus of the diaphragm is true?
    a. It is larger and longer than the left.
    b. It attaches the psoas muscle to the diaphragm.
    c. It is the frequent site of metastasis in lymphoma.
    d. It is shorter than the left.

111. Which of the following does not describe the pancreas?
    a. It lies within the peritoneal space.
    b. It is a retroperitoneal structure.
    c. It is nonencapsulated.
    d. It is a multilobulated gland.

112. Which of the following is the correct order of abdominal wall structures from the skin inward?
    a. linea alba, rectus muscle, subcutaneous fat
    b. subcutaneous fat, rectus sheath, rectus muscle, peritoneum
    c. peritoneum, linea alba, rectus sheath
    d. rectus muscle, peritoneum, linea alba

113. With aging, the pancreas becomes
    a. smaller and more echogenic
    b. larger and more echogenic
    c. smaller and less echogenic
    d. the same size but less echogenic

114. The most common posthepatic transplant vascular complication is
    a. portal vein thrombosis
    b. hepatic artery thrombosis
    c. portal hypertension
    d. hepatic vein thrombosis

115. The abdominal organ transplant most commonly performed is
    a. pancreas
    b. liver
    c. kidney
    d. heart

116. The aorta is named the "abdominal aorta" when it passes through the
    a. diaphragm
    b. Glisson's capsule
    c. spleen hiatus
    d. aortic arch

117. Atherosclerosis involves accumulation of lipids in the
    a. intima only
    b. media only
    c. intima and media
    d. adventitia only

118. The most common type of aneurysm is
    a. saccular
    b. mycotic
    c. fusiform
    d. pseudoaneurysm

119. A complication of pancreatitis is
    a. formation of islet cell tumor
    b. formation of pseudocyst
    c. formation of cystadenoma
    d. pancreatic carcinoma

120. The most common cause of aortic aneurysm is
    a. infection
    b. atherosclerosis
    c. trauma
    d. congenital

121. The spleen is a peritoneal structure lying between
    a. the right hemidiaphragm and the stomach
    b. the left hemidiaphragm and the stomach
    c. the hepatic flexure of the colon and the left kidney
    d. spleen is not peritoneal

122. The most echogenic organ or structure listed below is the
    a. liver
    b. spleen
    c. renal sinus
    d. pancreas

123. The remnant of the fetal umbilical vein is the
    a. main lobar fissure
    b. ligamentum venosum
    c. falciform ligament
    d. ligamentum teres

124. Focal calcifications seen in the spleen as small, bright, echogenic foci with or without shadow are often the result of
    a. metastasis
    b. primary neoplasm
    c. previous granulomatous infection
    d. hydatid disease

125. Splenomegaly may be associated with diffuse splenic disease that includes all of the following except
    a. sickle cell
    b. hereditary spherocytosis
    c. polycythemia vera
    d. abscess

126. The pancreas is both an exocrine and an endocrine gland. The endocrine function is to produce
    a. insulin
    b. lipase
    c. amylase
    d. trypsin

127. Mild to moderate splenomegaly most often is caused by all of the following except
    a. infection, portal hypertension, or AIDS
    b. metastatic disease
    c. trauma
    d. leukemia

128. A phlegmon of the pancreas represents
    a. an inflammatory process
    b. a malignant neoplasm
    c. a benign adenoma
    d. a functioning islet cell tumor

129. If a mass is found in the head of the pancreas, special attention should be directed to which of the following areas?
    a. the portal vein for portal hypertension
    b. the liver for fatty changes
    c. the spleen for splenomegaly
    d. the bile ducts for dilatation

130. When the gallbladder fundus is folded over on itself, it is called
    a. junctional fold
    b. Hartmann's pouch
    c. phrygian cap
    d. Morison's pouch

131. One sonographic method used to distinguish dilated bile ducts involves demonstrating the
    a. double-barrel shotgun sign
    b. Mirizzi syndrome
    c. Courvoisier's sign
    d. stop sign

132. A congenital insertion of the common bile duct (CBD) into the pancreatic duct causing a focal and abnormal dilatation of the CBD is called
    a. sclerosing cholangitis
    b. Courvoisier's gallbladder
    c. choledochal cyst
    d. biliary atresia

133. Adenomyomatosis of the gallbladder is
    a. proliferation and thickening of the epithelial layer with glandlike outpouchings in the wall
    b. an inflammation of the gallbladder wall
    c. strongly associated with a positive Murphy's sign
    d. always accompanied by dilated ducts

134. A 42-year-old female presents with right upper quadrant pain and nausea that comes and goes. Her sonogram reveals a normal-sized gallbladder with a slightly thick wall and contains a small echogenic focus that casts an acoustic shadow. This most likely represents
    a. choledochal cyst
    b. cholangitis
    c. cholelithiasis with chronic cholecystitis
    d. choledocholithiasis with intermittent jaundice

135. Nonshadowing, nonmobile echogenic foci attached to the gallbladder wall most likely represent
    a. calculi
    b. gravel
    c. sludge
    d. polyps

136. Thick, viscid bile ("sludge") within the gallbladder indicates
    a. obstruction of the intrahepatic ducts
    b. an incidental finding sometimes linked to gallbladder pathology
    c. the definite presence of calculi
    d. carcinoma of the gallbladder

137. All of the following describe the appearance of a gallbladder filled with stones except
    a. WES triad
    b. double-arc sign
    c. two parallel echogenic lines separated by a thin anechoic space with distal acoustic shadowing
    d. single echogenic line from the falciform ligament with posterior shadowing

138. The usual sonographic appearance of acute pancreatitis is
    a. hyperechoic with generalized decrease in size
    b. hypoechoic with generalized enlargement
    c. isoechoic with generalized enlargement
    d. isoechoic with increase in size

139. Focal gallbladder tenderness is referred to as
    a. Mirizzi syndrome
    b. Courvoisier's sign
    c. Klatskin's sign
    d. positive Murphy's sign

140. Perforation of the gallbladder is strongly associated with
    a. gangrenous cholecystitis
    b. acute cholecystitis
    c. chronic cholecystitis
    d. biliary atresia

141. With regard to bile duct dimensions after a cholecystectomy, the size of the CHD or CBD may be
    a. somewhat larger
    b. somewhat smaller
    c. slow to return to normal size for several months
    d. shortened

142. Jaundice is due to a buildup of _____ in the body.
    a. glycogen
    b. urea
    c. heparin
    d. bilirubin

143. One way to distinguish hepatic veins from portal veins is by
    a. size; the hepatic veins are much smaller than the portal veins
    b. tracing them to their points of origin
    c. noting the decrease in caliber as they approach the IVC
    d. visualizing the wall thickness of the vessels, knowing that hepatic veins have thicker walls

144. A patent umbilical vein may be found in the
    a. ligamentum venosum
    b. main labor fissure
    c. ligamentum teres
    d. intersegmental fissure

145. The portal veins can be distinguished from the hepatic veins by their
    a. thicker wall and echogenic rim surrounding them
    b. thin wall and echo-poor rim surrounding them
    c. close proximity to the periphery
    d. cluster-like appearance close to the hepatic periphery

146. The portal triad consists of
    a. portal vein, hepatic artery, bile duct
    b. left hepatic vein, middle hepatic vein, right hepatic vein
    c. common duct, cystic duct, pancreatic duct
    d. caudate lobe of liver, right lobe of liver, left lobe of liver

147. A high level of serum lipase would be most associated with
    a. liver disease
    b. dilated intrahepatic ducts
    c. pancreatitis
    d. insulinoma

148. Which of the following is the most common site for pseudocyst formation?
    a. iliac fossa
    b. lesser sac
    c. Morison's pouch
    d. pouch of Douglas

149. The celiac axis gives rise to all of the following vessels except
    a. splenic artery
    b. hepatic artery
    c. superior mesenteric artery
    d. left gastric artery

150. A linear echodensity that connects the gallbladder to the main portal vein is the
    a. ligamentum teres
    b. main lobar fissure
    c. ligamentum venosum
    d. coronary ligament

151. Chronic pancreatitis most often is caused by
    a. cholelithiasis
    b. ETOH abuse
    c. trauma
    d. choledocholithiasis

152. The vessel that can be seen posterior to the IVC is the
    a. right renal artery
    b. splenic artery
    c. pancreaticoduodenal artery
    d. left renal vein

153. Which of the following vessels courses between the SMA and the aorta?
    a. right renal vein
    b. right renal artery
    c. gastroduodenal artery
    d. left renal vein

154. Which of the following structures is seen in close relation to the anterolateral aspect of the head of the pancreas?
    a. common bile duct
    b. pancreaticoduodenal artery
    c. right gastric vein
    d. gastroduodenal artery

155. In the liver, the right and left hepatic ducts will join to form the
    a. cystic duct
    b. common bile duct
    c. valves of Heister
    d. common hepatic duct

156. Calcifications, pancreatic duct dilatation, and pseudocyst formation are most consistent with
    a. islet cell tumor
    b. acute and chronic pancreatitis
    c. cholelithiasis
    d. adenocarcinoma

157. Budd-Chiari syndrome may present sonographically as
    a. relative enlargement of the caudate lobe caused by hepatic vein thrombosis of the liver
    b. relative shrinkage of the caudate lobe caused by splenic vein thrombosis
    c. relative enlargement of the quadrate lobe caused by splenic vein thrombosis
    d. relative shrinkage of all lobes of the liver caused by IVC thrombosis

158. The liver is supplied with blood via the
    a. inferior vena cava and hepatic veins
    b. splenic artery and splenic vein
    c. abdominal aorta and iliac artery
    d. hepatic artery and portal vein

159. The normal echographic pattern of the liver is
    a. diffusely inhomogeneous throughout
    b. patchy areas of increased echogenicity
    c. decreased areas of echogenicity diffusely situated
    d. homogeneous throughout without interruption of the echo pattern

160. Lymphocele is a fluid collection caused by
    a. lymph duct obstruction secondary to inflammation
    b. agenesis of a lymphatic chain
    c. lymph-filled spaces secondary to surgery
    d. enlarged lymph nodes secondary to neoplasm

161. The segments of the right lobe of the liver are
    a. medial and lateral
    b. anterior and posterior
    c. cephalad and caudad
    d. caudad and quadrate

162. Loculations within ascites are most commonly the result of
    a. malignancy or inflammation
    b. benign conditions
    c. pedal edema
    d. pleural effusions

163. Riedel's lobe is a normal liver variant defined as a(n)
    a. elongated left lobe of the liver
    b. tonguelike extension of the caudate lobe of the liver
    c. tonguelike extension of the right lobe of the liver
    d. tonguelike extension of the quadrate lobe of the liver

164. Ascites is defined as accumulation of fluid in the
    a. abdominal wall
    b. peritoneal cavity
    c. retroperitoneal cavity
    d. any abdominal cavity

165. The visceral peritoneum refers to the surface that is in contact with the
    a. abdominal wall
    b. organs
    c. skin
    d. retroperitoneum

166. Ultrasound is capable of demonstrating the ligaments and fissures of the liver because
    a. they are hyperechoic
    b. collagen and fat are present within and around these structures
    c. they contain heparin, an echogenic substance
    d. they are perpendicular to the beam

167. Crohn's disease is an inflammatory bowel disease usually affecting the
    a. terminal ileum
    b. stomach
    c. pylorus
    d. esophagus

168. Compared with the adult adrenal gland, the neonatal adrenal gland
    a. appears larger and increased in medullary echogenicity
    b. appears smaller and hypoechoic
    c. appears no different
    d. cannot be seen

169. An echogenic linear echo located immediately anterior to the caudate lobe represents the
    a. main lobar fissure
    b. ligamentum venosum
    c. falciform ligament
    d. ligamentum teres

170. The segments of the left lobe of the liver are
    a. medial and lateral
    b. anterior and posterior
    c. cephalad and caudad
    d. caudate and quadrate

171. When longitudinal scans of the liver are performed with a subcostal approach, the patient is asked to take in a deep breath. This technique displaces the liver
    a. anteriorly
    b. posteriorly
    c. superiorly
    d. inferiorly

172. Sonographic visualization of the anterior wall of the appendix greater than _____ in an adult with RLQ pain is highly suggestive of acute appendicitis.
    a. 1.6 cm
    b. 16 mm
    c. 6 cm
    d. 6 mm

173. Portal vein obstruction may develop as an extension of
    a. hepatocellular carcinoma
    b. Budd-Chiari syndrome
    c. marked dilatation of the interhepatic veins
    d. fatty liver infiltration

174. Portal vein gas is an important diagnosis in the infant associated with
    a. right renal cell carcinoma
    b. ascites
    c. abdominal tumor
    d. necrotizing enterocolitis

175. The reflection of the liver above the diaphragm is due to
    a. reverberation
    b. mirror-image artifact
    c. reflection
    d. ring-down artifact

176. Metastatic lesions in the liver may appear sonographically as any of the following except
    a. anechoic with decreased transmission
    b. hyperechoic with decreased transmission
    c. hypoechoic
    d. anechoic with good transmission

177. Glycogen storage disease is associated with
    a. adenomas
    b. angiomyolipomas
    c. lipomas
    d. pancreatitis

178. An amebic abscess of the liver most frequently is located
    a. superior to the liver
    b. in the right lobe of the liver
    c. in the caudate lobe of the liver
    d. inferior to the liver, posterior to the right kidney

179. Which of the following disorders may not produce a complex sonographic pattern?
    a. infected cyst
    b. hemorrhagic cyst
    c. hematoma
    d. congenital cyst

180. All of the following structures form neighboring structures for the thyroid gland except
    a. superficial and deep fascia
    b. parotid muscle
    c. strap muscles
    d. sternocleidomastoid muscle

181. All of the following statements about thyroid cysts are true except
    a. Cysts account for 20% of all cold thyroid nodules.
    b. Lesions are usually multiple.
    c. The vast majority result from hemorrhage or degenerative changes in an adenoma.
    d. Incidence of carcinoma in cystic lesions less than 4 cm is less than 2%.

182. The most common sonographic finding of a thyroid goiter is
    a. lymph node enlargement
    b. rapidly enlarging mass
    c. fainting
    d. thyroid enlargement

183. All of the following details about thyroid carcinoma are true except
    a. has central sonolucent halo
    b. most common endocrine malignancy
    c. usually found in women older than 40 years of age
    d. rapid growth

184. The most descriptive sonographic finding in thyroid carcinoma is
    a. well-defined borders
    b. lesion is more hyperechoic than normal thyroid tissue
    c. solid complex mass with heterogeneous echo pattern and irregular margins
    d. lymph nodes of normal size

185. The most common feature of a thyroid adenoma is
    a. diffuse echogenicity
    b. hemorrhage
    c. peripheral sonolucent halo
    d. inhomogeneity

186. The most common cause of hyperparathyroidism is
    a. thyroid adenoma
    b. parathyroid adenoma
    c. parathyroid cyst
    d. parathyroid hemorrhagic cyst

187. Fat, Cooper's ligaments, connective tissue, blood vessels, nerves, and lymphatics are found
    a. in the retromammary region
    b. in the parenchyma
    c. in the subcutaneous layer
    d. in the subareolar area

188. The most important signs to look for in identifying a cystic lesion of the breast include all of the following except
    a. well-defined borders
    b. good through-transmission
    c. anechoic
    d. disruption of architecture

189. The most common solid benign tumor of the breast is
    a. cystosarcoma phyllodes
    b. fibroadenoma
    c. papilloma
    d. lipoma

190. A cystic enlargement of a distal duct filled with milk is called a
    a. galectostasis
    b. galactoma
    c. galactocele
    d. lacterrhea

191. The most common malignant neoplasm of the breast in women is
    a. lymphoma
    b. adenocarcinoma
    c. mucinous carcinoma
    d. cystosarcoma phyllodes

192. A breast lesion that presents with well-defined borders, low-level internal echoes, and moderate through-transmission most likely represents
    a. infected cyst
    b. simple cyst
    c. fibroadenoma
    d. cystosarcoma phyllodes

193. A linear stripe of variable thickness and echogenicity running through the testis in a craniocaudal direction represents the
    a. Cowper's fascia
    b. mediastinum testis
    c. epithelial fascia
    d. dartos muscle

194. The epididymis is located
    a. anterior and inferior to the testis
    b. anterior and superior to the testis
    c. posterior and inferior to the testis
    d. posterior and lateral to the testis

195. Which fact about undescended testes is false?
    a. The testis originates in the retroperitoneum at the level of the fetal kidney.
    b. All undescended testes are found in the inguinal canal.
    c. There is a 40% to 50% association with testicular malignancy.
    d. The incidence of infertility is increased.

196. Common causes of a secondary hydrocele include all of the following except
    a. trauma
    b. undescended testes
    c. infection
    d. neoplasm

197. Which of the following statements is false regarding varicocele?
   a. Varicoceles refer to dilated, serpiginous, and elongated veins of the pampiniform plexus.
   b. They are more common on the right side.
   c. Primary varicoceles result from incompetent valves in the spermatic vein.
   d. Secondary varicoceles develop from compression of the spermatic vein.

198. A common problem that is viral in origin and affects some adolescent and middle-aged men is
   a. epididymal cyst
   b. epididymitis
   c. spermatocele
   d. testiculitis

199. An infection that has spread to the testicle is
   a. epididymitis
   b. hydrocele
   c. orchitis
   d. spermatocele

200. Sonographic patterns of testicular neoplasms include all of the following except
   a. focal and well-defined homogeneous hypoechoic region
   b. diffuse and ill-defined region of decreased echogenicity
   c. complex mass with internal anechoic and echogenic areas
   d. anechoic pattern with increased transmission

# Obstetrics and Gynecology Review

*Select the answer that best completes the following questions or statements.*

1. The physiologic status of prepuberty is
   a. menarche
   b. menopause
   c. premenarche
   d. postmenarche

2. The bladder is considered adequately filled when
   a. it extends past the endometrial canal
   b. it extends past the uterine fundus
   c. it fills the true pelvic cavity
   d. it covers the fimbria

3. A routine transabdominal image protocol of the pelvis consists of longitudinal and transverse scans of
   a. uterus, cervix, adnexa
   b. cervix, right adnexa, left adnexa, uterus, rectouterine recess
   c. endometrial canal, cervix, adnexa
   d. cervix, uterus, fallopian tubes

4. If pelvic pathology is present, what other areas should be examined?
   a. renal
   b. subphrenic
   c. Morison's pouch, subphrenic, renal
   d. Morison's pouch, renal, pouch of Douglas

5. To image the cervix on the TV examination, the transducer should be
   a. inserted deep and angled anteriorly
   b. withdrawn and angled posteriorly
   c. withdrawn and angled anteriorly
   d. inserted deep and angled posteriorly

6. To image the fundus of the anteverted uterus on the TV examination, the transducer should be
   a. inserted deep and angled anteriorly
   b. withdrawn and angled posteriorly
   c. withdrawn slightly and angled anteriorly
   d. inserted deep and angled posteriorly

7. What muscle group is inserted on the pubic ramus and is called paired parasagittal straps in the abdominal wall?
   a. piriformis
   b. coccygeus
   c. obturator fascia
   d. rectus abdominis

8. What muscles may be identified in the true pelvis in the transverse plane with cephalic angulation of the transducer at the pubis?
   a. piriformis
   b. coccygeus
   c. obturator internus
   d. rectus abdominis

9. This muscle is best imaged in a transverse plane with caudal angulation at the most superior aspect of the bladder.
   a. levator ani
   b. rectus abdominis
   c. coccygeus
   d. piriformis

10. What muscle group may be seen in the false pelvis along the lateral side walls of the pelvis?
    a. obturator internus
    b. iliopsoas
    c. rectus sheath
    d. psoas major

11. The müllerian duct is important to development of the
    a. fallopian tube
    b. ovary
    c. female internal reproductive organs
    d. uterine canal

12. Bilateral support for the uterus is provided by the
    a. broad ligament
    b. round ligament
    c. uterosacral ligaments
    d. endometrial ligament

13. The ligament that occupies space between the layers of another ligament and occurs in front of and below the fallopian tube is the
    a. broad ligament
    b. uterosacral ligament
    c. round ligament
    d. tubal ligament

14. The texture of the myometrium of the uterus may be described as
    a. heterogeneous
    b. homogeneous with smooth borders
    c. heterogeneous with smooth borders
    d. homogeneous with irregular borders

15. The vessels seen in the periphery of the uterus are called the
    a. arcuate
    b. uterine
    c. ovarian
    d. tubal

16. The best way to measure the cervical-fundal length of the normal uterus is
    a. TA, longitudinal
    b. TV, sagittal
    c. TV, coronal
    d. TA, transverse

17. The normal length of the young adult uterus should measure
    a. 3 to 5 cm
    b. 2 to 3 cm
    c. 5 to 6 cm
    d. 6 to 9 cm

18. The endometrium changes during the menstrual cycle. When the three-line sign appears, this is the
    a. secretory phase
    b. early proliferative phase
    c. midproliferative phase
    d. late proliferative phase

19. The endometrial thickness is measured
    a. from inner to inner border
    b. from anterior to posterior layers
    c. from outer to outer layer, including fluid
    d. from inner to inner on TA only

20. The normal measurement of the endometrium should be _____ in a menstrual woman.
    a. 10 to 12 mm
    b. 1 to 2 mm
    c. 4 to 6 mm
    d. 4 to 12 mm

21. The structure that lies above the utero-ovarian ligaments, the round ligaments, and the tubo-ovarian vessels is the
    a. ovary
    b. fallopian tube
    c. broad ligament
    d. uterine artery

22. The ovary produces two hormones; estrogen is secreted by the _____, whereas progesterone is secreted by the _____.
    a. follicles, corpus luteum
    b. secretory, proliferative
    c. follicles, corpuscle
    d. corpus luteum, nabothian

23. The release of an egg from the ruptured mature follicle is
    a. menstruation
    b. corpus luteum
    c. ovulation
    d. follicle-stimulating hormone (FSH)

24. The ovary is located lateral to the _____ and anteromedial to the _____.
    a. round ligament, broad ligament
    b. uterus, internal iliac vessels
    c. external iliac vessels, piriformis
    d. obturator internus, internal iliac vessels

25. The posterior component of the pelvic cavity is occupied by all of the following except the
    a. rectum
    b. cervix
    c. colon
    d. ileum

26. Which statement is false regarding the ureter?
    a. It crosses the pelvic inlet anterior to the bifurcation of the common iliac artery.
    b. It runs in front of the internal iliac artery and posterior to the ovary.
    c. It runs forward and lateral under the base of the broad ligament.
    d. It runs forward and lateral to the vagina to enter the bladder.

27. The uterus is supported by the
    a. levator ani muscles and pelvic fascia
    b. obturator internus muscles
    c. iliacus muscles
    d. piriformis muscles

28. The ligaments of the uterus include
    a. broad, suspensory, round, ovarian
    b. broad, round, ovarian
    c. broad, fundal, round
    d. broad, fundal, piriformis

29. The texture of the ovary is
    a. less echogenic than the uterus
    b. more echogenic than the uterus
    c. more hypoechoic than the uterus
    d. less hypoechoic than the uterus

30. The failure of fusion that has two vaginas, two cervices, two uterine bodies is
    a. bicornuate uterus
    b. didelphys uterus
    c. bicornis unicollis uterus
    d. arcuatus uterus

31. The transvaginal technique may be contraindicated in all of the following except
    a. premenarche patients
    b. obese patients
    c. sexually inactive patients
    d. patients who refuse or cannot tolerate the examination

32. The Doppler indices used to evaluate the pelvic vessels include all of the following except
    a. A/B ratio
    b. Pourcelot resistive index
    c. Bernoulli's equation
    d. pulsatility index

33. The uterine vessels are found in the
    a. obturator internus
    b. broad ligaments
    c. piriformis
    d. aorta

34. The ovarian arteries and veins are found in the
    a. broad ligaments
    b. suspensory ligaments
    c. round ligaments
    d. oval ligaments

35. The three divisions of the fallopian tube are
    a. intramural, isthmus, ampullary
    b. intramural, ampullary, follicular
    c. isthmus, ampullary, follicular
    d. follicular, fimbriae, luteal

36. When only the body and the fundus of the uterus are flexed posteriorly, it is
    a. anteflexed
    b. anteverted
    c. retroflexed
    d. retroverted

37. The end of the fallopian tube that is open to the peritoneal cavity is called the
    a. isthmus
    b. frondosum
    c. ampulla
    d. fimbria

38. Hydrometra would appear sonographically as
    a. a sonolucent tubular structure in the adnexa
    b. an echogenic thickening of the endometrium
    c. a sonolucent fluid collection in the uterine canal
    d. a sonolucent fluid collection in the uterus, cervix, and vagina

39. The human chorionic gonadotropin (hCG) levels in gestational trophoblastic disease
    a. decrease in time
    b. increase at a markedly higher rate than in a normal pregnancy
    c. increase at a subnormal rate
    d. remain at an even level throughout the course of the disease

**523**

40. The hormone responsible for estrogen stimulation is
    a. FSH
    b. luteinizing hormone (LH)
    c. cortisone
    d. progesterone

41. Polycystic ovaries usually have cysts that are
    a. around the periphery of the ovary
    b. throughout the ovary
    c. large and septated
    d. infected

42. Sonographic evaluation of the pelvis in the patient with a suspected mass has several objectives. Which of the following is NOT one?
    a. to confirm the presence of a mass
    b. to determine its origin
    c. to provide a pathologic diagnosis
    d. to characterize its internal echoarchitecture

43. Which of the following is usually a preponderantly cystic mass?
    a. hydrosalpinx
    b. teratoma
    c. ovarian abscess
    d. mucinous cystadenoma

44. Teratomas are
    a. complex masses
    b. cystic masses
    c. always malignant
    d. lethal

45. The most common site of an ectopic pregnancy is
    a. the isthmus of the fallopian tube
    b. the abdomen
    c. the ovary
    d. the ampullary portion of the fallopian tube

46. A fluid collection in the endometrium that simulates the gestational sac of an early pregnancy is called
    a. decidual reaction
    b. endometritis
    c. pseudogestational sac
    d. hydrometra

47. Which of the following is NOT an adnexal structure?
    a. ovarian ligaments
    b. ovaries
    c. uterus
    d. broad ligaments

48. A dermoid is
    a. a large cystic mass with prominent septations
    b. a benign teratoma in which ectodermal elements are preponderant
    c. the most common large cystic mass, which may contain a lattice of internal thin-walled septations
    d. the largest of the functional cysts, associated with trophoblastic disease

49. The total sum of the measurement of the largest pocket of amniotic fluid in four quadrants is called the
    a. amniotic fluid volume
    b. amniotic fluid index
    c. amniotic pocket volume
    d. amniotic quadrant volume

50. A parovarian cyst is
    a. a large cystic mass with prominent septations
    b. a benign teratoma in which ectodermal elements are preponderant
    c. the largest of the functional cysts, associated with trophoblastic disease
    d. a cyst that arises from the broad ligament

51. Theca lutein cysts are
    a. large cystic masses with prominent septations
    b. benign teratomas in which ectodermal elements are preponderant
    c. the most common large cystic masses, which may contain a lattice of internal thin-walled septations
    d. the largest of the functional cysts, associated with trophoblastic disease or hyperstimulation of the hCG

52. Biparietal diameter can be used for fetal dating as early as
    a. 6 weeks
    b. 8 weeks
    c. 10 weeks
    d. 12 weeks

53. BPD measurement should be taken from the following borders:
    a. outer to outer
    b. outer to inner
    c. inner to inner
    d. inner to outer

54. A brachycephalic head describes a head that is
    a. round
    b. elongated
    c. abnormal
    d. small

55. The crown-rump length (CRL) measurement is the longest length of the embryo
    a. excluding the limbs
    b. including the limbs
    c. including the yolk sac
    d. including the femur

56. An intrauterine growth–restricted fetus is one that
    a. is always born with genetic defects
    b. has an abnormal heart rate
    c. is RH sensitive
    d. is born at or below the 10th percentile of weight for gestational age

57. The abdominal circumference should be taken at the level of
    a. the fetal stomach and the portal vein
    b. the fetal heart and ribs
    c. the fetal kidneys
    d. the umbilical cord insertion site

58. A(n) _____ is formed when an oocyte unites with a sperm cell.
    a. oocyte
    b. zygote
    c. corpus albicans
    d. morula

59. When the uterus empties itself of all products of conception, it is referred to as a(n)
    a. blighted ovum
    b. complete abortion
    c. impending abortion
    d. missed abortion

60. What is the approximate hCG level when a gestational sac is first observed (transabdominally)?
    a. 800 mIU/mL
    b. 1200 mIU/mL
    c. 1800 mIU/mL
    d. 2100 mIU/mL

61. All of the following statements regarding hydatidiform mole are true except
    a. A previous mole results in increased risk for recurrence.
    b. It is associated with markedly elevated hCG levels.
    c. The sonographic appearance is similar to that of a degenerating myoma.
    d. Although considered "tumors" of trophoblastic tissue, they are incapable of metastasizing.

62. Causes of polyhydramnios include all of the following except
    a. congenital abnormalities
    b. heart failure
    c. gastrointestinal anomalies
    d. amniotic bands

63. Higher than normal levels of hCG are seen in which of the following conditions?
    a. multiple gestation
    b. corpus luteum cyst
    c. ectopic pregnancy
    d. anembryonic gestation

64. Postmenopausal ovaries are difficult to recognize sonographically for all of the following reasons except
    a. They are no longer responsive to pituitary gonadotropins.
    b. They are smaller than premenopausal ovaries.
    c. The parenchymal tissue becomes hypoechoic as a result of atrophy.
    d. The blood supply to the ovaries is diminished.

65. Fusion of the amnion and the chorion normally occurs between
    a. 3 and 5 weeks
    b. 5 and 8 weeks
    c. 8 and 10 weeks
    d. 14 and 16 weeks

66. In the 8th to 9th week of gestation, the fetal heart rate on a transvaginal sonogram should measure
    a. 90 beats per minute
    b. 120 beats per minute
    c. 160 beats per minute
    d. 200 beats per minute

67. The most inaccurate measurement for fetal growth assessment is
    a. femur length
    b. biparietal diameter
    c. abdominal circumference
    d. head circumference

68. The fetal renal pelvis should be followed in utero if the measurement exceeds
    a. 1 to 2 mm
    b. 2 to 3 mm
    c. 4 to 5 mm
    d. 5 to 10 mm

69. If you are scanning a first-trimester pregnancy, documentation should be made of
    a. BPD
    b. crown-rump length
    c. head circumference
    d. abdominal circumference

70. To determine situs solitus, the following structures should be identified except
    a. stomach on left
    b. aorta on left, IVC right and anterior
    c. aorta on left, IVC right and posterior
    d. apex to left

71. A solid mass may exhibit all of the following except
    a. distal acoustic shadows
    b. distal acoustic enhancement
    c. irregular, poorly defined walls
    d. a heterogeneous interior

72. What type of cyst is commonly associated with pregnancy?
   a. a theca lutein cyst
   b. a parovarian cyst
   c. a corpus luteum cyst
   d. a follicular cyst

73. If an anterior abdominal wall mass is seen just to the right of the umbilical cord, the most likely diagnosis is
   a. gastroschisis
   b. omphalocele
   c. hernia
   d. limb–body wall defect

74. Trophoblastic disease, which extends outside the uterus and spreads to the lungs or brain, is called
   a. choriocarcinoma
   b. hydatidiform mole
   c. endometrioma
   d. lung-gestational molar

75. In what anatomic site does fertilization of the ovum usually occur?
   a. the vagina
   b. the uterine cavity
   c. the ovary
   d. the fallopian tube

76. A 22-year-old gravid patient presents with oligohydramnios. Which of the following would be least likely?
   a. anencephaly
   b. postterm pregnancy
   c. renal agenesis
   d. premature rupture of the membranes

77. A patient is GPA 8,2,1. How many abortions has she had?
   a. four
   b. eight
   c. two
   d. one

78. A near-term gravid patient lying face up for longer than 15 minutes sometimes will become ill with fainting and nausea. She is probably experiencing
   a. supine hypotensive syndrome
   b. supine hypertensive syndrome
   c. morning sickness
   d. hyperemesis gravidarum

79. Separation of the chorionic and amniotic membranes is normal
   a. after 24 weeks of gestation
   b. before 24 weeks of gestation
   c. after 16 weeks of gestation
   d. before 16 weeks of gestation

80. Which of the following is the appropriate description of gastroschisis?
   a. normal insertion of the umbilical cord, with herniation of the bowel occurring most often on the right side of the umbilicus
   b. herniation of the thoracic and abdominal contents, including the bowel and liver or spleen, with herniation at the base of the umbilical cord
   c. herniation of the umbilical cord
   d. herniation of bowel to the left of the umbilicus, containing spleen covered by peritoneum

81. A leiomyoma that deforms the endometrial cavity and may cause irregular or heavy menstrual bleeding is known as a(n)
   a. pedunculated fibroid
   b. subserosal fibroid
   c. submucosal fibroid
   d. intramural fibroid

82. Calcifications of fibroids may be secondary to all of the following except
   a. diabetes mellitus
   b. hypertension
   c. hypotension
   d. chronic renal failure

83. If the endometrium measures more than 14 mm without hormone replacement therapy, the sonographer should think of
   a. endometrial hyperplasia
   b. adenomyosis
   c. endometritis
   d. endometrioma

84. Clear evidence for endometrial carcinoma is
   a. light bleeding during the secretory phase
   b. myometrial invasion
   c. calcification of the arcuate arteries
   d. gestational trophoblastic disease

85. The most common cause of tubal obstruction is
   a. endometrioma
   b. hydrometrocolpos
   c. adenomyosis
   d. pelvic inflammatory disease

86. The function of the ovary is to
   a. produce testosterone
   b. produce follicles
   c. mature oocytes until ovulation
   d. manufacture corpus luteum

87. The normal follicle may enlarge to _____ before ovulation.
   a. 8 cm
   b. 24 mm
   c. 39 mm
   d. 78 mm

**529**

88. Increased levels of hCG may cause
    a. hemorrhagic cysts to develop
    b. teratomas
    c. theca lutein cysts
    d. polycystic ovaries

89. Cysts smaller than _____ are not likely to be malignant.
    a. 2 cm
    b. 3 cm
    c. 4 cm
    d. 5 cm

90. Another name for a chocolate cyst is
    a. dermoid tumor
    b. endometrioma
    c. hemorrhagic cyst
    d. adenoma

91. Cysts with thick septations and solid elements most likely are
    a. filled with blood
    b. filled with fluid
    c. malignant
    d. benign

92. The most common mass in young girls is
    a. polycystic ovary
    b. teratoma
    c. pelvic inflammatory disease
    d. Brenner tumor

93. Which statement regarding torsion of the ovary is false?
    a. The ovary becomes edematous, measuring more than 4 cm.
    b. Fluid is often found in the pelvis.
    c. Doppler shows increased blood surrounding the periphery of the ovary.
    d. The ovary is usually hypoechoic.

94. All of the following causes may mimic a pelvic mass except
    a. pelvic kidney
    b. omental cysts
    c. retroflexed ureter
    d. diverticular abscess

95. In an early gestation, the gestational sac
    a. represents the fluid-filled amniotic cavity
    b. surrounds the decidua capsularis and decidua parietalis
    c. can be visualized transvaginally by 4 weeks and transabdominally by 6 weeks
    d. cannot be correlated with hCG

96. The placenta develops from
    a. the portion of the trophoblast attached to the myometrium, the decidua basalis
    b. the portion of the trophoblast attached to the decidua capsularis
    c. the amnion before fusion with the chorionic cavity
    d. the double decidual sac

97. The echogenic walls of the secondary yolk sac is
    a. the first structure to be seen within the gestational sac
    b. not visualized in an ectopic gestation
    c. seen transabdominally at ±4 weeks after the LMP
    d. usually between 5 and 7 mm in diameter

98. During the first trimester, the developing embryo grows approximately _____ every day
    a. 2 to 3 mm
    b. 4 to 5 mm
    c. 1 to 2 mm
    d. 0.5 to 1 mm

99. On transvaginal imaging, by the end of the first trimester, the choroid plexus
    a. is not present and cannot be imaged
    b. can be imaged as a hyperechoic structure in the lateral ventricle
    c. can be imaged as a hypoechoic structure in the lateral ventricle
    d. is seen as a linear echogenic structure in the gestational sac

100. A corpus luteum of pregnancy
    a. is a functional cyst of the ovary
    b. precedes the formation of a follicular cyst
    c. becomes a corpus luteum cyst only if fertilization does not take place
    d. is found with a hydatidiform mole

101. The sonographer finds the cul-de-sac to contain a small amount of clear fluid. This is MOST likely to be evidence of
    a. a normal situation
    b. an ectopic pregnancy
    c. pelvic inflammatory disease
    d. vesicouterine reflux

102. A patient with a positive serum hCG test presents with some bleeding. The LMP indicates 5 to 6 weeks of gestation. Sonography does not reveal a fetal pole. The MOST likely diagnosis is a(n)
    a. hydatidiform mole
    b. complete spontaneous abortion
    c. ectopic pregnancy
    d. normal intrauterine gestation, but too early to detect the fetal pole

103. In a patient with a complete spontaneous abortion, the MOST likely finding is a(n)
    a. empty gestational sac with no evidence of decidua
    b. embryo with no evidence of a heartbeat
    c. complex mass in the cul-de-sac
    d. empty uterus with a decidual reaction

104. A patient presents with a closed cervical os and a distorted gestational sac in the lower uterine segment. This MOST likely represents a(n)

    a. blighted ovum

    b. complete spontaneous abortion

    c. threatened abortion

    d. inevitable abortion

105. With respect to ectopic pregnancies, which of the following is TRUE?

    a. An adnexal mass can usually be palpated.

    b. Implantation in the interstitial portion of the tube is a common occurrence.

    c. Cornual ectopic pregnancies may have dangerous prognoses.

    d. Ectopic pregnancies cannot be carried past the first trimester.

106. A succenturiate placenta is a(n)

    a. early matured placenta

    b. small placenta

    c. accessory lobe of the placenta

    d. benign tumor of the placenta

107. If a sonographer is unable to demonstrate the fetal urinary bladder, it is important to rescan the area in approximately

    a. 5 to 10 minutes

    b. 15 to 45 minutes

    c. 2 hours

    d. 24 hours

108. The normal fetal heart rate in the second and third trimesters generally ranges between

    a. 100 and 120 beats per minute

    b. 120 and 140 beats per minute

    c. 120 and 160 beats per minute

    d. 160 and 200 beats per minute

109. The fetal umbilical cord contains

    a. two arteries and one vein

    b. two arteries and two veins

    c. one artery and one vein

    d. one artery and two veins

110. Measurement of the cerebellum is BEST made at the level of the

    a. thalamus, hippocampus, midbrain, cavum septi pellucidi

    b. vermis, midbrain, cisterna magna

    c. sphenoid, temporal bone, pituitary stalk

    d. foramen magnum, pons, fourth ventricle

111. When measuring the ventricular system of the fetal head, the MOST accurate level to use is the

    a. frontal horn

    b. lateral ventricle parallel to the falx

    c. lateral ventricular atrium

    d. cisterna magna

112. A percentage of fetal blood from the IVC is shunted from
    a. left atrium to right atrium
    b. right atrium to left atrium
    c. ductus venosus to left atrium
    d. right atrium to ductus arteriosus

113. Visualization of a four-chambered heart within the fetal thorax enables determination of all of the following except
    a. position of the heart and size of the chambers
    b. mobility of the atrioventricular valves
    c. mobility of the semilunar valves
    d. visualization of the ventricular inflow tract

114. With respect to ultrasound of the fetal thorax, which of the following is TRUE?
    a. The diaphragm presents as a linear echoic band.
    b. Increased thickness of skin at the ventral aspect of the thorax usually indicates pathology.
    c. The long axis of the fetal heart is usually perpendicular to the long axis of the body.
    d. Visualization of fluid in the pleural space is normal.

115. An embryo presents with an outpouching from the anterior abdominal wall into the base of the umbilical cord. This is MOST likely to be
    a. gastroschisis
    b. omphalocele
    c. normal herniation of the fetal gut
    d. umbilical hernia

116. Which of the following statements is TRUE with regard to fetal bowel?
    a. Peristalsis can be seen in the small bowel, but not in the large bowel.
    b. Peristalsis can be seen in the large bowel, but not in the small bowel.
    c. The presence of echogenic meconium in the large bowel early in the second trimester is normal.
    d. Echogenic meconium may be distinguished from an amniotic bleed.

117. Which of the following statements is TRUE regarding the fetal bladder?
    a. If the bladder appears distended, pathology is always indicated.
    b. The fetus voids approximately once per hour.
    c. If the bladder is not seen, pathology is indicated.
    d. The sonographer should wait 10 minutes to rescan the fetal bladder.

118. Deoxygenated fetal blood enters the placenta through the
    a. umbilical vein
    b. umbilical artery
    c. spiral artery
    d. uterine artery

119. The most common tumor of the placenta is the
    a. choriocarcinoma
    b. subplacental hematoma
    c. chorioangioma
    d. placenta percreta

120. A single umbilical artery may indicate anomalies of all of the following systems except
   a. cardiovascular
   b. hepatobiliary
   c. central nervous
   d. genitourinary

121. Placenta previa is MOST likely to present in association with which of the following?
   a. increased maternal age, increased parity, or previous abortion
   b. second-trimester bleeding
   c. a distance from presenting part to maternal sacrum less than 1.5 cm
   d. a placenta extending to and covering the fundus

122. Regarding BPD measurement as a predictor of gestational age, which of the following is TRUE?
   a. BPD is more accurate than femur length in the late third trimester.
   b. BPD is more accurate than femur length in the second trimester.
   c. BPD is routinely measured at the level of the ventricles.
   d. BPD is more accurate than HC in the second trimester.

123. The largest transverse section of the abdomen is MOST likely found at the location of the
   a. umbilicus and stomach
   b. confluence of the umbilical and portal veins and stomach
   c. stomach and middle portal vein
   d. fetal kidneys

124. IUGR is best defined as a fetus
   a. that is below the 10th percentile in weight
   b. whose mother has hypertension
   c. at high risk of perinatal morbidity
   d. with known systemic disease

125. The type of twinning that occurs when two ova are fertilized is
   a. monozygotic twinning
   b. dizygotic twinning
   c. monochorionic and monoamniotic twinning
   d. monochorionic and diamniotic twinning

126. Which of the following complications is NOT associated with multiple gestations?
   a. IUGR of one or both twins
   b. increased incidence of preeclampsia
   c. increased third-trimester bleeding
   d. postterm labor

127. In a twin pregnancy, visualization of a septum greater than 1 mm in width is MOST likely to represent which type of twinning?
   a. dichorionic
   b. monochorionic
   c. diamniotic
   d. monoamniotic

128. Which of the following is LEAST LIKELY to be found in the fetus of a diabetic mother?

    a. IUGR

    b. microsomia

    c. skeletal and CNS anomalies

    d. cardiac anomalies

129. The presence of hypertension in the second or third trimester is NOT likely to increase the risk of

    a. fetal hydrops

    b. IUGR

    c. placental abruption

    d. toxemia

130. With the PUBS procedure, it is best to involve percutaneous sampling of the

    a. umbilical vein near the cord insertion at the placenta

    b. umbilical vein near the cord insertion at the umbilicus

    c. umbilical artery near the cord insertion at the placenta

    d. umbilical vessels within the placenta

131. Which of the following is MOST likely to cause postpartum hemorrhage?

    a. obesity

    b. increased age or parity

    c. prolonged labor

    d. delayed uterine involution

132. Prolonged severe oligohydramnios is MOST likely to lead to which of the following conditions?

    a. femur dysplasia

    b. pulmonary hypoplasia

    c. postterm pregnancy

    d. single umbilical artery

133. The Spalding sign is most often associated with

    a. fetal hydrops

    b. IUGR

    c. fetal demise

    d. pleural effusion

134. The term *fetus papyraceus* refers to a condition wherein the fetus

    a. is reabsorbed, leaving no detectable sign

    b. lacks normal bone structure

    c. lacks red blood cells, rendering it white as paper

    d. dies, but persists as a flattened structure with bones

135. A malformation that is characterized by the fourth ventricle defect of a retrocerebellar cyst communicating with the fourth ventricle is

    a. choroid plexus cyst

    b. Dandy-Walker malformation

    c. hydranencephaly

    d. holoprosencephaly

136. The MOST accurate method for evaluating hydrocephalus is to measure the diameter of the
    a. atrium of the lateral ventricle through the choroid plexus
    b. superior lateral ventricle from the falx to the lateral margin of the ventricle
    c. fourth ventricle at the level of the cerebellum
    d. frontal horns at the level of the thalami

137. A complex cystic mass appearing on either side of the fetal neck is most likely a
    a. meningomyelocele
    b. cephalocele
    c. cystic hygroma
    d. choroid plexus cyst

138. A spinal defect containing meninges and neural tissue is most likely to be a
    a. cephalocele
    b. spina bifida
    c. meningocele
    d. meningomyelocele

139. The "lemon" and "banana" signs are usually associated with
    a. Arnold-Chiari malformation
    b. Dandy-Walker malformation
    c. duodenal atresia
    d. renal agenesis

140. Sonographic visualization of a fluid-filled mass behind the left atrium and ventricle in the lower thorax most likely represents
    a. cystic adenomatoid formation
    b. congenital diaphragmatic hernia
    c. pleural effusion
    d. pericardial effusion

141. Oligohydramnios after week 16 of gestation most likely indicates which of the following?
    a. unilateral renal agenesis
    b. bilateral renal agenesis
    c. dominant polycystic renal disease
    d. unilateral multicystic renal disease

142. Which of the following is NOT likely to be seen as a fluid-filled mass in the RUQ?
    a. congenital duplication cyst
    b. choledochal cyst
    c. urachal cyst
    d. ascites

143. A fetus with findings of a narrow bell-shaped thorax, curved and shortened long bones, and a cloverleaf skull is most likely to have
    a. osteogenesis imperfecta
    b. achondroplasia
    c. VACTERL syndrome
    d. thanatophoric dysplasia

144. Failure of the atrioventricular valves to separate into mitral and tricuspid valves is part of
    a. tetralogy of Fallot
    b. atrioventricular canal defect
    c. hypoplastic heart syndrome
    d. Ebstein's anomaly

145. Sonographic findings of oligohydramnios, absent kidneys, IUGR, and pulmonary hypoplasia are most consistent with
    a. Meckel-Gruber syndrome
    b. Potter's syndrome
    c. amniotic band syndrome
    d. limb–body wall syndrome

146. Uterine contractions *throughout* pregnancy may be confused with
    a. leiomyoma
    b. Braxton Hicks
    c. Breus' mole
    d. hemangioma

147. Ovarian hyperstimulation syndrome may be associated with
    a. polycystic ovaries
    b. theca lutein cysts
    c. corpus luteum cysts
    d. mesenteric cysts

148. An allantoic duct cyst is most likely to be associated with which of the following intrauterine structures?
    a. gallbladder
    b. cystic duct
    c. umbilical cord
    d. hepatic vein

149. When placental tissue is seen to extend beyond the external uterine wall into the bladder, this condition is
    a. placenta previa
    b. placenta percreta
    c. placenta increta
    d. placenta accreta

150. What usually happens to the hCG levels in 48 hours in the presence of an ectopic pregnancy?
    a. hCG levels drop.
    b. hCG levels rise at a subnormal rate.
    c. hCG levels double.
    d. hCG levels rise at a markedly high rate.

151. The collection of watery fluid or mucus in the uterus is called
    a. decidual reaction
    b. endometritis
    c. hydrometra
    d. pseudogestational sac

152. In a nonstimulated cycle, the maximum normal size of the dominant follicle before ovulation is
    a. 5 mm
    b. 15 mm
    c. 25 mm
    d. 35 mm

153. Ovarian hyperstimulation syndrome typically occurs
    a. after the patient has received hCG and may be pregnant
    b. before the patient has received hCG
    c. after failed induction of ovulation
    d. after the patient has received intrauterine artificial insemination

154. The cervical os is usually about _____ cm long.
    a. 1 to 2
    b. 3 to 4
    c. 5 to 7
    d. 6 to 8

155. The cephalic index is defined as the ratio of biparietal diameter to
    a. femur length
    b. occipitofrontal diameter
    c. abdominal circumference
    d. binocular distances

156. The date of the last menstrual period indicates
    a. the date when fertilization occurred
    b. the date when menstrual bleeding ended
    c. the date when ovulation occurred
    d. the date when menstrual bleeding began

157. Which of the following is not a sonographic finding of a hydatidiform mole?
    a. theca lutein cysts
    b. grapelike clusters throughout the uterus
    c. homogeneous uterine texture
    d. low-impedance, high-flow Doppler pattern

158. How early can the site of the placenta be identified on sonography?
    a. 8 weeks
    b. 14 weeks
    c. 16 weeks
    d. 20 weeks

159. Amniotic band syndrome consists of
    a. adhesions of torn amniotic membranes wrapped around fetal parts and producing congenital amputations
    b. complications of placental abruption
    c. a syndrome that occurs after the fetus swallows too much fluid
    d. a and c

160. A 30-year-old gravid patient, 32 weeks by dates, now presents with painless vaginal bleeding that has lasted for 5 days. The first condition to rule out by sonography is
    a. ectopic pregnancy
    b. placenta previa
    c. ovarian cyst
    d. hydatidiform mole

161. The kidneys should be scanned transversely at a level
    a. superior to the hepatic veins
    b. inferior to the bladder
    c. superior to the falciform ligament
    d. inferior to the stomach

162. Ovulation occurs
    a. always after intercourse
    b. approximately on the 7th day of the menstrual cycle
    c. around the 14th day of the menstrual cycle
    d. approximately on the 2nd day of the menstrual cycle

163. The most common cause of painless vaginal bleeding in the second and third trimesters of pregnancy is
    a. trauma
    b. ectopic pregnancy
    c. placental abruption
    d. placenta previa

164. A growth-restricted fetus will show a Doppler pattern in the umbilical cord that is
    a. high resistance
    b. low resistance
    c. normal
    d. indicative of increased diastolic flow

165. The amount of amniotic fluid present increases the most during the
    a. embryonic period
    b. third trimester
    c. second trimester
    d. first trimester

166. What references should be used to document the biparietal diameter?
    a. thalamus, cavum septi pellucidi, falx
    b. thalamus, peduncles
    c. peduncles, cerebellum
    d. falx, cavum septi pellucidi, fourth ventricle

167. The age of conceptus from fertilization is called
    a. menstrual age
    b. embryonic period
    c. conceptional age
    d. zygotic period

168. The term that describes the transformed endometrial lining of the uterus during pregnancy is
   a. chorion
   b. decidua
   c. chorion laeve
   d. decidua basalis

169. The thin decidua overlying the portion of the gestational sac facing the endometrial cavity is the
   a. decidua capsularis
   b. decidua
   c. decidua basalis
   d. decidua vera

170. The formula used to calculate gestational age from CRL is
   a. GA = CRL + 6.5
   b. GA = CRL + 2.3
   c. GA = CRL + 5.6
   d. GA = CRL + 4.2

171. What occurs when there is death of the embryo or fetus, but the gestational parts remain in utero?
   a. incomplete or missed abortion
   b. spontaneous abortion
   c. blighted ovum
   d. ectopic pregnancy

172. Oligohydramnios means the AFI is
   a. less than 12 cm
   b. more than 9 cm
   c. less than 8 cm
   d. less than 5 cm

173. A bicornuate uterus may be identified by
   a. two cervices
   b. two vaginas
   c. two cornua
   d. two urethras

174. In a four-chamber view of the heart, the right side may be differentiated from the left by
   a. flap of the foramen ovale opening to the right
   b. foramen ovale, moderator band, apical position of tricuspid valve
   c. thebesian valve, eustachian valve, papillary muscles
   d. lack of trabeculations at the apex of the ventricle

175. The renal pyramids appear as _____ areas throughout the renal medulla.
   a. hyperechoic
   b. anechoic
   c. hypoechoic
   d. echogenic

176. A diabetic mother may have an increased incidence of delivering a fetus with
    a. neural tube or cardiac defect
    b. Potter's syndrome
    c. trisomy 18
    d. cystic hygroma

177. Hydrops fetalis is characterized by
    a. cystic masses within the lungs
    b. edema, ascites, pleural or pericardial effusion
    c. dilated ventricles
    d. pericardial effusion

178. When measuring AFI, the sonographer should use color Doppler to
    a. separate umbilical cord and uterine wall from fluid
    b. make sure the placenta does not have a tear
    c. look for a rupture in the membrane
    d. record cardiac activity

179. Evaluation of a(n) _____ would be required if intrauterine growth restriction in all its forms were to be detected.
    a. weight chart
    b. head circumference chart
    c. growth profile
    d. abdominal circumference

180. The biophysical profile documents all of the following except
    a. fetal breathing
    b. gross fetal movements
    c. AFI
    d. fetal position

181. Which broad muscle covers the anterior surface of the iliac fossa?
    a. piriformis
    b. iliacus
    c. obturator internus
    d. psoas

182. The broad ligament encloses all of the following except
    a. ovaries
    b. uterus
    c. uterine tubes
    d. bladder

183. The thickened fold of mesentery that supports and stabilizes the position of each ovary is the
    a. ligamentum teres
    b. fibrous ligament
    c. broad ligament
    d. round ligament

184. The pouch located between the uterus and the rectum is
   a. rectouterine
   b. rectovesicular
   c. Morison's
   d. uterine

185. The muscle that originates from the ilium and sacrum and passes through the great sciatic notch to insert on the greater trochanter is the
   a. obturator internus
   b. obturator externus
   c. piriformis
   d. coccygeus

*Select the answer that best completes the following questions or statements.*

1. The neural plate develops at
   a. 4.5 menstrual weeks
   b. 6 menstrual weeks
   c. 9 menstrual weeks
   d. 12 menstrual weeks

2. The conus medullaris is located at approximately the level of
   a. T12-L1
   b. L1-L2
   c. L2-L3
   d. L3-L4

3. What are the common clinical findings in a patient with appendicitis?
   a. RLQ pain, fever, nausea and vomiting
   b. nausea and projectile vomiting
   c. right flank pain and bile stasis
   d. abdominal pain radiating to the right shoulder

4. Early in development, the brain segments into three primary vesicles:
   a. prosencephalon, forebrain, midbrain
   b. prosencephalon, mesencephalon, rhombencephalon
   c. hindbrain, midbrain, rhombencephalon
   d. forebrain, midbrain, prosencephalon

5. What are the outgrowths on either side of the diencephalon?
   a. choroid plexus
   b. cerebral hemispheres
   c. midbrain
   d. pons

6. What structure invaginates into the lateral ventricles?
   a. pia
   b. forebrain
   c. choroid plexus
   d. subarachnoid

7. Extrahepatic obstruction in the neonate includes all except
   a. choledochal cyst
   b. biliary atresia
   c. hepatitis
   d. spontaneous perforation of the bile ducts

8. Dysgenesis of the fourth ventricle results in
   a. corpus callosum malformation
   b. cystic dilatation of the lateral ventricle
   c. Dandy-Walker malformation
   d. hypospadias

9. Define the measurement used to determine whether appendicitis is present.
   a. an outer diameter greater than 10 mm with compression
   b. an outer diameter less than 5 mm with compression
   c. an outer diameter greater than 12 mm without compression
   d. an outer diameter greater than 6 mm with compression

10. What structure forms between the corpus callosum and fornices?
    a. septum pellucidum
    b. Dandy-Walker
    c. fourth ventricle
    d. Sylvian fissure

11. The normal size of the lateral ventricle as measured in the axial plane should be less than
    a. 4 mm
    b. 10 mm
    c. 8 mm
    d. 6 mm

12. The cisterna magna gradually decreases with gestational age.
    a. True
    b. False

13. What pitfalls should be avoided when determining lateral ventricular size? (Choose two answers.)
    a. developing fetal cortical mantle
    b. choroid plexus
    c. echogenic subarachnoid space
    d. echogenic white matter

14. Approximately 30% of fetuses identified with hydrocephalus are associated with
    a. calcified cortex
    b. spina bifida
    c. subarachnoid hemorrhage
    d. agenesis of the corpus callosum

15. Which statement is false regarding the choroid plexus?
    a. The choroid plexus fills the lateral ventricle from side to side during the second trimester.
    b. With the development of hydrocephalus, the choroid plexus in the far ventricle separates from the medial wall of the lateral ventricle.
    c. Its texture is heterogeneous.
    d. The choroid plexus in the near ventricle separates from the lateral wall of the lateral ventricle.

16. The most characteristic finding of absence of the corpus callosum is
    a. complete or partial agenesis of the cerebellar vermis
    b. dilatation and superior displacement of the third ventricle
    c. enlargement of the fourth ventricle
    d. hydrocephalus

17. What term is used for any cavitation or CSF-filled cyst in the brain?
    a. hydranencephaly
    b. schizencephaly
    c. porencephaly
    d. encephalocele

18. What bony parts contribute to formation of the vertebral arch?
    a. two pedicles, two laminae, one spinous process, two transverse processes, two superior and two inferior articular processes
    b. one pedicle, two laminae, one spinous process, two transverse processes, two superior and two inferior articular processes
    c. one pedicle, two laminae, one spinous process, one transverse process, two superior and two inferior articular processes
    d. two pedicles, two laminae, two spinous processes, two transverse processes, one superior and one inferior articular process

19. A vein of Galen aneurysm is best imaged with color Doppler as
    a. disturbed flow within the structure
    b. disturbed flow surrounding the structure
    c. disturbed flow posterior to the structure
    d. absence of flow within the structure

20. Which phrase describes intussusception in the infant?
    a. occurs when bowel prolapses into more distal bowel and is propelled in an antegrade fashion
    b. occurs when one segment of bowel twists around another
    c. occurs in the presence of appendicitis
    d. occurs in utero only

21. What percentage of premature infants may have intracranial hemorrhage?
    a. 30
    b. 40
    c. 80
    d. 90

22. What clinical criterion is used to determine whether an infant has pyloric stenosis?
    a. jaundice
    b. frequent urination
    c. fever
    d. projectile vomiting

23. What soft tissue structure is seen to form a bridge of gray matter across the third ventricle when it is abnormal?
    a. mass intermedia
    b. thalamus
    c. hypothalamus
    d. cerebral peduncle

24. The lateral ventricles drain into the third ventricle via what structure?
    a. aqueduct of Sylvius
    b. medulla oblongata
    c. cerebellar vermis
    d. foramen of Monro

25. What measurements are used to evaluate a patient with pyloric stenosis?
    a. length greater than 16 mm, thickness greater than 4 mm
    b. length less than 16 mm, thickness greater than 4 mm
    c. length greater than 12 mm, thickness greater than 2 mm
    d. length greater than 13 mm, thickness greater than 6 mm

26. What connects the third and fourth ventricles?
    a. cerebral aqueduct
    b. aqueduct of Sylvius
    c. foramen of Monro
    d. foramen of nucleus

27. What anatomic landmark within the brain is used to find the middle cerebral arteries?
    a. vein of Galen
    b. aqueduct of Monro
    c. caudate nucleus
    d. Sylvian fissure

28. What is the most common age and gender for pyloric stenosis to occur?
    a. female, age birth to 3 months
    b. female, age 1 to 5 months
    c. male, age 3 to 6 weeks
    d. male, age 1 to 3 months

29. Name the four segments of the lateral ventricles.
    a. frontal horn, body, occipital and temporal horns
    b. anterior, medial, lateral, posterior
    c. anterior, body, frontal, temporal horn
    d. anterior, body, occipital, frontal horn

30. What is the "pseudokidney" or "sandwich" sign?
    a. the sign of a pelvic kidney
    b. sonographic finding in a patient with appendicitis
    c. sonographic finding in a patient with intussusception
    d. hydroureter with a pelvic kidney

31. Name the fontanelle through which the neonatal brain may be scanned in the coronal plane.
    a. posterior fontanelle
    b. occipital fontanelle
    c. temporal fontanelle
    d. anterior fontanelle

32. The layer of meninges closely adhering to the brain tissue is the
    a. dura mater
    b. pia mater
    c. arachnoid
    d. choroid plexus

33. A subependymal hemorrhage is found at what site?
    a. supraependymal germinal matrix
    b. subependymal choroid plexus
    c. subarachnoid plexus
    d. thalamic-caudate groove

34. In the pediatric ultrasound examination of the abdomen, all of the following are true except
    a. the right hepatic lobe should not extend more than 1 cm below the xiphoid process
    b. the common bile duct should measure less than 2 mm in infants up to 1 year of age
    c. the length of the gallbladder should not exceed the length of the kidney
    d. the texture of the pancreas is hypoechoic when compared with the liver

35. What is the most common site for a choroid plexus hemorrhage?
    a. anterior horn
    b. occipital horn
    c. lateral horn
    d. temporal horn

36. Where does the germinal matrix lie?
    a. between the midbrain and the forebrain
    b. superior to the caudate nucleus in the floor of the lateral ventricle
    c. lateral to the cerebral peduncles
    d. inferior to the cisterna magna

37. Which phrase defines acute periventricular leukomalacia?
    a. hemorrhagic germinal matrix with cavitation
    b. echogenic formations in the epidural cavity
    c. increased echogenicity in the subarachnoid space
    d. multiple foci or coagulation necrosis in periventricular white matter

38. Which two complications are seen in patients with periventricular leukomalacia? (Choose two answers.)
    a. anomalous myelination of the immature brain
    b. hydrocephalus
    c. agenesis of the corpus callosum
    d. abnormal neurologic development

39. Which is the best definition for hydrocephalus?
    a. marked separation of the anterior horns and bodies of the lateral ventricles
    b. enlargement of the ventricular system
    c. decreased production of cerebrospinal fluid
    d. displacement of the inferior part of the cerebellum through the foramen magnum

40. Which detail regarding ventriculitis is false?
    a. common complication of purulent meningitis in newborns
    b. caused by hematogenous spread of the infection to the choroid plexus
    c. ventricular shunt decreases the risk
    d. leads to compartmentalization of the ventricular cavities

41. The hip bones represent the fusion of all the following except
    a. ilium
    b. femur
    c. ischium
    d. pubis

42. Agenesis of the corpus callosum may indicate what malformation?
    a. Dandy-Walker malformation
    b. Arnold-Chiari malformation
    c. vein of Galen malformation
    d. choroid plexus cyst

43. When the hip is laterally and posteriorly displaced to the extent that the femoral head has no contact with the acetabulum and the normal U configuration cannot be obtained on ultrasound, this condition is
    a. frank dislocation
    b. dysplasia
    c. subluxation
    d. normal

44. The _____ nerve is the largest nerve in the body.
    a. cranial
    b. diaphragmatic
    c. sciatic
    d. optic

45. Passage of cerebrospinal fluid between the third and lateral ventricles is accomplished via the
    a. foramen of Magendie
    b. aqueduct of Sylvius
    c. foramen of Luschka
    d. foramen of Monro

46. What is the function of the hippocampus?
    a. taste
    b. smell
    c. memory
    d. motor control

47. Cerebrospinal fluid circulates between the
    a. pia mater and arachnoid
    b. dura mater and arachnoid
    c. pia mater and cerebral cortex
    d. dura mater and periosteum

48. The upper and lower vertebral notches of adjacent vertebrae meet to form the
    a. transverse foramina
    b. central canal
    c. intervertebral foramina
    d. apophyseal joints

49. The most inferior portion of the spinal cord, located at approximately the level of the first or second lumbar vertebra, is called the
    a. cauda equina
    b. filum terminale
    c. sacral plexus
    d. conus medullaris

50. The "ball on a spoon" refers to
    a. ilium and gluteus minimus
    b. femoral head and acetabulum
    c. ischium and pubis
    d. pectineus and iliacus

# Case Studies

Provide a short answer for each question after evaluating the images.

## CASE 1

A    B

A 62-year-old male with abdominal distention, pain, and hepatomegaly by physical examination presented to the internist for evaluation. Describe your sonographic findings.

_____

_____

_____

_____

Is this patient in right heart failure? Why or why not?

_____

_____

_____

_____

CASE 3

LIVER CYST

An incidental mass was noted on the abdominal ultrasound. Describe the sonographic features of the mass.

_____

_____

_____

_____

A 24-year-old female presented with several weeks of nausea. Describe the sonographic findings of the uterus.

_____

_____

_____

_____

## CASE 5

A 61-year-old male presented with right-sided pain. Describe the sonographic findings.

_____

_____

_____

_____

A

B

A 26-day-old male presented with a history of projectile vomiting suspicious for pyloric stenosis. Describe the sonographic findings.

_____

_____

_____

_____

CASE 7

A 39-year-old female presented with back pain, nausea, and vomiting that she had been experiencing whenever she drank too much alcohol. She had elevated lipase. Describe what you would look for and the sonographic findings in these transverse images of the pancreas.

_____

_____

_____

_____

A middle-aged woman presented with the feeling of "fullness in her neck" for several months. Describe your sonographic findings.

_____

_____

_____

_____

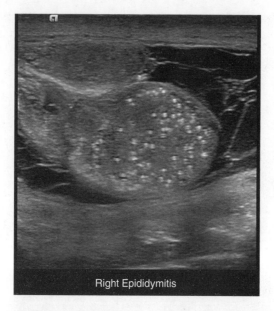

Right Epididymitis

A young male with hemophilia presented with swelling, fever, and tenderness in the right testicle following a tackle from a rugby match. Describe your sonographic findings.

_____

_____

_____

_____

Chin-ling-Sung is a 75-year-old female with a history of acute onset of chronic right upper quadrant pain. There was a previous history of jaundice, hepatitis, and fever. Hepatomegaly was present on physical examination. Describe your sonographic findings of the pancreas.

_____

_____

_____

_____

A 44-year-old obese, diabetic female with a history of alcohol abuse presented with right upper quadrant pain. Her liver function tests are mildly elevated, but otherwise her clinical information is unremarkable. What is your diagnosis based on sonographic evaluation of the gallbladder?

_____

_____

_____

_____

A premature infant with a difficult delivery was evaluated for neurologic changes and a drop in hematocrit. Describe your sonographic findings.

_____

_____

_____

_____

This is a middle-aged male with a history of recurrent urinary tract infections. Describe your sonographic findings.

_____

_____

_____

_____

## CASE 14

A 21-year-old graduate student with a fondness for refried beans and margaritas returned from an archaeology expedition in Baja California. He presented with fever, nausea, and vomiting for the past week. What would you expect to find on the sonogram? Describe the sonographic findings.

_____

_____

_____

_____

A 54-year-old female with mild right upper quadrant pain was ordered to undergo an abdominal ultrasound. What are your findings, and what maneuvers would you do as the sonographer?

_____

_____

_____

_____

## CASE 16

A young athlete presented with an enlarging left testicle. Describe the sonographic findings.

_____

_____

_____

_____

J.L. had lived as a ranch hand in Wyoming for 13 years on the Wrangle Peehs Ranch. He presented to the Mobile Medicine Man Clinic with right upper quadrant pain, abnormal liver function tests, and fever. Describe your sonographic findings.

_____

_____

_____

_____

## CASE 18

An elderly male was in the passenger seat of a car that was involved in a side-swipe automobile accident. He presented in the emergency department with left-sided pain. Describe your sonographic findings.

_____

_____

_____

_____

A young female presented with intense right lower pelvic pain. Describe your sonographic findings of this transvaginal image.

_____

_____

_____

_____

## CASE 20

What are the arrows pointing to on this sagittal view of the popliteal vein?

_____

_____

_____

_____

This is a middle-aged female with shortness of breath. What echocardiographic findings are present in this subcostal image?

_____

_____

_____

_____

CASE 22

The patient has a history of lymphoma. The ultrasound image of the spleen demonstrates what abnormality?

_____

_____

_____

_____

A second-trimester pregnancy was referred for further evaluation. Describe your sonographic findings in this image of the fetal abdomen.

_____

_____

_____

_____

## CASE 24

RIGHT BREAST 900 3 CMN AREA PALP

A young female presented in the emergency department after falling from her horse during the Grand Prix event and landing on her chest. What is found on the breast sonogram?

_____

_____

_____

_____

A 65-year-old male presented with a pulsatile abdominal mass. Describe your sonographic findings of these transverse and sagittal images.

_____

_____

_____

_____

**CASE 26**

How is the patient positioned, and what vascular structures are seen in this abdominal image?

_____

_____

_____

_____

A 49-year-old female with ovarian cancer presented to the emergency department with a 3-day history of tenderness and pain in her lower abdomen. Describe the sonographic findings.

_____

_____

_____

_____

**CASE 28**

A 34-year-old patient presented with right upper quadrant pain. What is your diagnosis based on the sonographic findings?

_____

_____

_____

_____

A 63-year-old female with a recent renal transplant was evaluated with ultrasound. What is your sonographic finding?

_____

_____

_____

_____

CASE 30

What findings are noted in this four chamber view of the fetal heart?

_____

_____

_____

_____